T0211695

Lecture Notes in Computer Science　　9085

Commenced Publication in 1973
Founding and Former Series Editors:
Gerhard Goos, Juris Hartmanis, and Jan van Leeuwen

More information about this series at http://www.springer.com/series/7409

Xiaoxia Yin · Kendall Ho
Daniel Zeng · Uwe Aickelin
Rui Zhou · Hua Wang (Eds.)

Health Information Science

4th International Conference, HIS 2015
Melbourne, Australia, May 28–30, 2015
Proceedings

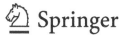 Springer

Editors
Xiaoxia Yin
Victoria University
Melbourne
Australia

Kendall Ho
Faculty of Medicine
University of British Columbia
Vancouver
British Columbia
Canada

Daniel Zeng
University of Arizona
Tucson
Arizona
USA

Uwe Aickelin
University of Nottingham
Nottingham
UK

Rui Zhou
Victoria University
Melbourne
Australia

Hua Wang
Victoria University
Melbourne
Australia

ISSN 0302-9743   ISSN 1611-3349   (electronic)
Lecture Notes in Computer Science
ISBN 978-3-319-19155-3   ISBN 978-3-319-19156-0   (eBook)
DOI 10.1007/978-3-319-19156-0

Library of Congress Control Number: 2015939173

LNCS Sublibrary: SL3 – Information Systems and Applications, incl. Internet/Web, and HCI

Springer Cham Heidelberg New York Dordrecht London
© Springer International Publishing Switzerland 2015

Printed on acid-free paper

Springer International Publishing AG Switzerland is part of Springer Science+Business Media
(www.springer.com)

Preface

The International Conference Series on Health Information Science (HIS) provides a forum for disseminating and exchanging multidisciplinary research results in computer science/information technology and health science and services. It covers all aspects of health information sciences and systems that support health information management and health service delivery.

The Fourth International Conference on Health Information Science (HIS 2015) was held in Melbourne, Australia, during May 28–30, 2015. Founded in April 2012 as the International Conference on Health Information Science and their Applications, the conference continues to grow to include an ever broader scope of activities. The main goal of these events is to provide international scientific forums for exchange of new ideas in a number of fields that interact in-depth through discussions with their peers from around the world. The scope of the conference includes: (1) medical/health/biomedicine information resources, such as patient medical records, devices and equipments, software and tools to capture, store, retrieve, process, analyze, and optimize the use of information in the health domain, (2) data management, data mining, and knowledge discovery, all of which play a key role in decision making, management of public health, examination of standards, privacy and security issues, (3) computer visualization and artificial intelligence for computer-aided diagnosis, and (4) development of new architectures and applications for health information systems.

The conference has solicited and gathered technical research submissions related to all aspects of the conference scope. All the submitted papers in the proceeding were peer-reviewed by at least three international experts drawn from the Program Committee. After the rigorous peer-review process, a total of 20 full papers and 5 short papers among 45 submissions were selected on the basis of originality, significance, and clarity and were accepted for publication in the proceeding. The authors were from 12 countries, including Australia, China, Finland, Germany, Malaysia, Morocco, Saudi Arabia, Sweden, Switzerland, Pakistan, the UK, and the USA. Some papers will be invited to submit the extended versions of their papers to a special issue of the Health Information Science and System Journal, published by BioMed Central (Springer) and the World Wide Web Journal.

The high quality of the program - guaranteed by the presence of an unparalleled number of internationally recognized top experts - can be assessed when reading the contents of the proceeding. The conference will therefore be a unique event, where attendees will be able to appreciate the latest results in their field of expertise, and to acquire additional knowledge in other fields. The program has been structured to favor interactions among attendees coming from many different horizons, scientifically, geographically, from academia and from industry.

We would like to sincerely thank our keynote and invited speakers:

- Professor Lei Wang, Deputy Director of the Institute of Biomedical and Health Engineering, Shenzhen Institutes of Advanced Technology, China;

- Associate Professor Jinyan Li, Faculty of Engineering and IT, University of Technology Sydney, Australia;

- Professor Rezaul Begg, College of Sport and Exercise Science, Victoria University, Australia;

- Professor Lizhu Zhou, Department of Computer Science and Technology, Tsinghua University, China;

- Professor Michael Steyn, UQ Centre for Clinical Research, University of Queensland, Australia

Our thanks also go to the host organization, Victoria University, Australia; the support of the following research funding Australian Research Council Linkage Project LP100200682 and National Natural Science Foundation of China. (No. 61332013). Finally, we acknowledge all those who contributed to the success of HIS 2015 but whose names were listed here.

May 2015

Xiaoxia Yin
Kendall Ho
Daniel Zeng
Uwe Aickelin
Rui Zhou
Hua Wang

Organization

General Co-chairs

Yanchun Zhang   Victoria University, Australia and
Fudan University, China

Michael Blumenstein   Griffith University, Australia

Program Co-chairs

Xiaoxia Yin   Victoria University, Australia

Kendall Ho   The University of British Columbia, Canada

Daniel Zeng   The University of Arizona, USA and
Chinese Academy of Sciences, China

Uwe Aickelin   The University of Nottingham, UK

Conference Organization Chair

Hua Wang   Victoria University, Australia

Industry Program Co-chairs

Jeffrey Soar   University of Southern Queensland, Australia

Lei Liu   Fudan University, China

Tutorial Chair

Xingshe Zhou   Northwestern Polytechnical University, China

Workshop Chair

Chaoyi Pang   Zhejiang University (NIT), China

Publicity Co-chairs

Xiaohui Tao   University of Southern Queensland, Australia

Jenna Reps   The University of Nottingham, UK

Panel Chair

Lei Wang   Shenzhen Institute of Advanced Technology,
Chinese Academy of Sciences, China

Conference Website Co-chairs

Zhangwei Jiang	Chinese Academy of Sciences, China
Rui Zhou	Victoria University, Australia

Publication Chair

Rui Zhou	Victoria University, Australia

Local and Financial Chair

Irena Dzuteska	Victoria University, Australia

Program Committee

Mathias Baumert	The University of Adelaide, Australia
Klemens Boehm	Karlsruhe Institute of Technology, Germany
Ilvio Bruder	Universität Rostock, Germany
Yunpeng Cai	Shenzhen Institutes of Advanced Technology, Chinese Academy of Sciences, China
Jeffrey Chan	The University of Melbourne, Australia
Song Chen	University of Maryland, Baltimore County, USA
Jan Chu	Flinders University, Australia
Xuan-Hong Dang	University of California at Santa Barbara, USA
Hongli Dong	University of Duisburg-Essen, Germany
Ling Feng	Tsinghua University, China
Yi-Ke Guo	University of Utah, USA
Xiao He	Tsinghua University, China
Zhisheng Huang	Vrije Universiteit Amsterdam, The Netherlands
Du Huynh	The University of Western Australia, Australia
Wenjing Jia	University of Technology, Sydney, Australia
Clement Leung	Hong Kong Baptist University, Hong Kong, China
Yidong Li	Beijing Jiaotong University, China
Xi Liang	IBM Research, Australia
Xiaohui Liu	Brunel University London, UK
Zhiyuan Luo	University of London, UK
Gang Luo	University of Utah, USA
Nigel Martin	University of London, UK
Fernando Jose Martin Sanchez	The University of Melbourne, Australia
Brian Ng	The University of Adelaide, Australia
Prema Sankaran	Thiagarajar School of Management, India

Contents

Reality Mining in eHealth 1
Peter Wlodarczak, Jeffrey Soar, and Mustafa Ally

Analysis and Comparison of the IEEE 802.15.4 and 802.15.6 Wireless
Standards Based on MAC Layer. 7
Renwei Huang, Zedong Nie, Changjiang Duan, Yuhang Liu,
Liya Jia, and Lei Wang

Securing Electronic Medical Record and Electronic Health Record Systems
Through an Improved Access Control 17
Pasupathy Vimalachandran, Hua Wang, and Yanchun Zhang

Supporting Frontline Health Workers Through the Use of a Mobile
Collaboration Tool 31
Jane Li, Leila Alem, and Weidong Huang

Canonical Document for Medical Data Exchange 37
Sanae Mazouz, Ouçamah Mohammed Cherkaoui Malki,
and El Habib Nfaoui

Identifying Candidate Risk Factors for Prescription Drug Side Effects
Using Causal Contrast Set Mining 45
Jenna Reps, Zhaoyang Guo, Haoyue Zhu, and Uwe Aickelin

Analyzing Sleep Stages in Home Environment Based
on Ballistocardiography 56
Hongbo Ni, Tingzhi Zhao, Xingshe Zhou, Zhu Wang,
Lei Chen, and Jun Yang

Heart Rate Variability Biofeedback Treatment for Post-Stroke
Depression Patients: A Pilot Study 69
Xin Li, Tong Zhang, Luping Song, Guigang Zhang, and Chunxiao Xing

A New Approach for Face Detection Based on Photoplethysmographic
Imaging 79
He Liu, Tao Chen, Qingna Zhang, and Lei Wang

Biometrics Applications in e-Health Security: A Preliminary Survey 92
Ebenezer Okoh and Ali Ismail Awad

Developing a Health Information Systems Approach to a Novel Student
Health Clinic: Meeting the Educational and Clinical Needs
of an Interprofessional Health Service............................ 104
*James Browne, Aileen Escall, Andi Jones, Maximilian de Courten,
and Karen T. Hallam*

A Stable Gene Subset Selection Algorithm for Cancers................ 111
Juanying Xie and Hongchao Gao

Toward Establishing a Comprehensive Public Health Service Platform
for Chronic Disease Management and Medication in China: A Practice
in Building a Smart Hypertension Medical System................... 123
Yuncheng Hua, Jue Xie, Lei Liu, and Anjun Chen

TeenChat: A Chatterbot System for Sensing and Releasing
Adolescents' Stress.. 133
*Jing Huang, Qi Li, Yuanyuan Xue, Taoran Cheng, Shuangqing Xu,
Jia Jia, and Ling Feng*

Ethical Quality in eHealth: A Challenge with Many Facets............ 146
Marjo Rissanen

Experiences in Developing and Testing an Ambient Assisted Living Course
for Further Education 154
*Ilvio Bruder, Andreas Heuer, Thomas Karopka, Juliane Schuldt,
and Kerstin Kosche*

Prognostic Reporting of p53 Expression by Image Analysis in Glioblastoma
Patients: Detection and Classification 165
*Mohammad F. Ahmad Fauzi, Hamza N. Gokozan, Christopher R. Pierson,
Jose J. Otero, and Metin N. Gurcan*

Identification of Schizophrenia-Associated Gene Polymorphisms
Using Hybrid Filtering Feature Selection with Structural Information 174
Yingying Wang, Zichun Zeng, and Yunpeng Cai

Mobile Clinical Scale Collection System for In-Hospital Stroke Patient
Assessments Using Html5 Technology 185
*Furu Xiang, Wenxuan Guan, Xingxian Huang, Xiaomao Fan,
Yunpeng Cai, and Haibo Yu*

Comparative Evaluation of Two Systems for Integrating Biometric
Data from Self-quantification................................... 195
Bibin Punnoose and Kathleen Gray

Investigating Various Technologies Applied to Assist Seniors 202
Pouria Khosravi, Amir Hossein Ghapanchi, and Michael Blumenstein

Characteristics of Research on the Application of Three-Dimensional
Immersive Virtual Worlds in Health   213
    Reza Ghanbarzadeh, Amir Hossein Ghapanchi, and Michael Blumenstein

Trend Prediction of Biomedical Technology by Semantic Analysis.   225
    Xiaomeng Sun, Kexu Zhang, Peng Nan, and Lei Liu

SMS for Life in Burundi and Zimbabwe: A Comparative Evaluation.   231
    Gerardo Luis Dimaguila

Healthcare Data Validation and Conformance Testing Approach
Using Rule-Based Reasoning   241
    Hira Jawaid, Khalid Latif, Hamid Mukhtar, Farooq Ahmad,
    and Syed Ali Raza

Author Index   247

Reality Mining in eHealth

Peter Wlodarczak$^{(\boxtimes)}$, Jeffrey Soar, and Mustafa Ally

University of Southern Queensland, West Street, Toowoomba Qld 4350, Australia
wlodarczak@gmail.com, {Jeffrey.Soar,Mustafa.Ally}@usq.edu.au

Abstract. There is increasing interest in Big Data analytics in health care. Behavioral health analytics is a care management technology that aims to improve the quality of care and reduce health care costs based capture and analysis of data on patient's behavioral patterns. Big Data analytics of behavioral health data offers the potential of more precise and personalized treatment as well as monitor population-wide events such as epidemics.

Mobile phones are powerful social sensors that are usually physically close to users and leave digital traces of users' behaviors and movement patterns. New Apps (application or piece of software) are emerging that passively collect and analyze mobile phone data of at-risk patients such as their location, calling and texting records and app usage, and can find deviations in a user's daily patterns to detect that something is wrong before an event occurs. Data mining and machine learning techniques are adopted to analyze the "automated diaries" created by the smart phone and monitor the well-being of people. The App first learns a patients daily behavioral patterns using machine learning techniques. Once trained, the App detects deviations and alerts carers based on predictive models.

This paper describes the techniques used and algorithms for reality mining and predictive analysis used in eHealth Apps.

Keywords: Reality mining · Big data · Machine learning · eHealth · Predictive analytics · Behavioral health analytics · Mobile sensing

1 Introduction

An important question for behavioral epidemiology and public health is to better understand how individual behavior is affected by illness and stress [3]. Someone who becomes depressed isolates himself and has a hard time to get up and go to work. He shows deviations from his normal behavioral patterns. Smartphones produce significant amounts of behavioral data. They are essentially off-the-shelf wearable computers. They can provide a convenient tool for measuring social connectivity features related to phone calls and text messages [1]. Users usually keep mobile phones physically close to themselves. The mobile sensor data thus reflects the same movement patterns as the user. Most Smartphones are equipped with accelerometers for motion detection, GPS (Global positioning system) monitor where a user visits and call logs record call duration. They are powerful social sensors for spatio-temporal data. Decreased movement detected by motion sensors or infrequent texts in the message log might be symptoms of depression. Shorter than usual calls might signal isolation.

© Springer International Publishing Switzerland 2015
X. Yin et al. (Eds.): HIS 2015, LNCS 9085, pp. 1–6, 2015.
DOI: 10.1007/978-3-319-19156-0_1

Real-time data collection and analysis of mobile phone data reveals information on the health state of a user and can be used to diagnose if a patient becomes symptomatic and prompt early treatment. Symptoms that can be detected are anxiety, stress, disease spread, and obesity [2, 3]. If symptoms are detected, a health care center can be alerted and a nurse can call the patient and check on his situation. This type of proactive healthcare is especially useful for high risk patients or patients susceptible of underreporting like mentally ill or elderly people.

2   Methodology

Reality mining refers to the process of collecting and analyzing machine sensed human behavioral data such as movement patterns, human interactions and human communication patterns, with the goal of detecting predictable behavioral patterns [18]. Reality mining comprises four phases. A data collection phase, a data pre-processing phase, a data mining phase and a post-processing phase. Sometimes a predictive analysis phase is added. Here the predictive step is considered part of the post-processing.

2.1   Data Collection

The data collection phase records a patient's behavioral data from interactions from electronic exchanges (call records, SMS logs, email headers) and contextual data (location information). Sometimes other data like face-to-face proximity for individuals has been collected too using the mobile phones Bluetooth connection [2]. The mobile phone is used to extract conversational partners and location of a user, that is, the total number of interactions, the diversity of interactions, and the diversity (entropy) of his behavior [2]. Smartphones provide APIs to access the underlying functionality such as GPS sensors or call logs programmatically.

2.2   Data Pre-processing

Not all data collected is useful. The data has thus to be relevance filtered first. Also the raw sensor data is not in a format that can be used by most ML algorithms. The data has to be transformed into a feature vector. A feature in a feature vector can represent the coordinates of a location or the call duration. Eigenvector analysis, commonly known as principal components analysis, is the optimal linear method for obtaining a low-dimensional approximation to a signal such as observations of user behavior [5]. Behavioral structure can be represented by the principal components of the spatiotemporal data set, termed eigen-behaviors [10]. The term eigenbehavior was introduced by Eagle and Pentland [11]. We represent this behavioral structure by the principal components of the complete behavioral dataset, a set of characteristic vectors we have termed eigenbehaviors [11]. Eigenbehaviors provide an efficient data structure for learning and classifying tasks.

To calculate the Eigenbehavior a person's behavior has to be measured, for instance the time sequence of their phone calls or text messages. For a group of M people, and the behaviors $\Gamma_1, \Gamma_2, \ldots, \Gamma_M$, the average behavior is:

$$\psi = \frac{1}{M} \sum_{n=1}^{M} \Gamma_n \qquad (1)$$

A set of M vectors, $\Phi_i = \Gamma_i - \Psi$, is defined to be the deviation of the normal behavior. Principle components analysis is subsequently performed on these vectors generating a set M orthonormal vectors, u_n, which best describes the distribution of the set of behavior data when linearly combined with their respective scalar values, λ_n [5]. The Eigenvector and Eigenvalues of the covariance matrix of Φ are calculated as:

$$C = \frac{1}{M} \cdot \sum_{n=1}^{M} \phi_n \cdot \phi_n^{T} = A \cdot A^{T} \qquad (2)$$

Where the Matrix $A = [\Phi_1, \Phi_2, \ldots, \Phi_M]$. A typical daily pattern is leaving the sleeping place in the morning, spending time in a small set of locations during office hours, and occasionally moving to a few locations in the evening and on the weekends. For typical individuals the top three Eigenbehavior components account for up to 96% of the variance in their behavior [5]. This means that a person's location context can be classified with high accuracy.

2.3   Data Mining

To make predictions about a person's health state, the behavioral data needs to be automatically classified into normal and deviant behavior. Machine learning (ML) techniques have been successfully applied for data classification problems. A given data set is typically divided into two parts: training and testing data sets with known class labels [8]. The class label is "normal" and "deviant" behaviour. The training data is the data collected during a training phase to learn a patient's normal behaviour as represented by the Eigenvector. It is used to train a model. The test data, the real-time behavioural data, is then applied against the trained model. The model analyses the data for any abnormalities and makes predictions about the health state. Typical supervised learning methods include naïve Bayes classification, decision tree induction, k-nearest neighbors, and support vector machines [4]. There are many more ML algorithms. Experience shows that no single machine learning scheme is appropriate to all data mining problems [9]. Usually several algorithms are trained and compared to determine which one gives the most accurate results for a given problem [6].

Ultimately we want to obtain a decision function f, that classifies the behavioral pattern h as normal (N), or deviant (D). If we denote the set of all behavioral patterns by H, we search for a function $f:H \rightarrow \{N,D\}$. We use the set of behavioral data collected during the training phase $\{(h_1, c_1), (h_2, c_2), \ldots, (h_n, c_n)\}$, where: $h_i \in H$, $c_i \in \{N, D\}$, to train the model. The naïve Bayes classifier is a family of simple probabilistic classifiers based on the Bayes theorem [6]. Decision tree learning creates decision trees, where a decision could be: did the patient go to coordinate x,y early in the morning, yes/no. Support Vector Machine (SVM) classifications are based on statistical learning theory and classifies data by separating them with a hyperplane. Which classification algorithm performs best can depend on the type of illness, but other factors such as the patient's normal behavior have an influence on the accuracy. Once the model is trained, it can be used for predictions based on real-time data collected through the mobile phone. ML techniques are well documented in literature [6,9,12] and are not further explored here.

2.4   Data Post-processing

Characteristic behavioral changes can be associated with symptoms based on the classification scheme from behavioral patterns. In the Susceptible, Infectious, Recovered or SIR model especially in the S(usceptible) to I(nfectious) transition phase user behavior changes [3] and can thus be used to improve prediction accuracy.

To analyze the temporal relationship of the behavior, Granger causality analysis has been used. The traditional linear Granger test has been widely used to examine the linear causality among several time series in bivariate settings as well as multivariate settings [14]. It is used to determine if one time series has predictive information for another. For a behavioral pattern a time series can be for instance the coordinates of places a patient frequently visited during the training phase, for instance the coordinates of his work place or favorite café. The second time series are the coordinates of places he visits over time during the testing phase.

The original Granger tests examined the linear causality among several time series in a bivariate and multivariate setting. However many real world applications are nonlinear and extensions have been developed [14, 16] to overcome this constraint. Recently the Phase Slope Index (PSI) has been preferred over Granger causality in some studies [3], [17]. PSI is a recently proposed spectral estimation method designed to measure temporal information flux between time series signals [3]. It is based on the assumption that the information flux between two signals can be estimated using the phase slope of the cross-spectrum of the signals. Independent noise mixing does not affect the complex part of the coherency between multivariate spectra, and hence PSI is considered more noise immune than Granger analysis [3]. The Phase Slope Index is defined as:

$$\Psi_{ij} = \Im(\sum_{f \in F} C_{ij}^{*}(f) C_{ij}(f + \delta f)) \tag{3}$$

Where C_{ij} is the complex coherency, $\delta f = 1/T$ is the frequency resolution, and $\Im(\cdot)$ denotes taking the imaginary part. PSI has been used to validate causal links between time series of symptom days where participants showed stress and depression symptoms [2].

3   Challenges and Ethical Issues

Behavioral patterns are highly personal and vary from individual to individual. Behavioral patterns of introverts, persons lacking social skills, lethargic or isolated persons show smaller variations when sick than active, sociable persons. Training and predictive models have to be enough granular to capture and detect deviant behavior of patients with a big variety of different behavioral patterns. There are many reasons why behavioral patterns change. Students before examinations spend more time studying and are less engaged in physical activities. Someone in a new relationship might change his behavioral patterns. The challenge of correctly classifying behavior and avoiding false positives based on misinterpretation like "work at home" interpreted as deviant behavior has to be addressed by any real-world application. Recording and analyzing the behavioral patterns of patients in real-time raises serious privacy issues. It represents a high level of surveillance where every movement and conversation is logged for analysis. There are also security issues. Announcing a person's location to the world can tip off burglars or stalkers.

4   Conclusions

While reality mining on mobile phones in the health care sector is still in its infancy, there are already promising applications. Modern societies face the challenge of caring for their aging population. Applications of reality mining using mobile phones might help elderly people, people with disabilities or diseases like Alzheimer's living safer and more independently and reduce health care costs. But there seems to be no boundary for further applications on the individual level as well as on the public health level. Reality mining has already been used to measure social interactions or movement patterns of populations to determine the spread of infectious diseases and studies have buttressed the effectiveness of cell phones for early detection of outbreaks of epidemics [1,2]. There are already projects studying the spread of diseases in Africa [7]. Our findings suggest that it might be possible to answer such questions in the near future and to begin planning how to influence the development of even greater health-sensing capabilities in smartphones [2].

Lastly reality mining has shown that humans are more predictable than believed and that it is thus possible to reveal the identity of a person even if the mobile phone data is anonymized. More research in anonymizing behavioral patterns in reality mining would be highly desirable especially when used in the eHealth area.

References

1. Chronis, I., Madan, A., Pentland, A.: SocialCircuits: the art of using mobile phones for modeling personal interactions. In: Proceedings of the ICMI-MLMI 2009 Workshop on Multimodal Sensor-Based Systems and Mobile Phones for Social Computing, Cambridge, Massachusetts, pp. 1–4 (2009)

2. Madan, A., Cebrian, M., Moturu, S., Farrahi, K., Pentland, A.: Sensing the "Health State" of a Community. IEEE Pervasive Computing **11**(4), 36–45 (2012)
3. Madan, A., Cebrian, M., Lazer, D., Pentland, A.: Social sensing for epidemiological behavior change. In: Proceedings of the 12th ACM International Conference on Ubiquitous Computing, Copenhagen, Denmark, pp. 291–300 (2010)
4. Gundecha, P., Liu, H.: Mining Social Media: A Brief Introduction. Informs **9**, 1–17 (2012)
5. Pentland, A.: Automatic mapping and modeling of human networks. Physica A: Statistical Mechanics and its Applications **378**(1), 59–67 (2007)
6. Wlodarczak, P., Soar, J., Ally, M.: What the future holds for Social Media data analysis. World Academy of Science, Engineering and Technology **9**(1), 545 (2015)
7. Big Data Gets Personal. MIT Technology Review **16**(4) (2013)
8. Tretyakov, K.: Machine learning techniques in spam filtering. In: U. o. T. Institute of Computer Science (ed.) Data Mining Problem-Oriented Seminar, p. 19 (2004)
9. Witten, I.H., Frank, E., Hall, M.A.: Data Mining, 3rd edn. Elsevier, Burlington (2011)
10. Sookhanaphibarn, K., Thawonmas, R., Rinaldo, F., Chen, K.-T.: Spatiotemporal analysis in virtual environments using eigenbehaviors. In: Proceedings of the 7th International Conference on Advances in Computer Entertainment Technology, Taipei, Taiwan, pp. 62–65 (2010)
11. Eagle, N., Pentland, A.: Eigenbehaviors: identifying structure in routine. Behavioral Ecology and Sociobiology **63**(7), 1057–1066 (2009)
12. Liu, B.: Sentiment Analysis and Opinion Mining. Morgan & Claypool (2012)
13. Liu, B.: Web Data Mining: Exploring Hyperlinks, Contents, and Usage Data, 2nd edn. Springer, Heidelberg (2011)
14. Bai, Z., Wong, W.-K., Zhang, B.: Multivariate linear and nonlinear causality tests. Mathematics and Computers in Simulation **81**(1), 5–17 (2010)
15. Diks, C., Panchenko, V.: A new statistic and practical guidelines for nonparametric Granger causality testing. Journal of Economic Dynamics and Control **30**(9–10), 1647–1669 (2006)
16. Hiemstra, C., Jones, J.D.: Testing for Linear and Nonlinear Granger Causality in the Stock Price- Volume Relation. The Journal of Finance **49**(5), 1639–1664 (1994)
17. Nolte, G., Ziehe, A., Krämer, N., Poupescu, F., Müller, K.-R.: Comparison of granger causality and phase slope index. In: NIPS 2008 Workshop on Causality, Canada (2008)
18. Simonite, T.: Smartphone Tracker Gives Doctors Remote Viewing Powers. Technology Review **116**(4) (2013)

Analysis and Comparison of the IEEE 802.15.4 and 802.15.6 Wireless Standards Based on MAC Layer

Renwei Huang, Zedong Nie$^{(\boxtimes)}$, Changjiang Duan, Yuhang Liu, Liya Jia, and Lei Wang

Shenzhen Institutes of Advanced Technology,
Chinese Academy of Sciences, Shenzhen, China
zd.nie@siat.ac.cn

Abstract. IEEE 802.15.4 and IEEE 802.15.6 are two kinds of wireless area network standards for short range communication applications. IEEE 802.15.4 is proposed for Wireless Person Area Network (WPAN) that provides low data rate, low power, and low cost applications in a short range. Meanwhile, IEEE 802.15.6 is the first international Wireless Body Area Network (WBAN) standard, which distributes nodes on or inside a human body, also operates in low power and short range, mainly provides real-time monitoring and human physiological data to judge the human physiological condition. In view of many similarities in both two standards, we analyzed the two standards mainly from the MAC frame format, MAC access mechanisms in this paper. In addition, some discussions of the differences of applications in the two standards were illustrated.

Keywords: WBAN · MAC · IEEE 802.15.4 · IEEE 802.15.6

1   Introduction

Nowadays, with the advancement of microelectronics technology, it becomes one of the most leading force to improve human existence and lifestyle through combing computer technology and communication technology. In this instance, the Wireless Sensor Networks (WSNs) with short distance, strong mobility, and high transmission rate is becoming more and more necessary and popular.

A WSN is composed of a large number of sensor nodes, and these nodes communicate with each other by self-organization and multi-hop [1]. A WSN is mainly used for monitoring physical or environmental conditions, such as temperature, sound, pressure, and to cooperatively pass their data through the network to a main location [2]. Earlier, several wireless communication standards have been formulated [3], such as the IEEE 802.11 [4], IEEE 802.15.1 [5], IEEE 802.15.4 [6] standards. However, these standards are not suitable for WBAN applications. The power consumption of 802.11 Wireless Local Area Network (WLAN) is too high to satisfy the wear WBAN requirements with a low power. In addition, the number of auxiliary nodes in IEEE 802.15.1 are limited. IEEE 802.15.4 is widely used in industrial sensors, smart grids

© Springer International Publishing Switzerland 2015
X. Yin et al. (Eds.): HIS 2015, LNCS 9085, pp. 7–16, 2015.
DOI: 10.1007/978-3-319-19156-0_2

and other areas of IOT (Internet of Things) [7], but it is not enough to support high data rate applications (data rate > 250 Kbps). In order to develop a low power consumption communication standard which is suitable for WBAN application [8], IEEE 802 established a task group for the standardization of WBAN called IEEE 802.15.6 in November 2007 [9]. WBAN is centered on the human body, which is composed of network elements (including personal terminal, independent nodes that are situated in the clothes, on the body or under the skin of a person, and communication equipment near human body within 3~5m) and so on [10]. WBANs provide unconstrained freedom of movement for patients suffering from chronic diseases, such as diabetes, heart disease [11]. The advantage is that a patient doesn't have to stay in bed, but can move everywhere freely, which improves the quality of life for patients and reduces hospital costs. In February 2012, the first version of IEEE 802.15.6-2012 was published.

IEEE 802.15.6 is a standard for short-range, wireless communications in the vicinity of, or inside, a human body (but not limited to humans) [9]. It defines a Medium Access Control (MAC) layer that works at lower sublayer of the data link layer of the OSI (Open System Interconnection) model [12], and offers unicast, multicast, or broadcast communication service. Unfortunately, more protocol details are hidden in current version of IEEE 802.15.6 standard, it is a better way to design a new WBAN system based on IEEE 802.15.4 standard, which is a mature protocol and has been applied in many fields. So far many research groups have studied the key issues of IEEE 802.15.4 and IEEE 802.15.6, the IEEE 802.15.6 MAC, PHY (Physical Layer), and security specifications were reviewed in [3]; the IEEE 802.15.4 security framework for WBAN was analyzed in [13]; the 802.15.4 MAC protocols for WBANs was introduced in [14]. However, few study was conducted to compare the similarities and differences between IEEE 802.15.4 and IEEE 802.15.6.

Analyzing and comparing 802.15.6 with 802.15.4 would help developers choose the better communication protocol to design new application systems and propose some approaches to optimize the 802.15.6 standard. In order to introduce the differences between the two standards, we discussed the MAC sublayer starting from the MAC format and access mechanisms, because the MAC sublayer plays an important role in providing guarantee for the reliable communication between SSCS (Service-Specific Convergence Sublayer) and PHY. The MAC sublayer concludes the MAC frame format, access mechanism and security services. The MAC frame format is used to indicate the frame types with different functions. The MAC access mechanism provides guarantee for the reliable communication. The security services make sure information safety. The MAC frame format and access mechanisms occupy an important position in the MAC sublayer, so we analyzed the two standards mainly from the MAC frame format, MAC access mechanisms in this paper.

The rest of the paper was organized into five sections. Section 2 presented the differences of the MAC frame format in the two standards. Section 3 introduced the different MAC access mechanisms between the two standards. A discussion of the differences of applications in the two standards was illustrated in section 4. The final section concluded our work.

2   Mac Frame Format of the Two Standards

A MAC frame is a sequence of fields in a specific order. The MAC frame format is composed of a MAC Header, a MAC Payload, and FCS both in IEEE 802.15.4 and IEEE 802.15.6. As depicted in Table 1.

Table 1. General MAC frame format

Octets: variable	variable	2
MAC Header	MAC Payload	FCS

If a device wants to transmit data to other devices in IEEE 802.15.4, it should contains a MAC Header with at least 9 octets length which is longer than those with 7 octets length in IEEE 802.15.6. These may result in many difficulties during the frames transmission and reception, such as increasing the burden of transceivers. In addition, the data rate will decrease and the transmission power will increase.

2.1   Frame Control field

Besides the intuitionistic difference of the length of MAC Header, there are many similarities and differences between the two frame control fields, as described in Table 2 and Table 3.

Table 2. Format of the Frame Control field in IEEE 802.15.4

Bits:0-2	3	4	5	6	7-9	10-11	12-13	14-15
Frame Type	Security Enabled	Frame Pending	ACK Request	PAN ID Compression	Reserved	Destination Addressing Mode	Frame Version	Source Addressing Mode

Table 3. Frame Control format of IEEE 802.15.6

Bits:1	2	2	1	1	1	4	2	1	1	8	3	1	4
Bit order:b0	b1-b2	b3-b4	b5	b6	b7	b0-b3	b4-b5	b6	b7	b0-b7	b0-b2	b3	b4-b7
Protocol Version	ACK Policy	Security Level	TK Index	BAN Security /Relay	ACK Timing/ EAP Indicator /First Frame On Time	Frame Subtype	Frame Type	More Data	Last Frame/ Access Mode/ B2	Sequence Number /Poll-Post Window	Fragment Number /Next	Non-final Fragment /Cancel/Scale /Inactive	Reserved

The Frame Type subfield of IEEE 802.15.4 is 3 bits in length and shall be set to one of the non-reserved values. 0b000, 0b001, 0b010, 0b011 respectively denote the beacon frame, data frame, response frame, MAC command frame, other values were reserved. The IEEE 802.15.6 describe the Frame Type by using not only Frame Type subfield but also Frame Subtype subfield. 0b00,0b01,0b10 of the Frame Type subfield represent management frame, control frame and data frame respectively, 0b11 is reserved. On the other hand, the Frame Subtype subfield refines the frame type with 4 bits data, which is helpful to classify different frames. For example, if a frame field carries security association information, it must be a management frame not a MAC command frame. In other words, a combination of Frame Type subfield and Frame Subtype subfield is more efficient than an independent use of Frame Type subfield. In addition, the IEEE 802.15.6 defines an UP (User Priority) to decrease collision possibility.

2.2   MAC Frame Body

In IEEE 802.15.4, the Frame Payload field has a variable length and contains information specific to individual frame types. The PHR (PHY header) frame length field identifies the length of the MAC frame, it is a byte long and the MSB of the PHR frame length field is not valid, so the length of the MAC frame can't exceed 127 bytes, which is not suitable to use the RTS/CTS mechanism. Nor is IEEE 802.15.6 with a variable length from 0 to 255 bytes of MAC Frame body. Because a RTS package with 20 bytes in length could account for about 20% of the MAC Frame body in IEEE 802.15.4 and 10% of those in IEEE 802.15.6 respectively, which lead to extra energy consumption, meanwhile, the RTS/CTS mechanism couldn't effectively restrain hidden conflicts [15]. In IEEE 802.15.6, when MAC Frame body has a nonzero length, it contains 1-bit Low-Order Security Sequence Number, a variable length of Frame Payload (Do not exceed pMaxFrameBodyLength) and 4-bit MIC (Message Integrity Code). The Low-Order Security Sequence Number field carries message freshness information required for nonce construction and relay detection. In addition, the last 32-bit MIC (Message Integrity Code) carries information about the authenticity and integrity of the current frame.

3   MAC Access Mechanism

As shown in in Figure 1, the IEEE 802.15.4 communication mode is represented.

In IEEE 802.15.4, the beacon-enabled with superframe uses a slotted ALOHA or slotted CSMA/CA in CAP and GTSs in CFP to exchange information between the coordinator and devices. In addition, unslotted CSMA/CA mechanism is used by non-beacon without superframe.

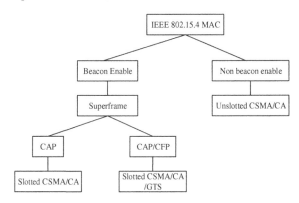

Fig. 1. IEEE 802.15.4 communication mode

Similarly, the IEEE 802.15.6 also employ the slotted ALOHA and CSMA/CA mechanism, what's more, there are two other protocols named improvised and unscheduled access mechanism and scheduled and scheduled-polling access mechanisms.

3.1   Random Access Mechanism

In EAP, RAP, and CAP periods of beacon mode with superframe boundaries of IEEE 802.15.6, as shown in Figure 2, the hub may employ either a slotted ALOHA or CSMA/CA protocol, depending on the PHY. To send data type frames of the highest UPs (User Priorities) based on CSMA/CA, a hub or a node may combine EAP1 and RAP1 as a single EAP1 and EAP2 and RAP2 as a single EAP2, so as to allow continual invocation of CSMA/CA and improve channel utilization. When using slotted ALOHA for high-priority traffic, RAP1 and RAP2 are replaced by another EAP1 and EAP2 respectively but not a continuation EAP1 and EAP2, due to the time slotted attribute of slotted ALOHA access.

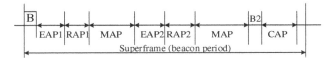

Fig. 2. Beacon mode with superframe boundaries in IEEE 802.15.6

In a slotted ALOHA protocol, the nodes access the channel using predefined UPs, as given in Table 4.

Table 4. Bounds for slotted-ALOHA and CSMA/CA protocols

| User | Slotted –ALOHA | | CSMA/CA | |
Priorities	CP_{max}	CP_{min}	CW_{max}	CW_{min}
0	1/8	1/16	64	16
1	1/8	3/32	32	16
2	1/4	3/32	32	8
3	1/4	1/8	16	8
4	3/8	1/8	16	4
5	3/8	3/16	8	4
6	1/2	3/16	8	2
7	1	1/4	4	1

Initially, the CP (Collision Probability) is selected according to the UPs. If Z≤CP, where Z is equal to a random number in the interval [0-1], the node obtains a contended allocation in the current ALOHA slot, during which data frames transmission occur. When the transmission is fail, the CP remains the same if the number of failures are odd or be cut in half if the number of failures are even.

The IEEE 802.15.4 protocol defines two versions of the CSMA/CA mechanism: slotted CSMA/CA mechanism for beacon mode with superframe and unslotted CSMA/CA mechanism for non-beacon network. In both cases, the algorithm is implemented using units of time called backoff periods, which is equal to aUnitBackoff-Period symbols. The CSMA/CA algorithm is controlled by three variables: NB (Number of Backoffs), CW (Content Window) and BE (Back off Exponent). Where NB is initialized to zero and the maximum value is 4. CW is decreased using units of backoff, the default value is 2 and the maximum is 31. BE is related to how many backoff periods a device shall wait before attempting to assess the channel and the scope of BE is 0~5, the default value is 3. The whole CSMA-CA algorithm is illustrated in Figure 3.

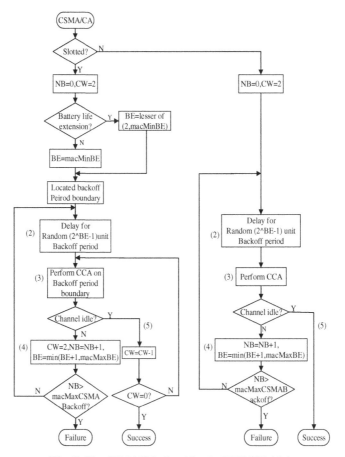

Fig. 3. The CSMA/CA algorithm in IEEE 802.15.4

In IEEE 802.15.6, the node initially sets BC (Backoff Counter) to a random inter that is uniformly distributed over the interval [1, CW], where CW $\in (CW_{min}, CW_{max})$. As shown in Table 4, the values of CW_{min} and CW_{max} are selected according to the

UPs. Before implementing the CSMA/CA algorithm, the CSMA slot boundary and pSIFS should be located, which each idle CSMA slot is equal to pCSMASlotLength and the default value of pSIFS is 75 μs. The m is the times of the node had failed consecutively. It is important to note that if double of the CW exceeds the CW_{max}, then the CW is CW_{max}. Figure 4 shows an example of the CSMA/CA algorithm.

Comparing the two CSMA/CA protocols in IEEE 802.15.4 and IEEE 802.15.6, it is found that there are some similarities and differences between them. First of all, since they are both CSMA/CA, so the node needs to detect the channel by using CCA (Clear Channel Access) before transmitting frames. CW is both used to implement backoff algorithm which is not the same in using. In IEEE 802.15.4, BE is related to how many backoff periods a device shall wait before attempting to assess the channel and the BEth backoff is randomly chosen from $\{0,1,\ldots,2^{BE}-1\}$, this is done to reduce the probability of the same backoff period for different nodes. However, owing to the less nodes, the shorter distance, the faster rate, the IEEE 802.15.6 defines UPs to decrease collision possibility. Different UPs mean different CW and BC, additionally, smaller CW and BC lead to low latency and higher channel utilization. All these designs are adopt to IEEE 802.15.6 network topology.

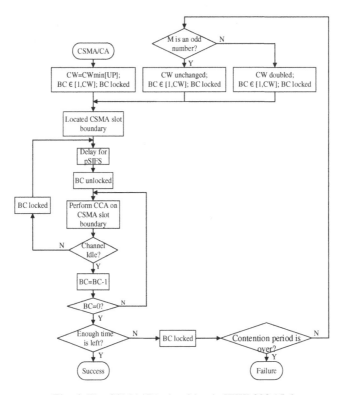

Fig. 4. The CSMA/CA algorithm in IEEE 802.15.6

3.2   Improvised and Unscheduled Access Mechanism

Besides the slotted ALOHA protocol and the CSMA/CA mechanism both in IEEE 802.15.4 and IEEE 802.15.6, there are another two access mechanisms in IEEE 802.15.6. The hub may use improvised access to send poll or post commands without advance reservation in beacon or non-beacon modes with superframe boundaries. Figure 5 illustrates an example of immediate polled allocations.

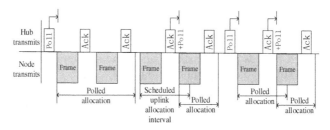

Fig. 5. Immediate polled allocations

The hub may also use an unscheduled access mechanism to obtain an unscheduled bilink allocation to apply for some specific condition, such as emergency communication service. In beacon or non-beacon modes with superframe, unscheduled bilink allocations may be 1-periodic, where frames transmission every superframe, or m-periodic, where frames transmission every m superframes. An m-periodic bilink allocation is helpful to reducing power consumption because nodes could sleep in m-periodic allocation.

3.3   Scheduled and Scheduled-Polling Access Mechanism

Unlike unscheduled allocation, a node and a hub may employ scheduled access to obtain scheduled uplink, downlink, and bilink allocations. In addition, the scheduled polling is used for polled and posted allocations. These allocations may be 1-periodic or m-periodic, but not the both in the same BAN. Figure 6 illustrates an example of scheduled 1-periodic allocations.

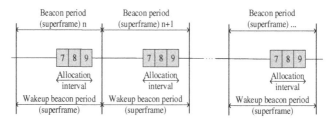

Fig. 6. Scheduled one-periodic allocation

4   A Discussion of Differences of Applications

The standards are described differ by which frequencies they used and the data rate and range they covered. According to Table 5, 802.15.6 (BAN) has a much shorter range than 802.15.4, which proves to be an advantage. Shorter range communication means lower power requirements. In addition, due to the short distance in the vicinity of, or inside, a human body only, it's more secure than 802.15.4. The lower consumption of the IEEE 802.15.6 not only comes from the sleep mode as same as IEEE 802.15.4, but also the shorter distance and less interference. In addition, it enables equipment to be smaller and frequency reuse to be better. The data rate of 802.15.6 is up to 15.6 Mbps, which is much faster than 802.15.4 with a max data rate 250 kbps [16]. All of these are good for BAN since the design of original intention is to make it unobtrusive, you can put it in the clothes, attach or implant into the human body, such as wearable devices.

Table 5. Comparison of the two wireless standards

Standard Project	802.15.4	802.15.6
MAC frame type	beacon frame, data frame response frame and command frame	management frame, control frame and data frame
MAC access mechanism	Slotted CSMA/CA Unslotted CSMA/CA	CSMA/CA mechanism Improvised and unscheduled access mechanism Scheduled and scheduled-polling access mechanism
Data Rate (Max)	20kbps,40kbps/250kbps	15.6Mbps
Transmission Range	75m	3~5m
Applications	Low data rate, industrial sensors, smart grid	Wearable devices

The major reason in increasing data rate is that the transmission medium is the human body, which with little interference. Coupling with new modulation techniques, making it possible that the data transfer rate of IEEE 802.15.6 is much higher than IEEE 802.15.4. In a word, IEEE 802.15.6 defines a new wireless communication technology for low power, high data rate, short range, high safety which is especially suitable for wearable device applications.

5   Conclusions

This paper presented the most significant features of comparison of MAC between IEEE 802.15.6 and IEEE 802.15.4 standard. An analysis of differences of MAC format and access mechanisms of the two standards were presented. At last, starting from the aspects of frequency, data rate and range, the superiority of 802.15.6 in BAN communication was discussed. We believed that this paper could be used to quickly understand the key feature of MAC sublayer of IEEE 802.15.4 and IEEE 802.15.6. Besides, it also helped you to develop the potential application of IEEE 802.15.6 on the basis of IEEE 802.15.4.

Acknowledgment. This study was financed partially by National Natural Science Foundation of China (Grant No.61403366), Shenzhen Basic Research Project Fund (JCYJ2014041711 3430695), the National 863 Program of China (Grant No. 2012AA02A604), the Next generation communication technology Major project of National S&T (Grant No. 2013ZX03005013).

References

1. Heragu, A., Ruffieux, D., Enz, C.: The design of ultralow-power MEMS-based radio for WSN and WBAN. In: Frequency References, Power Management for SoC, and Smart Wireless Interfaces, ed , pp. 265-280. Springer (2014)
2. Rawat, P., Singh, K.D., Chaouchi, H., Bonnin, J.M.: Wireless sensor networks: a survey on recent developments and potential synergies. The Journal of Supercomputing **68**, 1–48 (2014)
3. Ullah, S., Mohaisen, M., Alnuem, M.A.: A review of ieee 802.15. 6 mac, phy, and security specifications. International Journal of Distributed Sensor Networks (2013)
4. T. W. G. f. W.: Standards. IEEE WLAN (2012). http://www.ieee802.org/11/
5. IEEE WPAN Task Group 1 (2012). http://www.ieee802.org/15/pub/TG1.html
6. IEEEStd.802.15.4:WirelessMedium Access Control(MAC) and Physical Layer (PHY) Specifications for Low Data Rate Wireless. IEEE Std 802.15.4™-2006 (2006)
7. Gubbi, J., Buyya, R., Marusic, S., Palaniswami, M.: Internet of Things (IoT): A vision, architectural elements, and future directions. Future Generation Computer Systems **29**, 1645–1660 (2013)
8. Nie, Z.D., Ma, J.J., Ivanov, K., Wang, L.: An investigation on dynamic human body communication channel characteristics at 45MHz in different surrounding environments. In: Antennas and Wireless Propagation Letters, p. 1. IEEE (2014)
9. IEEE Standard for Local and metropolitan area networks - Part 15.6: Wireless Body Area Networks, IEEE Std 802.15.6-2012, pp. 1-271 (2012)
10. Chávez-Santiago, R., Khaleghi, A., Balasingham, I., Ramstad, T. A.: Architecture of an ultra wideband wireless body area network for medical applications. In: 2nd International Symposium on Applied Sciences in Biomedical and Communication Technologies, ISABEL 2009, pp. 1-6 (2009)
11. Kim, T.-H., Kim, Y.-H.: Human effect exposed to UWB signal for WBAN application. Journal of Electromagnetic Waves and Applications, 1-15 (2014)
12. Kumar, M. G., Roy, K.S.: Zigbee Based Indoor Campus Inventory Tracking Using Rfid Module
13. Saleem, S., Ullah, S., Kwak, K.S.: A study of IEEE 802.15. 4 security framework for wireless body area networks. Sensors **11**, 1383–1395 (2011)
14. Ullah, S., Shen, B., Islam, S.M., Khan, P., Saleem, S., Kwak, K.S.: A study of MAC protocols for WBANs. Sensors (Basel) **10**, 128–145 (2010)
15. Barroca, N., Borges, L. M., Velez, F.J., Chatzimisios, P.: IEEE 802.15. 4 MAC layer performance enhancement by employing RTS/CTS combined with packet concatenation. In: 2014 IEEE International Conference on Communications (ICC), pp. 466-471 (2014)
16. Nie, Z., Ma, J., Li, Z., Chen, H., Wang, L.: Dynamic propagation channel characterization and modeling for human body communication. Sensors **12**, 17569–17587 (2012)

Securing Electronic Medical Record and Electronic Health Record Systems Through an Improved Access Control

Pasupathy Vimalachandran$^{(\boxtimes)}$, Hua Wang, and Yanchun Zhang

Centre for Applied Informatics, College of Engineering and Science,
Victoria University, Melbourne, Australia
Pasupathy.Vimalachandran@live.vu.edu.au,
{hua.wang,yanchun.zhang}@vu.edu.au

Abstract. During the last two decades, modern technology is increasingly being used in the healthcare sector in order to enhance the quality and the cost efficiency of the healthcare services. In this process, Electronic Medical Record (EMR) has been introduced to collect, store and communicate patient's medical information. The EMR systems enable efficient collection of meaningful, accurate and complete data to assist improved clinical administration through the development, implementation and optimisation of clinical pathways. While its cost and time savings are encouraging for transition, it does not come without inherent challenges. Inadequate policy development in the areas of data security and privacy of health information appear to be the major weakness. In this paper, we present a secure access control model for the EMR and Electronic Health Record (EHR) to provide acceptable protection for health sensitive data retained at healthcare organisations. We systematically analyse four existing access control mechanisms that have been proposed in the past, and present a combined more secure model for the EMR and EHR for healthcare provider organisations in Australia.

Categories and Subject Descriptions: Security and protection – access control

General Terms: Security · Access control · EMR · EHR · PCEHR

1 Introduction

25 years ago, patient records were on 8 x 5 inch cards, receipts were done using the Kalamazoo system, suture material was okay to reuse if soaked in antiseptic solution, and the only transfer of information was by telephone or mail [1]. Times have now changed. 98% of general practitioners now have a computer on their desk and 70% to 94% use computers to the level of regularly documenting progress notes/clinical records [2]. In most parts of the developed world, healthcare has evolved to a point where patients have more than one healthcare provider. This may include general practitioners, specialists, allied health services and hospitals to service their diverse medical needs. As a result, medical records have been found scattered throughout the entire healthcare sector, from primary care - general practices and clinical laboratories, to

© Springer International Publishing Switzerland 2015
X. Yin et al. (Eds.): HIS 2015, LNCS 9085, pp. 17–30, 2015.
DOI: 10.1007/978-3-319-19156-0_3

pharmacies and specialist practices. This has resulted in the growing need to create an integrated infrastructure for the collection of diverse medical data for healthcare professionals, where the adoption of standardised Electronic Health Record (EHR) has become imminent.

The distinction between EMR and EHR can be quite confusing. The EMR consists of electronic information about a patient recorded in an individual clinic, and performs a similar function to that previously performed by the paper record. The EHR, on the other hand, is a summary of health events (usually drawn from several EMRs) and may consist of the elements that are eventually shared in a national EHR [1]. An online EHR enables patients to manage and contribute to their own medical notes in a centralised way which greatly facilitates the storage, access and sharing of personal health data. It is clear that storing medical records digitally on the cloud offers great promise for increasing the efficiency of the healthcare system. As a result, a national EHR was introduced to Australia in 2012 and the Government has invested $467 million to build key components of the Personally Controlled Electronic Health Record (PCEHR) to improve health outcomes and reduce costs in the country [3].

The setting up of the PCEHR system faces many challenges which ultimately impede its wider adoption. Privacy and confidentiality of patients' health information is crucial. Once patients' personal health data are stored in the cloud or local server with EMR or EHR, it is not quite clear who else can access it other than the patient's usual doctor. For example, with the current system, in a healthcare provider organisation, all other healthcare providers working for the organisation can access patient clinical information. There are also instances where administration staff may access patients' clinical information for improving the business (e.g. targeting chronic disease high risk or pap smear patients who are due for a reminder).

Healthcare organisations are inherently complex and dynamic environments [4], [5] which makes it difficult for administrators to define access control policies [6]. EMR and EHR user privileges are therefore often defined at a coarse level to minimise workflow inefficiencies and maximise flexibility in the management of a patient. The consequence of such practice is that EMR systems are left vulnerable to potential abuse from insiders who are authenticated within the organisation, which ultimately can compromise patient confidentiality. Furthermore, Information Technology (IT) technical staff or the system operators who maintain the IT systems and the databases also may access patients' clinical information. This leads to risk of intentional or unintentional leakage, despite privacy and confidentiality agreements. However, these agreements do not eliminate leaks occurring, they mitigate the risk, based on the person's professional integrity. This demonstrates that information stored in EMR and EHR databases or cloud servers face significant risk of exposure. This potential for internal abuse must be addressed. It is also important to acknowledge and investigate these challenges and shortcomings associated with the current electronic health information system and determine possible solutions to ensure its wide adoption and success of the PCEHR system in Australia.

In this paper, we discuss four different existing access control strategies and eight different spectrums of attack or misuse that have been identified in the past and we present a combined and improved access control mechanism with a security model to the health industry.

2   Related Work

There are different access control strategies for EHR and EMR that have been developed in the past [4].

According to one Forrester study, 80% of data security and privacy breaches involve insiders, employees or those with internal access to an organisation, putting information at risk [5]. With health sensitive data, this risk becomes more prominent. Many researchers have proposed various resolutions to solve the security and privacy problems associated with the EMRs and EHRs. These problems mainly refer to access control. The term "access control" is simply defined as "the ability to permit or deny the use of something by someone" [5]. The key objective of access control mechanisms is to permit authorised users to manipulate data and thus maintain the privacy of data [6]. There are different access control mechanisms that have been identified in the literature review. The basic models of the access control principles are i) Discretionary Access Control (DAC), ii) Mandatory Access Control (MAC), iii) Role Based Access Control (RBAC) and iv) Purpose Based Access Control (PBAC). However, the development is not satisfactory enough to fulfil the privacy requirements of EMRs and EHRs [7].

DAC uses access restriction set by the owner and restricts access to the objects. However a user who is allowed to access an object by the owner of the object has the capability to pass on the access right to other users without the involvement of the owner of the object [8]. Because of this granting, read access transitive, the policies are open for Trojan Horse Attack [9].

MAC is a set of security and privacy policies constrained according to system classification, configuration and authentication. The policies made by a central authority [10]. Compared to DAC, MAC policy can prevent a Trojan Horse Attack and the integrity of the data objects can be protected by using the "Read Up" and "Write Down" Rules. In MAC, the individual owner of an object has no right to control the access. Therefore, MAC policy fails to preserve the privacy requirement for EHRs of the patients [11].

In RBAC [9], each user's access right is determined based on user roles and the role-specific privileges associated with them. RBAC policy uses the need-to-know principle to assign permissions to roles and to fulfil the least privileged condition by the system administrator. However, RBAC does not integrate other access parameters or related data that are significant in allowing access to the user [12]. PBAC is based on the notion of relating data objects with purposes [13]. Many researchers have identified that greater privacy preservation is possible by assigning objects with purposes [14]. However, Al-Fedaghi describes [15] that PBAC leads to a great deal of complexity at the access control level.

In addition to access control mechanisms, it is also important to identify the spectrum of attacks or misuse that could be performed by attackers. A wide range of attacks have been documented in the literature. It is essential to know the different possible attacks for health based databases, in order to design a suitable health data security system. To achieve this goal the literature review has been performed to discuss different main attacks that health based databases currently face.

In the British Computer Society website at http://www.bcs.org/server.php?
show=ConWebDoc.8852, Amichai Schulman and Imperva say "enterprise database
infrastructures, which often contain the crown jewels of an organisation, are subject to
a wide range of attacks" [16].

A review of previous attacks has revealed the following main methods utilised to
obtain sensitive health information.

1. Excessive privilege granted to staff
2. Privilege abuse
3. Unauthorised privilege elevation
4. Platform vulnerabilities
5. SQL injection
6. Weak audit
7. Weak authentication
8. Exposure of back-up data

With excessive privilege, healthcare organisation application users are granted privileges that may exceed the requirements of their role.   As an example, a reception/
administrative staff member whose job requires name, contact details and time of the
appointments of a patient, may be able to view clinical notes of patients.

Healthcare application users may abuse legitimate data access privileges for unauthorised purposes. This is known as 'privilege abuse'.

Unauthorised privilege elevation means that the attackers may take advantage
of vulnerabilities in health based cloud software systems to convert low-level
access privileges to high-level access privileges. For instance, an attacker may take
advantage of cloud based system buffer overflow vulnerability to grant administrative
privileges.

Platform vulnerability is taking advantage of the vulnerabilities in underlying operating systems, which may lead to unauthorised data access or corruption. The blaster
worm took advantage of a Windows 2000 vulnerability to take down target servers
[17].

Users may take advantage of vulnerabilities in front-end web applications and
stored procedures to send unauthorised database queries. This is known as "SQL injection".

Weak audit policy and technology represents risks in terms of compliance, deter-
rence, detection, forensics and recovery.   In other words, the cloud based health system software provides weak audit solutions itself. These products very rarely log the
detail about what application was used; the source IP address and what queries failed.

Weak authentication allows attackers to assume the identity of legitimate database
users. Most of the time, the users use their name, personal identification, meaningful
words or plain text as a password.

In most situations, people protect the main cloud based health database, not actual
back-ups. With exposure of back-up data, attacks have involved theft of database
backup tapes and hard disks.

3   Secure EMR and EHR Through an Improved Access Control Mechanism

The system operator of the PCEHR who manages the system or practice staff in a healthcare provider organisation, may intentionally leak patients' clinical information. The access control currently in use does not prevent this kind of breach.

In a healthcare provider organisation or an organisation that manages an EHR system, it is not clear who accesses what information in that organisation. In a general practice (medium or large) environment in Australia, organisations normally use two types of software systems to deal with patients. One is the Patient Management System (PMS) that assists with appointment and billing related tasks. This is also known as the 'billing system'. The other is for managing clinical tasks and information and is called the 'clinical system'. Most general practice software systems are integrated with both tasks. In some cases, the same product has two software systems which are compatible and work together. If an organisation uses different software systems for billing and clinical, then assigning access control is easier. For instance, reception staff have access to the billing system and not the clinical system. On the other hand clinicians including doctors and nurses access both clinical and PMS but not billing. However if an organisation uses an integrated one system for both billing and clinical, then the issues associated with access control becomes complicated. However there are situations, where healthcare organisations manage this issue by giving permission levels based on the roles and purposes. These permission controls are managed by the software itself.

In healthcare organisations, there are non-clinical staff, such as administration staff who may need to access clinical related information to target patients to increase the organisation's business. For example; the practice follows up with health checks due and reminds mainstream patients or identified chronic disease high risk patients of the need for consultations. In these circumstances, administration staff may access clinical information. This access may lead to internal abuse. Therefore, administration staff accessing clinical information is a risk. However, considering the financial benefit to the organisation, it cannot just be ignored. Hence the access must carefully be monitored and controlled to maintain the privacy and confidentiality of patients to mitigate this risk.

The healthcare organisation's software systems use DAC and MAC access control principles. RBAC is also used in those systems however PBAC is not in use in many healthcare systems because of the complexity at the access level. Furthermore, considering the current privacy and security issues associated with health records, a single access control principle is inadequate to protect the highly sensitive information. Thus, it is crucial to use a combination of more than one access control principles in this environment. When administration staff access clinical information from the system where RBAC is switched on, the purpose of the access is not mentioned. To solve this issue, an authorisation from an authority must be given to access the information.

Then a combination of RBAC and PBAC must be applied for a secure access. This means, if an administration staff wants to access the clinical information, a high level management staff must give permission every time. High level management staff might be a doctor or a nurse or practice manager who has high level privilege to access all parts of the health record. This will require both access control principles RBAC and PBAC for access.

In computer security, access control covers authentication, authorization and audit. Access control systems provide the important services of identification, authentication, authorization and accountability to enter into an application or system. Identification and authentication determine who can log into a system (the system may be an application or even an operating system). Authorization provides different privileges for a system (usually categorized high-level, medium-level and low-level) in accordance with employee's role in a healthcare organisation. Finally the accountability identifies the subject a user worked on during his or her log-in.

The Security Engineering Guide (SEG) explains the term as "Access control is the traditional centre of gravity of computer security. It is where security engineering meets computer science" [18].

The security engineering guide also discusses how the access control works at a number of levels and describes the following different levels in Figure 1.

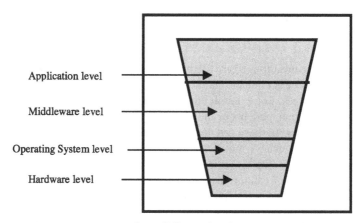

Fig. 1. Access *controls at different levels in a system* [18]

Authentication, authorization and audit ability and their levels of permission vary on different levels of access control for a system.

4   Proposed Model ("HighSec System")

After considering several aspects of access control mechanisms through literature research, it was realized that there is a real need to put more control on this level of security. This led to developing a mechanism called "log-in pair" which will be an ideal answer to minimise the potential for misuse or abuse of health data within a healthcare organisation. If this concept can be followed with well-planned pair design within a healthcare organisation, it will be one of the better options for maintaining high security.

In many instances, health sensitive and confidential data (e.g.; clinical notes / medical conditions) are stored in databases of clinical software systems. These data are susceptible to internal abuse as they can be viewed by anyone in the internal setting. Hence this sensitive data needs to be protected from internal abuse. The "log–in pair" is a technique which may achieve this objective.

Log-in pair: To access data through this system, an employee who has top level privilege (super user) has to give authorisation to a user to access health sensitive data. Hence, the super user keeps track of what the user does with the sensitive data. Every user is made aware that once they log in, the super user follows them, and keeps track of what is being accessed. It is like a counter check. The responsibility and the accountability are shared. This concept will ensure high security.

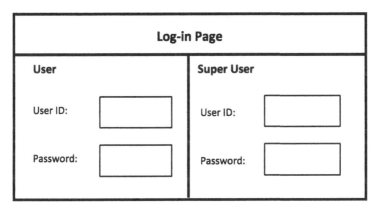

Fig. 2. Sample log-in page

When the pairs are set-up, the following main factors need to be considered; the physical location of the users and super users (e.g.; sharing the same office), job discipline of users (employees who are working in a similar discipline are paired) and the frequency and time an employee enters and uses the system (e.g.; an employee who needs to use the system for the whole day, all seven days a week should be paired with another employee who also uses the system for the whole day, all seven days a week rather than with an employee who only needs to access the system for a few hours in a week).

As Figure 2 illustrates, every user has his or her own individual user id and password to enter into the system. In this pair log-in concept, see table 1 below, for user A to enter into the system the super user D should enter his or her user id and password as well. Consider a healthcare organisation with three users (A, B and C) and three super users (D, E and F).

Table 1. Basic pair design

Pair	Users & Super Users
1	A & D or E or F
2	B & D or E or F
3	C & D or E or F

The log-in page must be designed to accept inputs for two users with separate user identification and password.

The security assurance in this system is that one person cannot function on his or her own. If one user wants to enter into the system, he or she must be given super user permission. Hence, it mitigates users abusing the system.

This system has its own problems:

1) If all super users are absent (from above example, if D, E and F are on leave) a user cannot enter into the system or perform routine jobs.
2) The system cannot prevent both user and super user as a pair deciding to abuse the data.
3) Having someone else to log in the same time as another user creates potential sources of bottleneck and make user frustrated with the system.
4) If doctors and nurses are potential "gatekeepers" (the authoring login), these professions are already extremely busy, and likely to create users circumventing the system.
5) If authorising persons consistently logon and give the login credentials to users, then this defeats the aim of the system.

To overcome the first problem, a super user may be able to give permission through the internet or networking as a future development. Alternatively doctors will also be considered as super user who can give permission for users to work on sensitive data.

However, it is very difficult to overcome the second problem. A system monitoring facility may be developed as a part of this system to monitor the users and super users. A system audit and/or quality improvement process may mitigate this risk.

The system itself must be notified and does not give access to other users to avoid bottlenecks and unnecessary delays in logging on the system over the network at that point in time.

In practice, doctors and nurses are extremely busy and difficult to contact to gain their login in order to access the system. However, they are the people who have got authorisation to access clinical information in healthcare organisation environment. To resolve this issue in creating users circumventing the system, alternative non-clinical top level staff can be appointed (i.e.; practice manager, assistant practice manager).

Super user authorisation is a crucial part of this method. Therefore login credentials of super users must be strong and changed periodically. Considering super users availability, the system can be configured to send an auto creating password to the super user through email or as a text message to mobile phone weekly. One option may be that the super user can login to the system using their member password (which is different to authorisation password) and view the weekly authorisation password.

5   Construction of the Proposed Model

When designing the pairs, the healthcare organisation internal workflow, organisation chart and the management inputs can also be considered. The log-in page must be designed to accept inputs for two users with separate user identification and password.

This can be accomplished using the same computer or different computers which are networked. The users should log-in one after another within 90 seconds. If the second user fails to login within 90 seconds of the first user logging-in, the permission to enter into the system will be refused.

The following specification and Figure 3 explain the construction of the proposed model.

Specification:
1. *Item – text box. Input into user_pw.u_id.*
2. *Item – text box. Input into user_pw.u_pw*
3. *Item - check box. Value (Y/N). If Value = 'Y' open Block 2 and enable. If value = 'N' hide Block 2.*
4. *Item - push button. On press open the main form.*
5. *Item – push button. On press exit from the application*
6. *Item – text box. Input into Block2.new_password.*
7. *Item – text box. Input into Block2.confirm_password.*
8. *Item - push button.*
    On press check that, if (New password =   confirm password)
    alter table user_pw
    setu_pw = new_password;
    commit change.
9. *Item - push button. On press clear item new_password, confirm_password.*
    Hide block 2.

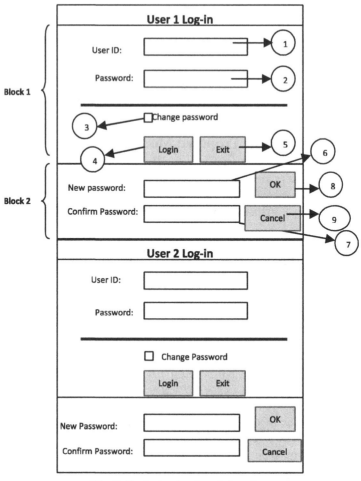

Fig. 3. Designing log-in pair interface

6   Conclusion and Future Suggestions

In this paper, we have introduced a new concept called 'log-in-pair' in access control. Even though access control is the first and basic security level for any computer system, it is important to make sure that the level of protection is high. This may be an ideal answer to minimise misuse or abuse within healthcare organisations. Though the proposed method seems easy to implement, in practice, there will be more concerns when this concept is in progress.

However, we are sure, if this concept could be followed with well-planned pair designing through education, policies and procedures within an organisation, it would be one of the better solutions in maintaining and practicing a high security system in a healthcare environment.

Log-in pair, the concept sounds good, but needs additional consideration in making pair users. There are number of factors/criteria that should be developed to satisfy this level of security. The physical location of the user of the pair user, discipline of the user, work load and purpose are some of them. A System Monitoring Facility (SMF), with log-in pair, which will observe the user activities with the EMR and EHR systems, and log audits after a user has entered into the system. This kind of SMF would definitely be beneficial in increasing the level of security for access control. Hence, an appropriate policy and procedure documentation in creating user pair and a SMF in monitoring users' could be considered for future development. Multiple login and logout over a day must be considered and resolved.

References

1. Pearce, C.: Electronic medical records - where to from here?. Professional Practice, Melbourne (2009)
2. McInnes, D.K., Slatman, D.C., Kidd, M.R.: General practitioners' use of computers for prescribing and electronic health records: results from a national survey, Australia (2011) http://www.clinfowiki.org/wiki/index.php/General_practitioners%27_use_of_computers_f or_prescribing_and_electronic_health_records:_results_from_a_national_survey (accessed September 12, 2014)
3. Department of Health Aging , Get your personal eHealth record now, Canberra: Department of Health Aging (2013) www.ehealth.gov.au (accessed June 28, 2013)
4. Bosch, M., Faber, M.J., Cruijsberg, J., Voerman, G.E., Leatherman, S., Grol, R.P., Hulscher, M., Wensing, M.: Review article: Effectiveness of patient care teams and the role of clinical expertiseand coordination: A literature review. Med. Care Res. and Rev. (2009)
5. Kannampallil, T.G., Schauer, G.F., Cohen, T., Patel, V.L.: Considering complexity in healthcare systems. J.Biomed. Informatics (2011)
6. Malin, B., Nyemba, S., Paulett, J.: Learning relational policies from electronic health record accesslogs. J. Biomed. Informatics (2011)
7. Motta, G.H.M.B., Furuie, S.S.: A contextual role-based access control authorization model for electronic patient record. IEEE Transactions on Information Technology in Biomedicine
8. Symantec Corporation, Strengthening Database Security (2006) http://www.federal newsradio.com/pdfs/StrengtheningDataBaseSecurityWP.pdf (accessed June 30, 2013)
9. Barua, M., Liang, X., Lu, R., Shen, X.: An efficient and secure patient-centric access control scheme for eHealth care system. In: IEEE Conference on Computer Communications Workshops (2011)
10. Santos-Pereira, C., Augusto, A.B., Cruz-Correia, R.: A secure RBAC mobile agent access control model for healthcare institutions. In: IEEE 26th International Symposium on Computer-Based Medical Systems (CBMS) (2013)
11. Gajanayake, R., Iannella, R., Sahama, T.: Privacy oriented access control for electronic health records. Presented in Data Usage Management on the Web Workshop at the Worldwide Web Conference. ACM, Lyon Convention Center, Lyon, France (2012)
12. Ferraiolo, D.F., Kuhn, D.R., Chandramouli, R.: Role-based access control, 2nd edition. Artech house (2003); Bauer, F.L.: Decrypted Secrets, 2nd edition. Springer (2000)
13. Sandhu, R.S., Samarati, P.: Access control: principle and practice. IEEE Communications Magazine (1994)
14. Motta, G.H.M.B., Furuie, S.S.: A contextual role-based access control authorization model for electronic patient records. IEEE Information Technology in Biomedicine (2003)
15. Evered, M., Bögeholz, S.: A case study in access control requirements for a health information system. In: Proceedings of the second Australian Information Security Workshop, AISW 2004, Dunedin, New Zealand (2004)

16. Byun, J.-W., Bertino, E., Li, N.: Purpose based access control of complex data for privacy protection. In: Proceedings of the Tenth ACM Symposium on Access Control Models and Technologies, New York, USA (2005)
17. Naikuo, Y., Howard, B., Ning, Z.: A purpose-based access control model. Journal of Information Assurance and Security (2007)
18. Al-Fedaghi, S. S.: Beyond purpose-based privacy access control. In: Proceedings of the Eighteenth Conference on Australasian Database, vol. 63. Australian Computer Society, Inc, Ballarat, Victoria, Australia (2007)
19. Schulman, A.: Top 10 database attacks, U. K (2007). http://www.bcs.org/server.php?show=ConWebDoc.8852
20. NoWires Research Group, University of Bergin , Introduction to Database Security, Bergin, July 2007. http://www.kjhole.com/WebSec/PDF/Database.pdf
21. Espiner, T.: Security Threats Toolkit: Security expertscrticise government database plans, U.K, January 2007. http://news.zdnet.co.uk/security/0,1000000189,39285536,00.htm
22. Wang, H., Cao, J., Zhang, Y.: A Flexible Payment Scheme and Its Role-Based Access Control. IEEE Transactions on Knowledge & Data Engineering **17**(3), 425–436 (2005)
23. Wang, H., Zhang, Y., Cao, J.: Access control management for ubiquitous computing. Future Generation Computer Systems **24**(8), 870–878 (2008)
24. Kabir, E., Wang, H., Bertino, E.: A conditional purpose-based access control model with dynamic roles. Expert Systems with Applications **38**(3), 1482–1489 (2011)

Appendix: Implementation of the Proposed Model

The following sample coding has been tested to validate the system using Visual Basic.6 programming language.

```
Function checkdata() As Boolean
bcheck = True
    If txtuser.Text = "" Then
MsgBox "Enter user name", , "HighSec System"
txtuser.SetFocus
bcheck = False
        Exit Function
    End If
    If txtpassword.Text = "" Then
MsgBox "Enter Password", , "HighSec System"
txtpassword.SetFocus
bcheck = False
        Exit Function
    End If
     If cmbUsertype.Text = "Normal" Then
        If cmbManager.Text = "Select" Then
MsgBox "Select Manager", , "HighSec System"
txtpassword.SetFocus
bcheck = False
            Exit Function
        End If
     End If
checkdata = bcheck
End Function

Private Sub cmbUsertype_Click()
    If cmbUsertype.Text = "Normal" Then
        Frame1.Visible = True
    Else
        Frame1.Visible = False
    End If
End Sub
```

Coding I – New user registration

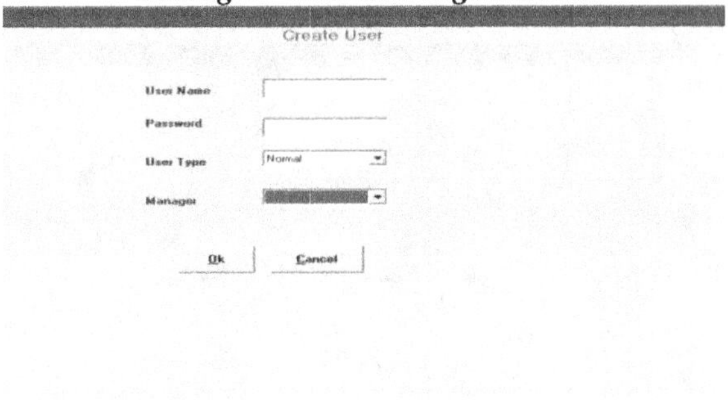

Fig. 4. System interface for new user registration

```
Private Sub cmdok_Click()
bcheck = checkdata
usertype = Left(cmbUsertype.Text, 1)
 If bcheck = checkdata Then
rs.Open "select * from usertable where userid='" + txtuser.Text + "'", cn
        If Not rs.EOF And Not rs.BOFThen
MsgBox "This user already exists", , "HighSec System"
        Else
newpwd = encryptdata(txtpassword.Text, newkey)
newpwd = txtpassword.Text
ssql = "insert into usertable (userid,pwd,usertype) values('" + txtuser.Text + "','" +
newpwd + "','" + usertype + "')"
 InputBox "", ,ssql

cn.Executessql
        If usertype = "N" Then
ssql = "insert into groupuser (user1,user2) values('" + txtuser.Text + "','" +
cmbManager.Text + "')"
cn.Executessql
        End If
ans = MsgBox("User created succesfully. " + vbCrLf + " Do you want to close this
window?", vbYesNo)
            If ans = vbYes Then
                Unload Me
            Else
txtuser.Text = ""
txtpassword.Text = ""
        End If
    End If
rs.Close
    End If
End Sub


Private Sub Form_Load()
ssql = "select * from usertable where usertype='M'"
rs.Openssql, cn
While Notrs.EOF
cmbManager.AddItemrs(0)
rs.MoveNext
Wend
rs.Close
cmbUsertype.ListIndex = 0
End Sub
```

Coding II – Creating super (pair) user and the verification process

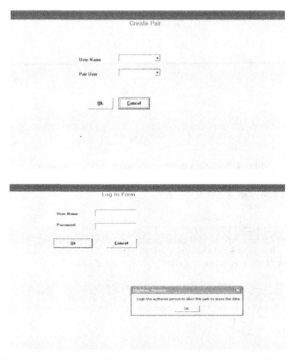

Fig. 5 and 6. System interfaces for creating new user and the verification process

Supporting Frontline Health Workers Through the Use of a Mobile Collaboration Tool

Jane Li[1(✉)], Leila Alem[2], and Weidong Huang[3]

[1] CSIRO Digital Productivity Flagship, P.O. Box 76, Epping, NSW 1710, Australia
jane.li@csiro.au
[2] University of Technology, Sydney, Australia
Leila.Alem@uts.edu.au
[3] University of Tasmania, Hobart, TAS, Australia
Tony.Huang@utas.edu.au

Abstract. This paper presents our work in exploring the design of a mobile collaboration tool to support frontline health workers who deliver healthcare services at local communities and patients' homes. Our design addresses their collaboration needs when they discuss patient cases with remote clinicians during the home visits. The tool is tablet-based and supports real-time communication and information sharing between health workers and clinicians and also asynchronous information exchange between them through the recording of rich media annotations. We present preliminary results from a pilot study examining the usability of the tool.

1 Introduction

Frontline health workers are those directly providing services to patients in area where they are most needed, particularly in remote and rural areas. Due to the shortage of skilled clinicians (e.g. medical specialist, general practitioner, specialist nurse), frontline health workers play a pivotal role in assisting the delivery of healthcare services at the local communities and patients homes. They are trained to manage patients' chronic conditions, common infections and other basic health needs. They also help identify conditions which require higher levels of care and provide a link to other healthcare service providers who work with them as a team for the care of patients.

Empowering frontline health workers and providing them with means to access clinical expertise when needed are important for them to deliver services to their patients. We have engaged with a group of clinicians and health workers and identified two collaboration needs. Frontline health workers may need to discuss patient cases in real time with remote clinicians to make decisions regarding the care of the patients during the home visits. As clinicians are not necessarily available, frontline health workers may also need to engage with clinicians by using asynchronous communication - health workers capture and save information collected during the home visits and share it with clinicians who review it at convenient time for assessment offline.

We have explored the design of a mobile collaboration tool. Our design work has been informed by the two collaboration needs of frontline health workers.

X. Yin et al. (Eds.): HIS 2015, LNCS 9085, pp. 31–36, 2015.
DOI: 10.1007/978-3-319-19156-0_4

This work is a preliminary contribution to the research in the field of telehealth which focuses on remote collaboration in healthcare. There are two traditional modes of collaboration in telehealth. One is real-time telehealth and the other is stored-and-forward or asynchronous telehealth which has been commonly used when real-time collaboration is not practical. Recently studies have suggested that a "hybrid" approach which integrates real-time and asynchronous telehealth fits well with clinicians' work flow and improves the efficiency of their practices [1, 2].

Our design has been inspired by the recent development in social media communication and cross time zone collaboration in which the boundary between synchronous and asynchronous interactions is blurred [3, 4]. Researchers have explored the design of rich media contents - combining the recordings of audio and video of interactions (e.g. annotation) over artefacts, as proxies for asynchronous communication [3, 4]. Annotation over video and still images provides rich support for real time collaboration [5, 6]. Our work extends the work of [3, 4] by incorporating the feature of recording annotation over video content.

Real-time telehealth relies on audio-video communication and sharing a range of medical information to support healthcare professionals to discuss patient diagnoses and treatment plans. Mobile and tablet devices have been increasingly used in telehealth [7]. One of our attentions is directed to how to appropriately integrate and configure audio-video communication space with information sharing space in mobile tablet devices to address the complexity of interactions in telehealth.

In this paper we first outline the technical design of the collaboration tool. We then present preliminary results of a pilot study that examined the usability of tool. We will finish with a discussion of potential future work.

2   Design

In this section we will briefly introduce the design of the mobile collaboration tool (ReColl). Hand-held table device is used as hardware interface for ReColl as it is portable for health workers to carry it around. The tablet used for the current version of the prototype of ReColl is iPad with 9.7 inch display. Same interface is facilitated at the clinician side and it can be adapted to other types of platforms.

ReColl supports the following *real-time* interactions between health workers and remote clinicians:

- Video conferencing by using the built-in cameras, microphone and speaker
- Using cameras to show patient details (e.g. skin color, wound) to the clinicians
- Sharing medical information, including patient records (e.g. medical images) in medical record systems, cloud-based information systems (e.g. patient monitoring data) and patient images captured by the iPad cameras
- Annotating over shared information

ReColl also enables the *asynchronous* information sharing to be used when the case is not urgent and when clinicians are not available for real-time interactions. The asynchronous mode allows the creation of a rich media annotation composed of

annotated images and videos to be shared for asynchronous discussion and information exchange. When a health worker annotates a patient record or an image of a patient, a short video with the audio of the health worker can be captured by the iPad
and recorded together with the patient record or image and annotations (Fig.1). This
rich media annotation is then sent to a clinician who can review it at a convenient
time and may respond with their own annotations of the content.

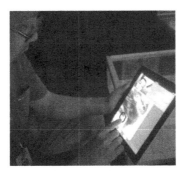

Fig. 1. Recording a rich media annotation

3   User Study

A pilot study has been conducted in our laboratory to test the functionality and usability of ReColl. The study was conducted using an initial prototype and has been part of
the on-going iterative design processes. While our future work includes testing these
tools in a real world setting, the focus of the study has been to improve the design by
observing how users communicate and interact in collaborative tasks designed to
mimic the typical activities of information sharing in telehealth.

We tested the use of the rich media recording for asynchronous communication
and the use of real-time interaction functionalities. 10 university students, 2 software
engineers and 2 researchers participated in the study. There were 10 males and 2 females. Each session included two randomly assigned participants who were located in
two separated rooms. Each pair of participants worked together to complete two collaborative negotiation tasks. Participants filled in a questionnaire at the end of the
session and this was followed by a debrief session between the participants and us.

In each session, participants were required to first review a pre-recorded and annotated video explaining the problem to be solved, in this case the need to plan a picnic
party in a park. The pre-recorded message consisted of the video recording of the
instructor explaining the scenario, a map image of the park and a video recording of
his annotations on the map as he explaining the constraints and context of the picnic.
After this the pair engaged in two real time negotiation tasks. One was to agree on a
location of the party. Each participant was allowed to annotate the map of the park
when putting forward their individual suggestions. The second task was to create
games to entertain the people attending the party. Each participant had a number of
physical objects they could draw on to create a game. The objects were put on a table

34   J. Li et al.

in front of them. Participants were allowed to use the rear camera of their iPads to
show the objects they had, or take still images of these objects, annotate them and
share them with their partners. Our aim was to understand how users perceived the
rich media annotations in the asynchronous mode when receiving the instructions
(Fig. 2) and how the real time interaction functionalities, including annotation, were
used to support the collaboration.

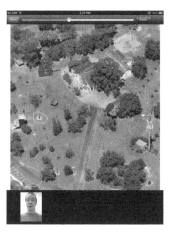

Fig. 2. Pre-recorded rich media annotation message

The questionnaire included six questions about participants' experience with rich
media recording and ten questions about real-time collaboration using ReColl. Fig 3
shows the specific aspects of the questions for rich media recording and Fig. 4 shows
those for real-time collaboration. Participants rated the extent to which they agreed
with the questionnaire statements based on a scale of 1 to 7, with 1 being "strongly
disagree" and 7 being "strongly agree".

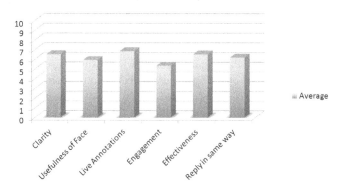

Fig. 3. Average usability ratings for rich media recording mess

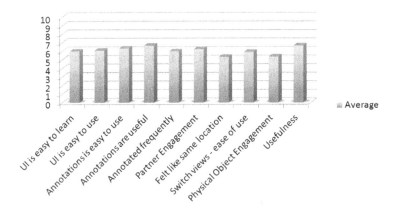

Fig. 4. Average usability ratings for real-time collaboration using ReColl

As shown in Fig. 3, participants felt that the rich media recording was an effective way of getting instructions. They also found that seeing a video of the instructor as they annotate the map was very useful. They would like to be able to reply to the message by doing their own annotations. The usefulness of the instructor's face view and the feeling of engagement were rated as neutral and the scores were lower than the scores of the other aspects.

Participants were positive about the functionalities of the real-time collaboration in ReColl (Fig. 4). In particular, the usefulness of the annotation tool had the highest rating. Participants were satisfied with the ease of use, partner engagement and switching between different views while the sense of being together with remote partner was rated just neutral.

The preliminary prototype of ReColl used for the study allows participants to select either person view or document view to be displayed in full-mode by clicking on the thumbnails at the lower part of the iPad screen. We found that participants switched between different views depending on different interaction activities. During the first task most of the participants kept the map image as their primary view for full mode display. In the second task participants switched between different cameras and different views more frequently. Some of them switched to use the rear camera of iPad to show the objects on the table. Some of them took a photo of the objects on the table, shared the photo to their partners and drew on the photo to indicate objects of interest. They switched between the local workspace view and remote workspace view during the discussion. During the debrief sessions, some participants suggested a side-by-side view of the two workspaces and the ability to annotate on both views.

4   Discussion

Supporting both synchronous and asynchronous interactions in a hybrid way [1] has been one of the design considerations of ReColl. In particular, our solution of recording rich media annotation adds an additional level of rich information to support asynchronous communication. The use of rich media annotation has been tested in our pilot study which has shown positive results. Researchers have pointed out that hybrid telehealth and the approach of using video recording in consultation and reviewing video data at another time could be one of the future trends of telehealth [2]. Our research contributes to this field by exploring the design of integrating synchronous and asynchronous functionalities in mobile devices to support flexible and rich communications in healthcare delivery.

We are aware of the limitations of the pilot laboratory study. Although the study has received positive results, we plan to get feedback from actual users and investigate the tool in real healthcare setting. There is a need to understand how to support the integration of medical information sharing with video conferencing for different collaboration scenarios. The mobile collaboration tool can be considered as a complex interaction space that users may switch between or combine different views, such as live video conferencing between health workers and clinicians, interactive annotatable view of medical data and videos of patients. One of our future directions is the flexible configuration of this interaction space. We have also explored the security issues when using ReColl for collaborations [8].

We believe the design of ReColl provides us with an opportunity to further explore mobile solutions and new collaboration support of value to healthcare.

References

1. Pan, E., Cusack, C., Hook, J., Vincent, A., Kaelber, D.C., Bates, D.W., Middleton, B.: The value of provider-to-provider telehealth. Telemedicine and e-Health **14**(5), 446–453 (2008)
2. Yellowlees, P., Nafiz, N.: The psychiatrist-patient relationship of the future: Anytime, anywhere? Harvard Rev Psychiatry **18**, 96–102 (2010)
3. Tang, J., Marlow, J., Hoff, A., Roseway, A., Inkpen, K., Zhao, C., Cao, X.: Time travel proxy: using lightweight video recordings to create asynchronous, interactive meetings. In: Proc. CHI 2012, pp. 3111-3120
4. Churchill, E.F., Nelson, L.: From media spaces to emplaced media: Digital poster boards and community connectedness. In: Media Space 20+ Years of Mediated Life, pp. 57–73 (2009)
5. Fussell, S.R., Setlock, L.D., Yang, J., Ou, J., Mauer, E., Kramer, A.D.I.: Gestures over video streams to support remote collaboration on physical tasks. Human-Computer Interaction **19**, 273–309 (2004)
6. Alem, L., Huang, W.: Developing mobile remote collaboration systems for industrial use: some design challenges. In: Campos, P., Graham, N., Jorge, J., Nunes, N., Palanque, P., Winckler, M. (eds.) INTERACT 2011, Part IV. LNCS, vol. 6949, pp. 442–445. Springer, Heidelberg (2011)
7. Olwal, A., Frykholm, O., Groth, K., Moll, J.: Design and evaluation of interaction technology for medical team meetings. In: Campos, P., Graham, N., Jorge, J., Nunes, N., Palanque, P., Winckler, M. (eds.) INTERACT 2011, Part I. LNCS, vol. 6946, pp. 505–522. Springer, Heidelberg (2011)
8. Jang-Jaccard, J., Li, J., Nepal, S. & Alem, L.: Security analysis of mobile-based collaboration tools in health applications. In: The 9th IEEE International Collaborative Computing: Networking, Applications and Worksharing (Collaboratecom), Austin, pp. 553–562 (2013)

Canonical Document for Medical Data Exchange

Sanae Mazouz[✉], Ouçamah Mohammed Cherkaoui Malki, and El Habib Nfaoui

Department of Computer Science, Faculty of Science, Dhar El Mahraz, Fez, Morocco
sanae.mazouz@gmail.com

Abstract. In the healthcare domain, the number of heterogeneous standards and medical applications is large. In consequence, the decision about which system and standard are more appropriate is difficult. The most widely deployed healthcare standard is Health Level Seven. Unfortunately, this standard has problems. The version 3 has seen slow adoption and the version 2.x had interoperability problems because of the variety of implementations by healthcare providers. To reduce the health interoperability problem between health information systems, we propose a canonical document for exchanging medical information. This document will be used as mediator between healthcare systems and shall allow health providers to share data among healthcare institutions without any adjustment or requirements. As result, the proposed mediator can make the exchange of health data simpler and efficient.

Keywords: Health information system · Interoperability · Health Level Seven · Canonical document · Mediator

1 Introduction

Exchanging information across healthcare stakeholders is a hard task. The existence of various Health Information Systems (HIS) [5] makes the exchange of Electronic Health Record (EHR) [3] very difficult. Many standards are created to enable the exchange of patient medical information such as HL7 [1], openEHR [4], DICOM [2], etc. The most deployed healthcare standard is Health Level Seven (HL7), adopted by more than 55 countries around the world. There are two major HL7 versions, HL7 v2.x and HL7 v3. The version 3 introduces new technologies like Extensible Markup Language[1] (XML) and Unified Modeling Language2 (UML) languages, which makes it more extensible and open. However, most medical applications use HL7 v2.x. The reason is the incompatibility between HL7 v2.x versions and the large number of implementations. Also, the use of standards requires changing the structure of existing patient's records.

Several countries have created and developed their own EHR for example: France "DMP", Canada "Health Infoway", Taiwan "TMT", UK "NHS", and Australia "NHETA"; and they are engaged to standardize a national Electronic Health Record. These efforts did not attempt the objective.

---

[1] http://www.w3.org/XML/
[2] http://www.uml.org/

© Springer International Publishing Switzerland 2015
X. Yin et al. (Eds.): HIS 2015, LNCS 9085, pp. 37–44, 2015.
DOI: 10.1007/978-3-319-19156-0_5

Therefore, there is an important need to communicate all systems through a simple and easy solution without any requirements or adjustment.

In this context, we propose a canonical document used as a mediator between healthcare systems. Our objective is to provide a health document mediator for exchanging health information across healthcare systems using XML language to encode the documents. The structure of the canonical document is simple and can be read by a non-expert. The mediator does not impose any training or adjustment on the system architecture. The use of the canonical document mediator will reduce the number of interfaces between HIS from $[n \times (n-1)/2]$ interfaces to (n) interfaces.

This paper summarizes some standards to deal with the problem of interoperability in healthcare domain and explains the mediator structure.

The paper is structured as follows. In the next section, we summarize some standards used to build interoperability into healthcare domain. Section 3 contains a review of related works. In section 4, we describe the structure of the mediator. Section 5 gives some experimental. Finally, section 6 concludes our paper.

2   Standards for Healthcare Interoperability

Aguilar [10] defines interoperability as the ability of two or more systems or components to exchange information and to use the information that has been exchanged. Interoperability depends upon two important concepts: syntax and semantics.

- Syntactic interoperability: is the ability of systems to communicate the structure of information basing on rules for spelling and grammar.
- Semantic interoperability: is the ability for information shared by systems to be correctly interpreted on the receiving end.

2.1   Standards

Standards for healthcare were created by a variety of organizations for various types or categories of interoperability in HIS. These standards allow HIS to communicate in the same way across system. Below is a summary of key standards at the syntactic and semantic level.

- **Health Level 7 (HL7)** [1] - is a standard for the exchange of data between healthcare applications. There are two major HL7 Versions, HL7 V2.x and HL7 V3. The Version 3 introduces a new approach to clinical information exchange: the Clinical Document Architecture (CDA), the Reference Information Model (RIM), and Clinical Context Object Workgroup (CCOW). The CDA is a document markup standard that specifies the structure and semantics of clinical documents. However, even with the innovations of the version 3 it has a seen slow adoption. In addition, the version 2.x had interoperability problems because of the variety of implementations by healthcare providers.

- **Digital Imaging and Communications in Medicine (DICOM)** [2] - is an international standard for the communication of medical images in radiology, cardiology, dentistry, and pathology. Developed by the DICOM Standards Committee and under the umbrella of National Electrical Manufacturers Association (NEMA).

- **International Statistical Classification of Diseases (ICDx)** [7] - is an international standard for epidemiology, health management, and clinical purposes. Used to identify diseases, signs, symptoms, abnormal findings, complaints, and social circumstances for billing purposes list by the World Health Organization (WHO)[3].

- **Clinical Context Object Workgroup (CCOW)** [11] – is a standard for providing comprehensive view and single sign-on capability across systems without integrating databases. CCOW specify technology-neutral architectures, component interfaces, and data definitions as well as an array of interoperable technology-specific mappings of these architectures, interfaces, and definitions. It is an independent vendor developed by the HL7 organization

- **OpenEHR** [4] - is an open international standard specification in health informatics describing the health data in EHRs.

- **Logical Observation Identifiers Names and Codes (LOINC)** [6] - is a universal standard for identifying individual laboratory results and clinical observations. It facilitates the exchange of test results for clinical care, healthcare management, and research.

- **National Council for Prescription Drug Programs (NCPDP)** [9] - is a standard for transmitting prescription requests and fulfillment from pharmacies to payers.

- **Clinical of Care Document (CCD)** [11] - is a standard for specifying the encoding, structure, and semantics of a patient summary clinical document for exchange. CCD allows physicians to send electronic medical information to other providers without loss of meaning and enabling improvement of patient care. CCD is a US version of CDA.

2.2   Classification of Healthcare Standards

In healthcare domain, a number of standards were created to address the requirements of interoperability problems at both semantic and syntactic layer. These standards are organized into six categories [12]. Table 1 provides a complete classification of these standards.

Table 1. Classification of healthcare standards

Functional and Syntactic level			Semantic level		
Messaging standards	Terminology standards	Document standards	Conceptual standards	Application standards	Architecture standards
HL7	LOINC	CDA	RIM	CCOW	OpenEHR
DICOM	ICDx	CCD			
NCPDP					

---

[3] www.who.int

• **Messaging standards** – outline the structure, content and data requirements of electronic messages to enable the effective and accurate sharing of information.

• **Terminology standards** – provide specific codes for terminologies and classifications for clinical concepts such as diseases, allergies and medications. Terminology systems assign a unique code or value to a specific disease or entity.

• **Document Standards** – indicate the type of information included in a document and also the location of the information.

• Conceptual standards – allow the transmission of information between systems without losing meaning and context.

• **Application standards** – determine the implementation rules for software systems to interact with each other. For example, application standards using single sign-on allow users to logs into multiple information systems within the same environment.

• **Architecture standards** – define a generic model for health information systems. They allow the integration of health information systems by providing guidance to aid the planning and design of new systems and also the integration of existing systems.

3   Related Works

Many pervious works have proposed solution to promote interoperability in healthcare domain. Bicer et al [13] proposed semantic mediation of exchanged messages. He demonstrates how to mediate between HL7 V2.x and HL7 V3 messages. First, messages exchanged in the healthcare domain are in EDI (Electronic Data Interchange) or XML format. They are transformed into OWL (Web Ontology Language) ontology instances. Then they are mediated through an ontology-mapping tool named OWLmt, which is used to reason over the source ontology instances while generating the target ontology instances according to the graphically defined mapping patterns. Lopez et al [15] proposed a framework as a set of principles and guidelines as well as methodologies and techniques for realizing semantic interoperability in Health Information Systems using Rational Unified Process (RUP) and formal software processes engineering methods. To achieve this objective, he analyzed approaches for information systems architecture and he harmonized them towards the framework. Jian et al [14] reported a national level standard called Taiwan Electronic Medical Record Template (TMT) that aims to achieve semantic interoperability in EHR exchanges. The TMT provides a basis for building a portable, interoperable information infrastructure for EHR exchange in Taiwan.

These projects are limited to a specific use. Therefore, the need to build a new solution for general use and without any requirement or adjustment is an urgent priority.

4   System Description

Traditional information systems reach a functional interoperability but not semantic. This means that the information arrives at its destination, but it is not understood. To reach semantic interoperability, terminological references are indispensable [16].

Our mediator includes these terminological standards such as SNOMED CT [18], LOINC and ICDx. Therefore, data coded with distinct terminologies can be related to each other.

Figure 1 illustrates the class diagram of our mediator. It is based on the canonical model [19, 20]. We have extracted the more prominent classes for mediation, and we propose a new canonical class diagram [8].

The canonical model contains three elements: (i) Post Production of Medical Information (PPMI) (ii) Medical Activity, and (iii) Pathological Case. The PPMI element contains the classes (MatrialPost, Team, and Actor) responsible for the production of medical information. The Medical Activity element include the classes (MedicalAction, ReferenceActivity, and MedicalActivity) used to represent the care plan realized by the PPMI. Finally, the Pathological Case consists of the classes (Patient and Pathology) that show the association between patient and their historical records.

The advantage of this representation is that the internal structure of each of the component can be left to the free conceptual choice of each healthcare system. In addition, this canonical model will be the basis for the creation of the canonical health document.

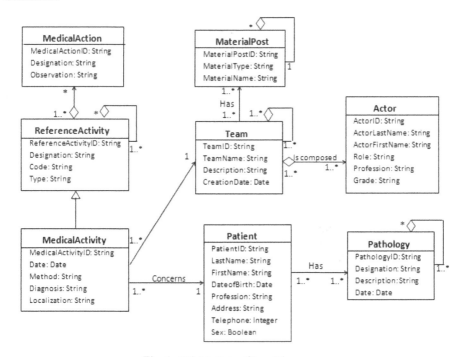

Fig. 1. HIS Mediator Class Diagram

The classes of our mediator are:

- Medical Activity represents information about diagnosis and treatment;
- Reference Activity contains description of methods of execution and the site on which it takes place;
- Medical Action is the simplest action of Medical Activity such as a question during a medical check;
- Patient is an individual awaiting or under medical care and treatment;
- Pathology contains historical diseases related to the patient.
- Actor describes the medical personnel;
- Team is a group of Actors that intervene in a Medical Activity.
- Material Post is the equipment used by Team to practice a Medical Activity.

Figure 2 illustrates the architecture of our mediator. The canonical transformer component will enable data to be converted into a canonical document. It transforms the message to a common canonical format. This canonical transformation requires the use of auxiliary information: thesaurus. Our mediator supports two types of thesaurus; terminological thesauri: WordNet [21] and biomedical thesauri: UMLS [17].

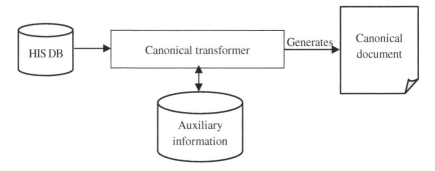

Fig. 2. The Mediator Architecture

5   Experiment

To demonstrate the simplicity of our mediator, we chose to work with HL7v 2 standards. The reason for this choice is that HL7 is the most popular standard in healthcare domain. Figure 3 shows an example of HL7 message in both versions.

It is clear that we should be an expert to understand HL7 version 2 message; even if it is the most widely used standard in the world today. Figure 4 shows message after canonical transformation.

The HL7 v2 message is converted to the canonical document using the canonical transformation. As result, the message can now easily be read by human eye and the content is understandable. Therefore, the use of the canonical mediator facilitates the exchange of medical data across healthcare systems.

```
<?xml version="1.0" encoding="UTF-8"?>
<ORU_R01>
  ...
  <ORU_R01.PATIENT>
   <PID>
    <PID.3>
     <CX.1>010-11-1111</CX.1>
    </PID.3>
    <PID.5>
     <XPN.1>
      <FN.1>Estherhaus</FN.1>
     </XPN.1>
     <XPN.2>Eva</XPN.2>
    </PID.5>
    <PID.7>
     <TS.1>19720520</TS.1>
    </PID.7>
    <PID.8>F</PID.8>
<XAD.1>
      <SAD.1>256 Sherwood Forest.</SAD.1>
     </XAD.1>

    ...
   </PID>
  ...
<CE.2>GLUCOSE</CE.2>
     <OBX.5>175</OBX.5>
     <OBX.6>
      <CE.1>mg/dl</CE.1>
     </OBX.6>
  ...
</ORU_R01>
```

```
...
<MedicalActivity>
    <MedicalActivityID>948642</MedicalActivityID>
    <Diagnosis>GLUCOSE</Diagnosis>
    <Date>200502150730</Date>
    <Patient>
     <PatientID>010-11-1111</PatientID>
     <LastName>Estherhaus</LastName>
     <FirstName>Eva</FirstName>
     <DateofBirth>19720520</DateofBirth>
     <Sex>F</Sex>
     <Adress>256 Sherwood Forest 70809</Adress>
     <Telephone>(225)334-5232</Telephone>
    </Patient>
    <Team>
     <Actor>
      <ActorID>020-22-2222</ActorID>
      <ActorLastName>Levin-Epstein</ActorLastName>
      <ActorFirstName>Anna</ActorFirstName>
      <Role>Ordering Provider</Role>
      <Grade>MD</Grade>
     </Actor>
    ..
    <MedicalAction>
      <MedicalActionID>1554-5</MedicalActionID>
      <Designation>GLUCOSE </Designation>
      <Observation>175 mg/dl </ Observation >
    </MedicalAction>
    </ReferenceActivity>
</MedicalActivity>
  ...
```

Fig. 3. HL7 v2 message   **Fig. 4.** HL7 version 2 message after transformation

6   Conclusion

In this paper, we briefly summarized standards used to support interoperability in healthcare domain. It is clear that the number of standards in health domain is large. However, it is extremely difficult to except the use of a single worldwide standard without further integration, and development. In this context, we propose a canonical document to mediate between health information systems.

The proposed mediator is simple and for general use. It does not impose any requirement or adjustment on the system architecture. Also, it is open, flexible, and platform independent.

References

1. HL7. http://www.hl7.org/
2. DICOM. http://dicom.nema.org/
3. Hoerbst, A., Ammenwerth, E.: Electronic health records. Methods Inf Med **49**(4), 320–336 (2010)
4. Kalra, D., Beale, T., Heard, S.: The openEHR foundation. Studies in health technology and informatics **115**, 153–173 (2005)
5. Haux, R.: Health information systems–past, present, future. International journal of medical informatics **75**(3), 268–281 (2006)

6. Mcdonald, C.J., Huff, S.M., Suico, J.G., et al.: LOINC, a universal standard for identifying laboratory observations: a 5-year update. Clinical chemistry **49**(4), 624–633 (2003)
7. Steindel, S.J.: International classification of diseases, clinical modification and procedure coding system: descriptive overview of the next generation HIPAA code sets. Journal of the American Medical Informatics Association **17**(3), 274–282 (2010)
8. Mazouz, S., Malki, M.O.C., Nfaoui, E.H.: An XML-based mediator for health information systems. Int. J. Medical Engineering and Informatics (accepted)
9. Liu, H., Burkhart, Q., Bell, D.S.: Evaluation of the NCPDP Structured and Codified Sig Format for e-prescriptions. Journal of the American Medical Informatics Association, p. amiajnl-2010-000034 (2011)
10. Aguilar, A.: Semantic interoperability in the context of eHealth. In: Research Seminar, DERI Galway, December 15, 2005. The Continuity of Care Document. Changing the Landscape of Healthcare Information Exchange. Corepoint Health (2009)
11. Seliger, R.: Overview of HL7's CCOW Standard. Health Level Seven, Inc (2001). http://www.hl7.Org/library/committees/sigvi/ccow_overview_2001.doc
12. Kim, K.: Clinical data standards in health care: Five case studies. California HealthCare Foundation Julio (2005)
13. Bicer, V., et al.: Artemis message exchange framework: semantic interoperability of exchanged messages in the healthcare domain. ACM Sigmod Record **34**(3), 71–76 (2005)
14. Jian, W.S., Hsu, C.Y., Hao, T.H., Wen, H.C., Hsu, M.H., Lee, Y.L., Li, Y.C., Chang, P.: Building a portable data and information interoperability infrastructure—framework for a standard Taiwan Electronic Medical Record Template. Computer methods and programs in biomedicine **88**(2), 102–111 (2007)
15. Lopez, D.M., Blobel, B.G.: A development framework for semantically interoperable health information systems. International journal of medical informatics **78**(2), 83–103 (2009)
16. Frandji, B., et al.: Interopérabilité des données de santé : comment passer à l'acte ?. 13èmes Journées Francophones d'Informatique Médicale Qualité, Risques, Information et Informatique de Santé 28, 29 et 30 avril 2009 - Nice, France
17. Bodenreider, O.: The unified medical language system (UMLS): integrating biomedical terminology. Nucleic acids research **32**(suppl 1), D267–D270 (2004)
18. Elkin, P.L., Brown, S.H., Husser, C.S., et al.: Evaluation of the content coverage of SNOMED CT: ability of SNOMED clinical terms to represent clinical problem lists. In: Mayo Clinic Proceedings, pp. 741–748. Elsevier (2006)
19. Cherkaoui, M.M.O., Doukkali, D., El Azami, I., Tahon, C.: Communication de l'activite medicale entre SIH: une representation canonique et un modele de patron. In: La Conférence Internationale GISEH 2008 Lausanne en Suisse, September 4–6, pp. 1–7. EPFL (2008)
20. Azami, I.E.: Ingéniérie des Systèmes d'Information Coopératifs, Application aux Systèmes d'Information Hospitaliers Ressource électronique. [S.l.] : [s.n.] (2012)
21. Miller, G.A.: WordNet: a lexical database for English. Communications of the ACM **38**(11), 39–41 (1995)

Identifying Candidate Risk Factors for Prescription Drug Side Effects Using Causal Contrast Set Mining

Jenna Reps[✉], Zhaoyang Guo, Haoyue Zhu, and Uwe Aickelin

School of Computer Science, University of Nottingham,
Nottingham NG8 1BB, UK
jenna.reps@nottingham.ac.uk

Abstract. Big longitudinal observational databases present the opportunity to extract new knowledge in a cost effective manner. Unfortunately, the ability of these databases to be used for causal inference is limited due to the passive way in which the data are collected resulting in various forms of bias. In this paper we investigate a method that can overcome these limitations and determine causal contrast set rules efficiently from big data. In particular, we present a new methodology for the purpose of identifying risk factors that increase a patients likelihood of experiencing the known rare side effect of renal failure after ingesting aminosalicylates. The results show that the methodology was able to identify previously researched risk factors such as being prescribed diuretics and highlighted that patients with a higher than average risk of renal failure may be even more susceptible to experiencing it as a side effect after ingesting aminosalicylates.

1 Introduction

Longitudinal observational data potentially hold a wealth of information, however we are currently limited in the ability to efficiently extract causal relationships from this form of data due to bias and confounding [1]. In randomised clinical trials confounding can be overcome by manipulating the variables and mixing the potential confounders equally between the group given the drug and the control group. Unfortunately, this is not possible for observational data as the data are passively observed. As a consequence, spurious results are common when analysing observational data due to the various forms of bias in the data. In the medical field the gold standard for causal discovery are randomised clinical trials [2]. However, these are costly and sometimes unethical [3]. If medical longitudinal observational data could be successfully analysed and the results used to complement randomised trials for causal discovery, then this would address these issues. This would enable a greater understanding of various medical mechanisms and enhance current knowledge.

Bayesian causal discovery techniques that learn complete causal models have often been used to identify causal relationships in longitudinal observational

© Springer International Publishing Switzerland 2015
X. Yin et al. (Eds.): HIS 2015, LNCS 9085, pp. 45–55, 2015.
DOI: 10.1007/978-3-319-19156-0_6

data[4]. Due to scalability issues the recent focus has shifted towards constraint based methods [5]. Although the constraint based methods have performed well in some domains, they rely on numerous assumptions [6] that may not always hold true and may still be inefficient for data with high volume and high variety. A recent approach for identifying causal association rules included a two step method, of firstly mining association rules and secondly implemented a cohort study to filter out those that are likely to be causal. This was accomplished by identifying controls that had the antecedent and matched specific attributes of the cases. The odds ratio was then used as the filter, as only the rules with a significant deviation between how often the consequence occurred for the cases and controls were kept [7]. In this paper we attempt a similar approach for identifying causal contrast sets but use logistic regression as a filter. Rather than using the odds ratio, we use the p-values of the logistic regression variables to indicate how significant having the antecedent is for the occurrence of the consequence. As the logistic regression can consider covariates such as age, and gender into the model, we can filter contrast set rules that are caused by observed confounders.

In this paper we present a proof-of-concept candidate risk factor detection algorithm based on causal contrast set mining. Causal contrast set mining is a term we use to define the discovery of causal association rules that identify differences between various groups. The algorithm firstly identifies interesting rules consisting of sets of events that commonly precede a user specified event and then investigates how often these interesting rules occur in general. Rules that occur more often before the user specified event are then investigated via a logistic regression model. This reduces age/gender confounding and highlights the most interesting rules. We implement the methodology to a real word dataset. The dataset we use is a UK general practice database containing complete medical and drug prescription records for millions of patients within the UK. Our focus is towards identifying risk factors for patients' experiencing prescription drug side effects for the drug family aminosalicylates (5-ASAs). These drugs are often given to treat inflammatory bowel disease but are known to cause renal failure with an incidence rate of 0.17 cases per 100 patients per year [8]. The purpose of this research is to investigate a new technique for mining contrast set causal relationships efficiently and evaluate its potential for identifying candidate risk factors of patients experiencing side effects to prescribed medication.

2   Materials and Methods

2.1   The Health Improvement Network

The Health Improvement Network (THIN) database (www.thin-uk.com) is a large longitudinal observational database containing medical records for millions of patients within the UK. There are over 600 general practices within the UK that are registered to the scheme consisting of over 3.5 million active patients. For each patient within THIN, their demographics such as age, gender and location are known, as well as their complete medical and therapy record histories during the period of time they are registered at a participating practice. The suitability of this database for epidemiological study has been investigated and the results show it is reasonably representative of the general UK population [9]. It is worth highlighting that the database does have some potential issues, such as not containing over the counter prescriptions, only containing data that patients have told their doctors about and delays in the recording of medical event into the database. A common problem with the database is historical event dropping, when a patient moves general practices, it is common for the patient to have historical illnesses/events recorded shortly after registering. To prevent this biasing analyses, it is standard to exclude the first year of a patient's records after moving to a new general practice [10]. This preprocessing was implemented in this study.

The READ code system is the coding system used within UK primary care to record medical events [11]. Each READ code corresponds to a medical event (e.g., a diagnosis, an administrative event, a laboratory result or a symptom). The READ codes consist of 5 alphanumeric digits and have a hierarchal tree structure based on the level of detail of the corresponding medical event being recorded. The level of a READ code corresponds to how many non dot digits it contains, for example the READ code 'A10..' is a level 3 READ code, whereas the READ code 'A....' is a level 1 READ code. A level 2 READ code is the child of a level 1 READ code if the READ codes have the same first digit. This is generalised to a level $n \in \{2, 3, 4, 5\}$ READ code being the child of the level $n - 1$ READ code if the first $n - 1$ digits of both READ codes are the same. The advantage of this hierarchal structure is that a child READ code represents a more specific version of its parent READ code's corresponding medical event. For example, the READ code 'A....' corresponds to the description 'Infection' and is the parent of the READ code 'A1...' corresponding to 'Tuberculosis', which is the parent of the READ code 'A11..' corresponding to 'Pulmonary tuberculosis'.

Prescriptions are recorded into THIN using a drug code and each prescription also contains the drug's British National Formula (BNF) code [12]. The BNF code groups drugs into similar families. Each prescription can be linked to up to three BNF codes.

2.2   Algorithms

Association Rules Mining. Association rules mining [13] is a method for discovering relations between variables in large databases. It was originally designed to identify relationships between items that are commonly purchased together (occur in the same shopping baskets). The relations are normally of the form {antecedent events } → {consequence}, meaning that if we find all of the antecedent events in a shopping basket, then we have a good chance of finding the consequence. An example of an association rule is {milk, butter} → {bread}, which means shoppers that buy milk and butter are also likely to buy bread.

The search space for identifying association rules can be extremely large with big datasets. Therefore it is common to restrict the search to only include rules containing sets of items that appear frequently in baskets. This is accomplished by specifying a minimum support threshold, and only items/itemsets that occur more often than the support are considered. These are referred to as frequent itemsets.

Formally, let $I = \{i_1, i_2, ..., i_n\}$ be a set of n items and $t = X \subset I$ be a transaction containing a set of items. We denote the database by $D = \{t_1, t_2, ..., t_m\}$. This is a set of m transactions. The support of an itemset X is the proportion of transactions within the database that contain X,

$$supp(X) = |\{t_i \in D | X \subset t_i\}|/m \tag{1}$$

An itemset X is said to be frequent if its support is greater than a given threshold $supp(X) > \omega$, where ω is called the minimum support.

The confidence of an association rule $X \rightarrow Y$ is the fraction of baskets that contain both X and Y ($supp(X \cup Y)$) divided by the number of baskets containing X ($supp(X)$),

$$conf(X \rightarrow Y) = supp(X \cup Y)/supp(X) \tag{2}$$

this is similar to the conditional probability of Y given X. In general, the association rules $X \rightarrow Y$ are identified such that the support and confidence of $X \rightarrow Y$ are greater than the minimum support and confidence thresholds.

There are various methods for identifying contrast set rules, including discovering emergent patterns by considering the ratio of two supports [14], using a suitable search technique combined with statistical hypothesis testing [15] or creatively using a classifier [16]. Emergent pattern discovery is suitable for simple problems that only require contrasting two groups. This is what we will do to identify candidate risk factors, as we just need to compare the patients that experienced the adverse drug reaction with those that did not.

Logistic Regression. Logistic regression [17] is a method that expresses the log odds of belonging to a class as a linear combination of the features,

$$ln(P(Y|\mathbf{X})/(1 - P(Y|\mathbf{X}))) = w_0 + \sum_i w_i X_i \tag{3}$$

The parameters w_i are found using maximum likelihood. This is re-arranged to give the conditional probability of belonging to each class as,

$$\begin{aligned} P(Y = 0|\mathbf{X}) &= \frac{exp(w_0 + \sum_i w_i X_i)}{1 + exp(w_0 + \sum_i w_i X_i)} \\ P(Y = 1|\mathbf{X}) &= \frac{1}{1 + exp(w_0 + \sum_i w_i X_i)} \end{aligned} \tag{4}$$

therefore, class 0 is chosen when $exp(w_0 + \sum_i w_i X_i) > 1$ and 1 is chosen otherwise. The parameter w_i and its standard error of the logistic regression tell us how significant the ith feature, X_i, is in determining the class. In this paper we use a significance level of 5%.

2.3   Methodology

The proposed candidate risk factor identification methodology consists of four steps. The first step is creating two different databases based on whether a patient who was prescribed a 5-ASA experienced renal failure or not. The second step is to identify frequent itemsets for the patients who experience renal failure after 5-ASAs and calculate whether these itemsets occur more often for these patients than for the patients prescribed 5-ASAs in general. This identifies any potential risk factors that are common (occur in more than 5% of the patients). The third step is to identify whether these potential risk factors are a significant influence on experiencing renal failure after a 5-ASA when accounting for age and gender confounding. The final step is presenting the frequent itemsets that occur more than in general for the patients who experience renal failure after a 5-ASA ordered by the p-value indicating the significance of the itemset's presence in predicting the chance of renal failure after a 5-ASA.

Step 1: Partition Databases Similar to market baskets, patients medical baskets can be constructed based on the records they have in the THIN database and frequent itemset mining can be applied to find frequent medical events sets. Due to the number of possible itemsets being very large, frequent itemset mining is often restricted so that only interesting itemsets are discovered.

   To generate association rules for the THIN database we consider the items to be all the medical events and all the drugs recorded within the THIN database. So the THIN items are $I = \{$all the medical events and all the drugs$\}$ and a transaction is $X \subset I$. Then we generated two databases from the THIN database: $D1$ contains the itemsets of patients that took 5-ASA but did not suffer from renal failure within a month and $D2$ contains the itemsets of patients that took 5-ASA and suffered from renal failure within a month. For each transaction, $t_i^{D1} \in D1$ or $t_i^{D2} \in D2$, the transaction consists of all the items within the THIN database that are recorded for the ith patient in the database.

   For example, if a patient had renal failure recorded within a month of a 5-ASA and only had the READ codes 681.., 8CB.., 9R8.., 246.. and H33..00 recorded in THIN, then his corresponding transaction in $D2$ would be {681..,8CB..,9R8.., 246.., H33..}.

Step 2: Calculating Support Ratio In general the THIN data is sparse and the majority of items have a low support. However, to identify risk factors for renal failure after ingesting a 5-ASA we only need to investigate the itemsets that are frequent in the patients that took 5-ASA and suffered from renal failure (frequent itemsets in $D2$). Then we need to find which of these frequent itemsets from $D2$ have a higher support than within $D1$, as this indicates itemsets that are more common in the 5-ASA patients who experience renal failure compared to all the 5-ASA patients. Therefore, we apply frequent itemset mining to the database $D2$ with minimum supports of $\omega = 0.05$ and for each frequent item we also calculated its support in $D1$. We then calculate the support ratio for each frequent itemset X from $D2$,

$$suppRatio(X) = [|\{t_i \in D2 | X \subset t_i\}|/m_2]/[|\{t_i \in D1 | X \subset t_i\}|/m_1] \quad (5)$$

where m_1 and m_2 are the number of patients that took 5-ASA but did not suffer from renal failure and took 5-ASA and suffered from renal failure, respectively. The value $\omega = 0.05$ was chosen as this means that any identified risk factors occur for at least 5% of the patients experiencing renal failure after 5-ASA. Therefore we are identifying common risk factors, however this value can be adjusted.

After applying the association rules, we will get a table containing the frequent itemsets of $D2$ and their support in both D1 and D2. The rate of each frequent itemset corresponds to the ratio of two support values (support(X, ASA→RF) / support(X,ASA→ ¬RF)), see Table 1. The itemsets with a suppRatio greater than 1 are considered potential risk factors that will be further evaluated using logistic regression.

Table 1. Example of how to calculate the suppRatio for each frequent itemset

Itemset (X)	Support(X,ASA→RF)	Support(X,ASA→ ¬RF)	suppRatio(X)
{G2...}	0.15903	0.056378	2.820757
{G3...}	0.080863	0.028041	2.883717
{6781.,G2...00}	0.067385	0.023302	2.891863
{D21z.}	0.067385	0.029588	2.277463
{65E..}	0.078167	0.036105	2.165022
...			

Step 3: Logistic Regression We then applied logistic regression with the independent variables: presence of potential risk factor, presence of 5-ASA, age and gender and dependant variable indicating renal failure. This identified whether the potential risk factors are in fact significant risk factors for experiencing renal failure after 5-ASAs when accounting for age/gender confounding.

To apply the logistic regression we needed to consider a set of cases (the patience with renal failure recorded in THIN) and a set of controls (the patients with no renal failure recorded in THIN). For each patient experiencing renal failure we selected 5 controls who did not. Increasing the number of controls per case is a technique that can increase the power of the analysis and 5 controls per case were chosen as we have a large number of controls available but only a limited number of cases. For each case, the age used in the logistic regression is considered as the age when the case first suffered from renal failure in life. Each control was selected by picking a random non-renal failure patient and a random point in the time while the patient is active in THIN such that the age/gender distributions of the cases and controls were the same.

Then, for each potential risk factor frequent itemset identified in step 2 (each X) we created the case/control data as displayed in Table 2, where the variable X is True if the patient's itemset up to their specified age contains X, the

Table 2. Example of the data used for each logistic regression

PatientId	Age	Gender	X	ASA	RF
1	45	1	True	True	True
2	50	2	False	True	False
3	45	1	False	True	True
4	59	2	False	True	False
5	22	2	True	False	True
...					

variable ASA is True if the patient was prescribed a 5-ASA before the specified age and RF is True if the patient has renal failure recorded in THIN and False otherwise. The logistic regression with RF as the dependant variable was then applied considering the independent variables: age, gender, X, and ASA. The interaction between the ASA variable and the X variable was also included.

Step 4: Ranking The p-value of the interaction between the frequent itemset and 5-ASA was calculated to evaluate whether the frequent itemset is a risk factor of experiencing renal failure after 5-ASA. The smaller the p-value is, the greater the confidence that the frequent itemset corresponds to a risk factor. The p-value of each frequent itemset is extracted and listed in the result table. The results are returned ordered by the p-values in ascending order. The final output of the methodology is this ranked list of frequent itemsets as illustrated in Table 3.

Table 3. Example of the output of the methodology

Itemset (X)	P-value(Age)	P-value(Gender)	P-value(ASA*Rules)
{9N1O.}	8.25E-8	3.08E-1	2.78E-18
{G33..}	1.87E-8	2.06E-1	2.28E-44
...			

2.4 Software

We use SQL to manage the data and R [18] to perform the analysis. The package arules [19] was used to identify the frequent itemsets.

3 Results and Discussion

The top 30 antecedents that occur significantly more often for patients who experience renal failure after ingesting a 5-ASA, ordered by the logistic regression p-value, are presented in Table 4. The results suggest that some potential risk factors for experiencing renal failure after ingesting a 5-ASA are hypertension, diuretics, pain, arthritis, diabetes, influenza vaccination, anaemia, dehydration and antibiotics.

Table 4. The results of the candidate risk factor identification for the occurrence of renal failure after 5-ASA

Description	RFsupp (val $\times 10^{-2}$)	noRFsupp (val $\times 10^{-2}$)	suppRatio	p-value	Potential Link
Hypertensive disease	15.9	5.64	2.82	1.62×10^{-30}	Hypertension
Furosemide tabs	11.9	3.21	3.70	7.86×10^{-30}	**Diuretics** [20]
BP reading	8.63	2.16	3.99	1.69×10^{-24}	Hypertension
Co-proxamol tabs	28.3	17.4	1.63	1.16×10^{-23}	Pain
Rheumatoid arthritis	24.5	14.1	1.74	1.3×10^{-23}	Arthritis
Blood pressure reading	9.70	2.92	3.32	1.42×10^{-23}	Hypertension
Furosemide & Co-proxamol tabs	6.74	1.38	4.89	3.07×10^{-23}	Diuretics & Pain
Diabetes mellitus	8.36	2.14	3.91	8.22×10^{-23}	Diabetes
Influenza inactivated split virion vaccine	9.43	2.70	3.50	1.1×10^{-22}	Influenza vaccination
Co-proxamol tabs & Hypertensive disease	7.01	1.82	3.84	4.62×10^{-21}	Pain & Hypertension
Pain	11.9	5.03	2.36	2.31×10^{-18}	Pain
Osteoarthritis	11.1	4.65	2.38	1.1×10^{-17}	Arthritis
Co-proxamol tabs & Pain	7.82	2.70	2.89	4.41×10^{-16}	Pain
Ischaemic heart disease	8.09	2.80	2.88	4.51×10^{-16}	Hypertension
Co-proxamol tabs & Rheumatoid arthritis	10.2	4.48	2.29	2.31×10^{-15}	Pain & Arthritis
Health education offered & Hypertensive disease	6.74	2.33	2.89	2.45×10^{-14}	Hypertension
Influenza inactivated surface antigen vaccine	9.97	4.52	2.21	5×10^{-14}	Influenza vaccination
Atenolol tabs	10.2	4.68	2.19	5.4×10^{-14}	Hypertension
Screening-health check	9.16	4.17	2.20	1.66×10^{-13}	
Amoxicillin caps & Hypertensive disease	6.20	2.21	2.80	4.02×10^{-13}	Antibiotic & Hypertension
Essential hypertension	12.9	7.58	1.71	2.59×10^{-12}	Hypertension
Pain & Screening-general	6.47	2.47	2.62	5.03×10^{-12}	Pain
Influenza vaccination	7.82	3.61	2.17	5.95×10^{-12}	Influenza vaccination
Arthritis	11.1	6.12	1.81	2.68×10^{-11}	Arthritis

Anaemia unspecified	6.74	2.96	2.28	5.94×10^{-11}	Anaemia
Loperamide caps	7.28	3.42	2.13	1.27×10^{-10}	**Dehydration** [20]
Cardiac disease monitoring	7.01	3.11	2.25	1.79×10^{-10}	Hypertension
Amoxicillin caps & Pain	6.20	2.63	2.36	1.85×10^{-10}	Antibiotic & Pain
Paracetamol tabs	15.4	10.5	1.46	2.33×10^{-10}	Pain
Screening-general & Rheumatoid arthritis	7.28	3.46	2.10	4×10^{-10}	Arthritis

The results identified some known risk factors. However, in general there is little information about the risk factors making the evaluation difficult. This highlights the importance of a new methodology for discovering risk factors. In a previous study it was observed that diuretics and dehydration may be risk factors [20]. The diuretic drug furosemide was ranked second by the methodology and patients with a history of furosemide were 3.7 times more likely to experience renal failure after 5-ASAs. We found that those with a history of co-proxamol and furosemide were 4.89 times more likely to experience renal failure after 5-ASAs. The drug loperamide was also identified as a risk factor by the method. This drug is used to treat diarrhoea and may indicate that the patients who experienced renal failure after loperamide and 5-ASAs were dehydrated.

Hypertension is a general risk factor for developing renal failure. Interestingly, this research suggests that 5-ASAs increase hypertension suffering patients' susceptibility to renal failure. Therefore 5-ASA may need to be prescribed more carefully to patients who are already susceptible to renal failure. It is common for side effects to occur in patients that have a higher background risk of the event, so this is not unexpected.

Some painkillers and drugs used to treat hypertension are known to cause renal failure. The identification of pain and hypertension as risk factors may indicate an interaction between these drugs and the 5-ASAs that results in the side effect of renal failure. Therefore the methodology may highlight indirect risk factors. This does highlight one limitation of this methodology, it is difficult to identify whether the medical event or the drugs used to treat the medical event may be risk factors. Additional work will be required to determine whether the identified potential risk factor is a direct or indirect risk factor.

It is worth highlighting that this methodology cannot definitively determine the risk factors of known adverse drug reactions. Any results obtained need to be validated via formal epidemiological studies. However, this method can highlight the most likely risk factors and can be considered to be a filter. Therefor this methodology may lead to more efficient discovery of unknown risk factors by identifying which candidate risk factors should be investigated further. Effectively this methodology is an ADR risk factor filter.

In this paper we chose to use a minimum support of 0.05 as this ensured any identified risk factors occurred for more than 5% of the patients who experienced the side effect. This value may need to be adjusted based on the type of risk factors of interest or based on how common the side effect being investigated is.

4   Conclusions

In this paper we have presented a proof-of-concept of a novel methodology for identifying causal contrast set rules in big longitudinal observational data. The methodology was able to identify known risk factors for patients experiencing renal failure after ingesting a 5-ASA drug. However this methodology cannot be considered to definitively identify risk factors. Rather, it acts as a filter for highlighting the most interesting.

Potential areas of future work are developing a way to tune the minimum support used to identify the frequent itemsets and applying the methodology to a range of known prescription side effects to determine its robustness.

References

1. Giordano, S.H., Kuo, Y.-F., Duan, Z., Hortobagyi, G.N., Freeman, J., Goodwin, J.S.: Limits of observational data in determining outcomes from cancer therapy. Cancer **112**(11), 2456–2466 (2008)
2. Cochran, W.G., Rubin, D.B.: Controlling bias in observational studies: A review. Sankhyā: The Indian Journal of Statistics, Series A, 417–446 (1973)
3. Black, N.: Why we need observational studies to evaluate the effectiveness of health care. British Medical Journal **312**(7040), 1215–1218 (1996)
4. Cooper, G.F., Herskovits, E.: A bayesian method for the induction of probabilistic networks from data. Machine learning **9**(4), 309–347 (1992)
5. Silverstein, C., Brin, S., Motwani, R., Ullman, J.: Scalable techniques for mining causal structures. Data Mining and Knowledge Discovery **4**(2–3), 163–192 (2000)
6. Heckerman, D., Meek, C., Cooper, G.: A bayesian approach to causal discovery. Computation, causation, and discovery **19**, 141–166 (1999)
7. Li, J., Le, T.D., Liu, L., Liu, J., Jin, Z., Sun, B.: Mining causal association rules. In: 2013 IEEE 13th International Conference on Data Mining Workshops (ICDMW), pp. 114–123. IEEE (2013)
8. Van Staa, T.P., Travis, S., Leufkens, H.G., Logan, R.F.: 5-aminosalicylic acids and the risk of renal disease: a large british epidemiologic study. Gastroenterology **126**(7), 1733–1739 (2004)
9. Lewis, J.D., Schinnar, R., Bilker, W.B., Wang, X., Strom, B.L.: Validation studies of the health improvement network (THIN) database for pharmacoepidemiology research. Pharmacoepidemiology and Drug Safety **16**(4), 393–401 (2007)
10. Lewis, J.D., Bilker, W.B., Weinstein, R.B., Strom, B.L.: The relationship between time since registration and measured incidence rates in the General Practice Research Database. Pharmacoepidemiology and Drug Safety **14**(7), 443–451 (2005)
11. Stuart-Buttle, C., Brown, P., Price, C., O'Neil, M., Read, J.: The read thesaurus-creation and beyond. Studies in health technology and informatics **43**, 416–420 (1996)
12. Committee, J.F.: British national formulary, vol. 65. Pharmaceutical Press (2013)

13. Agrawal, R., Imieliński, T., Swami, A.: Mining association rules between sets of items in large databases. In: ACM SIGMOD Record, vol. 22, no. 2, pp. 207–216. ACM (1993)
14. Dong, G., Li, J.: Efficient mining of emerging patterns: discovering trends and differences. In: Proceedings of the Fifth ACM SIGKDD International Conference on Knowledge Discovery and Data Mining, pp. 43–52. ACM (1999)
15. Bay, S.D., Pazzani, M.J.: Detecting group differences: Mining contrast sets. Data Mining and Knowledge Discovery **5**(3), 213–246 (2001)
16. Novak, P.K., Lavrač, N., Webb, G.I.: Supervised descriptive rule discovery: A unifying survey of contrast set, emerging pattern and subgroup mining. The Journal of Machine Learning Research **10**, 377–403 (2009)
17. Hosmer Jr., D.W., Lemeshow, S.: Applied logistic regression. John Wiley & Sons (2004)
18. Team, R.C., et al.: R: A language and environment for statistical computing (2012)
19. Hahsler, M., Gruen, B., Hornik, K.: arules - A computational environment for mining association rules and frequent item sets. Journal of Statistical Software **14**(15), 1–25 (2005). http://www.jstatsoft.org/v14/i15/
20. De Jong, D., Tielen, J., Habraken, C., Wetzels, J., Naber, A.: 5-aminosalicylates and effects on renal function in patients with crohn's disease. Inflammatory bowel diseases **11**(11), 972–976 (2005)

Analyzing Sleep Stages in Home Environment Based on Ballistocardiography

Hongbo Ni[1], Tingzhi Zhao[1(✉)], Xingshe Zhou[1], Zhu Wang[1], Lei Chen[1], and Jun Yang[2]

[1] School of Computer Science, Northwestern Polytechnic University, Xian, China
{nihb,zhouxs}@nwpu.edu.cn, bmtingzhi@163.com,
transitwang@gmail.com, losemyheaven@126.com
[2] Aeromedicine Institute of P.L.A, Beijing, China
marrow@sina.com

Abstract. Currently, a number of people have various sleep disorders, and sleep stages play an important role in assessment of sleep quality and health status. This paper proposes an effective approach of analyzing the sleep stages based on ballistocardiography (BCG), which can be continuously detected with micro-movement sensitive mattress (MSM) in this work, during non-intrusive sleep in home environment. This paper focuses on extracting features from BCG from the following three aspects: multi-resolution wavelet analysis of the heartbeat intervals based time-domain features, Welch's power spectrum estimation based frequency-domain features and the detrended fluctuation analysis (DFA) value for long term correlation based features. Moreover, the support vector machine (SVM) with or without the factor of sleep rhythm, and recurrent neural network (RNN) are adopted to build the classifiers, and both the personal model and self-independent model are investigated for different scenarios. Experimental result of 56 subjects [25 women and 31 men, aged from 16 to 71] was evaluated applying the proposed method and compared to the result provided by professional visual scoring by ECG and EEG. The SVM with the factor of sleep rhythm shows better performance with an average accuracy between 73.21%~83.94% in the personal model, and the self-independent model also achieves a satisfactory level with an average accuracy of 73.611~78.78% for male and 73.99%~79.46% for female.

Keywords: Heartbeat interval · BCG · Wavelet analysis · Sleep stage

1 Introduction

Sleep staging is very important and effective to estimate clinical and health status of people: the sleep rhythm including time possession of each stage and its variances are related to sleep quality assessment; People in slow wave sleep, i.e. deep sleep shows harder to be wakened and will be more drowsy when awake; Sleep-related disorders serve as an significant contributor to poor health and are closely associated with sleep disease, such as Insomnia, Obstructive Sleep Apnea-hypopnea Syndrome (OSAS), Parkinson's disease, etc.[1,2,3]. Thus sleep staging has drawn a great attention to health care and medical community.

© Springer International Publishing Switzerland 2015
X. Yin et al. (Eds.): HIS 2015, LNCS 9085, pp. 56–68, 2015.
DOI: 10.1007/978-3-319-19156-0_7

In sleep medicine, PSG has been the golden standard to divide sleep time into Not Rapid Eye Movement(NREM) and Rapid Eye Movement(REM) by visual scoring, the REM is further subdivided in stages 1,2,3,4,with a set of rules in Rechtshaffen and Kales science 1968[4]. However, PSG demands the subject to be attached with complicate and numerous electrodes during the recording of the perceived bio-signals, and it really disturbs the subject's natural sleep. Comparatively speaking, ECG is more convenient to record cardiovascular and respiratory information, and based on the detected heart interval series, the analysis of heart rate variability(HRV) has be widely applied in sleep staging, but the electrodes are still not suitable for continuously monitoring in daily living environment[5,6]. Actigraphy is a useful tool to track the motion of a subject for longitudinal sleep monitoring with a wrist-worn accelerometer [7]; A wearable health care system based on knitted integrated sensors had been presented for the sleep data acquisition [8]; Moreover, some researchers designed sleep monitoring systems with smart phones, using the built-in sensors to monitor stage-related presentations, such as subjects acoustic event, body movement and illumination condition [9]. Unfortunately, all of them are insufficient to get physiological parameters for the fine-grained sleep staging.

The BCG is a vital signal which is caused by the movements of the heart and blood [10]. In home environment, it can be acquired unobtrusively through pressure-sensitive sensors integrated into mattress.

With BCG signal, diverse approaches offer fine properties of non-stationary time series in extracting features, some of them are Wavelets analysis, Empirical Mode Decomposition, Time-Frequency analysis and Time-Varying Autoregressive Model (TVAM) analysis [11]. The methods based on machine learning and artificial neural network have also be widely used to construct the classifiers for different sleep stage. In paper[12,13], the Time-Varying Autoregressive Models (TVAMs) serve as feature extractor from the bio-signals, and the Hidden Markov Models (HMM) is chosen to be a sequential classifier; Fast Fourier Transform(FFT) is used as a main feature extraction tool in paper[14] and a feed forward artificial neural network as a classifier; And in paper[15], the Hilbert-transform-based is adopted to derive RR-based features and the quadratic discriminant classifier (QDC) based on Bayes' rule is also used to be the classifier.

In this paper, we present a systematic approach to assess the stage of sleep by BCG signal, which is obtained non-intrusively by the pressure-sensitive oil tubes embedded in the MSM. In section2, we briefly describe the data acquisition platform and data sets. In section3, the methodology is presented for designing classification models, as shown in Fig.1. Firstly, in order to mining features as complete as possible, we consider from the following respects: multi-resolution wavelet analysis is used for heartbeat interval based features, Welch spectrum estimation is applied to both initial BCG and the detected sequence of heartbeat intervals, DFA draws imply patterns in long term correlation analysis serving as an effective factor for sleep staging. Secondly, eliminating the redundant and irrelevant features by the principal component analysis (PCA) algorithm, we adopt SVM and RNN as the main classifiers for sleep staging. Finally, we design personal model and self-independent model adapting to different scenarios. Section 4 evaluates our approach by investigating the gap between true sleep stages and estimated results.

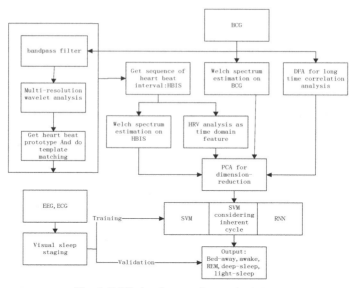

Fig. 1. BCG signal processing methodology

2   Data Acquisition

The non-intrusive sleep sensing system consists a micro-movement sensitive mattress, the analog-digital (AD) converter and a terminal PC. The mattress is embedded with two Hydraulic pressure sensors (oil tubes), one is located at upper part of the mattress (i.e. chest area) to sense the pressure of the heartbeat, and can make sure there is enough area for various subjects' physical sizes; the other is placed at the leg region. The original pressure will be recorded and amplified, converting to digital signal by the AD converter, and then we apply 16 bit resolution to sample these digital signals at the rate of 100 Hz. In this work, we pay more attention to the cardiac vibrations of subjects, so we only analyze BCG signal from chest area. There are 56 subjects participated in the experiment (25 women and 31 men, aged from 16 to 71), and for each subject we have recorded the sleeping data at least three nights, and the time duration is usually from approximately 8 pm to 10 am at the following day. Since wearing too many electrodes in PSG recording would disturb people's sleep, we only detected EEG and ECG which could record subjects' brain activity and cardiac physiology. They have been widely used for sleep staging, and then the expert clinicians score EEG and ECG data with the outputs: bed-away, awake, REM, deep-sleep, and light-sleep.

3   Methodology

3.1   Signal Pre-processing

The acquired BCG data not only includes the information of heartbeat, breath, body movement, but also includes environment noise, so it is necessary to remove the noise from the sensing data before BCG analysis. In this work, we applied Butterworth Low Pass Filter to filter the signal higher than 20 Hz, the BCG signal is retained.

As we know, many research have been done to do sleep staging from BCG signal, in this paper, we come up from the angle of heartbeat interval's detecting, and extract time domain features from it.

3.2   Multi-resolution Wavelet Analysis

Multi-resolution wavelet analysis is one of the most popular candidates of the time-frequency-transformations, benefiting from its great ability in analyzing signals at multiple scales, even in the presence of non-stationarity [16, 17]. This method has been successfully used to detect heartbeat interval from bio-medical signal [18, 19]. According to the scale-dependent property, we can refine detailed information by the standard deviation of wavelet coefficients, which has been demonstrated to be better than the scale-independent measures.

In heartbeat interval detection, we just focus on identifying the approximate shape of the heartbeats, but not take care of the details. Based on the advantage of wavelet analysis, fine-grained information contains the details, and the remained is coarse-grained information which describes the prime tendency and structure of the signal. Thus, it is adopted in the processing of BCG signal. When determining the optimal layers, we prefer to choose only one particular layer rather than reconstructing on several layers. While choosing a specific layer, smaller layers existing many glitches increase our difficulty for heartbeat detection, while larger layers make the signal "more smooth", leading some heartbeats missed or misjudged for its over distortion. Fig.2(a) shows a segment of pre-processed BCG, nearly 27 seconds, high-frequency noise mixed in our expected shapes, and from Fig.2(C), we find the signal is too smooth to distort the shape 'W' into 'v' at the third seconds.

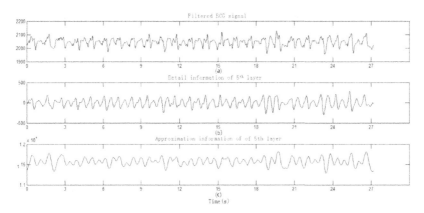

Fig. 2. multi-layer wavelet analysis plot

After a series of experiments, we observed that the detail information of 5th layer (shown on Fig.2 (b)) could satisfy our requirement, which not only depicts the overall shape of heart beat, but also fairly smooth for the interval detection. After that, we calculate the extreme points and the distance among them, and then get the heart beat profile by k-means clustering algorithm on a short segment. The average value calculated by this method is then regarded as the representative template of the BCG for further processing. In detail, do template matching between the prototype segment and the remained signal for peak position finding. Then we adopted both Euclidean distance and auto correlation function in the procedure, and the corresponding maximal position and maximal position indicate highest heartbeat response [20]. Fig. 3 shows the detected sequence of heart beat intervals (HBIS) during 30 minutes.

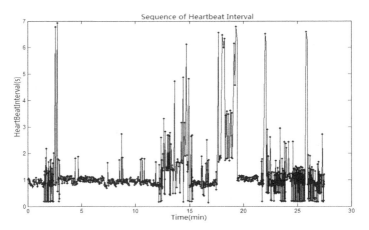

Fig. 3. The intervals of the detected HBIS

From Fig.3,we can see that during 0~2min and 4~12min, the subject has a normal heartbeat with interval around 1sec; At around 3min, 23min~27min, the heartbeat interval fluctuate up and down in a narrow range, representing that the subject's cardiac condition is a little unstable. In the period of 13~15min and 18~19min, the intervals show big fluctuation implying body movements on the bed. For a large amount of information can be gained from HBIS, it's necessary to extract features for sleep staging.

3.3   Features Based on HBIS

Time-domain analysis is obviously optimal to be adopted, because it's usually applied in the HRV analysis and it contains plentiful information of heart, blood vessels and nervous-humoral regulation [21]. Thus, based on HBIS, the properties of HRV [22] are reliable to be treated as time-domain features for sleep stage classifications, and they are shown in Table 1.

Table 1. Time domain features calculating from HBIS

Feature	Explanation
MI	The mean values of heartbeat intervals.
SDNN	The standard deviation of successive heartbeat intervals, estimating the overall variation within the total sequence.
SDANN	The standard deviation on average, reflecting the slow variation.
RMSSD	The root mean square of successive difference, reflecting the rapid variation.
RMSSD	The root mean square of successive difference, reflecting the rapid variation.

3.4   Welch Spectrum Estimation

The power distribution and central frequency of the spectral components vary a lot depending on the central nervous system rate, so power spectral density(PSD) of the bio-medical signal has been widely used in application of frequency representations[23,24]. Welch method is a good choice to calculate PSD due to the improved periodogram, since it shows much smoothness of the signal's spectrum curve [25, 26]. Specifically, the original signal is separated into equivalent digitalized segments, overlap with the Hamming sliding windows, and calculate the PSD with FFT. Fig.4 depicts the PSD of both HBIS and the original BCG by Welch, and after exploring the PSD of each segment of signal have little difference with others, we choose several frequency band and calculate its integral power for every band as the features of the segment. Then for each segment, we can get the frequency features in the fixed frequency band.Table2 depicts 12 frequency features from HBIS and BCG for each segment.

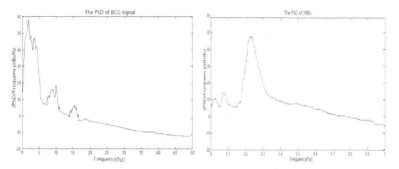

Fig. 4. The PSD of BCG and HBIS

Table 2. Frequency Features calculating from HBIS and BCG

HBIS	BCG
T_S: total power of segment	T_B: total power of the segment
VLF_S: power between 0.01-0.05hz band	VLF_B: power between 0-5hz band
LF_S: power between 0.05-0.15hz band	VHF_B: power between 5-11hz band
HF_S: power between 0.15-0.4hz band	VHF_B: power between11-17hz band
RLH_S: ratio between low and high	RLH_B: ratio between low and high

3.5   DFA

Besides the time and frequency domain analysis on short term, long term correlation analysis would reveal the implied patterns for each stage. DFA shows great advantages in analyzing the tendency components in the data series. It is based on the theory of random process and chaotic dynamics, and has an amendment with root mean square to the theory of random walk, so DFA is good at detecting the physical essence of time series [27]. In detail, the process flow is: segmenting a sequence firstly, removing the mean value, and calculating the summation-sequence, secondly, dividing the summation-sequence into sub-sequences with same length, finally, removing the trend of each sub-sequence and regarding the average for the square of all the sub-sequences as the DFA fluctuation value.

3.6   Feature Subset Selection

In each short term, we can extract 5 time-domain features and 12 frequency-domain features, and in long term, we can also get DFA value as a feature. Every long-term contains multiple short-term leading multi-group short-term features. However, with various classifiers in statistical methods, machine learning, and neural network, the addition of feature containing little or no relevant information in the classification process will not increase the performance of the classifier, but could increase the complication feature matching and consume system resources. Thus, before constructing the model, we should remove the redundant and irrelevant features by finding some effective subset combination, and these subsets make most of contributions for the classifiers or mapping the initial features into lower dimensions by linear transformation. In this paper, we adopted principal component analysis (PCA) algorithm [28] to demonstrate the discriminatory power for eigenvectors detecting, and make contribution rate cumulatively to 95%.

3.7   Classifiers

SVM: Support vector machine (SVM) is a powerful machine learning technique. Based on statistical learning theory and minimum structure risk, its purpose is to seek compromise between model complexity and autonomous learning ability-predictive accuracy [29]. SVM shows great advantages in resolving problems about small-sample set, non-linear and high dimensions by separating data with an optimized hyper plane and maximizing the margin between two classes. It appears in many sleep staging applications with various bio-medical. Besides, SVM has been expanded to resolve multi-class problem, such as building classifier for a certain class and the rest classes (one-versus-set), building classifiers for any two classes (one-versus-one) and building hierarchical support vector machines (H-Svms). In this paper, we employed the Matlab toolkit-Libsvm, which is implemented by the one-versus-one, to resolve our multi-class problem.

SVMps: The transition among Wake-NREM-REM stages gives information related to the sleep quality since this transition pattern is highly affected by sleep disorders and daily activities. However, SVM ignores the inherent temporality or the recognized patterns in the REM-NREM cycle, the features are only extracted by the current segment of data but not considering the transitions in adjacent segments. To avoid this weakness, we append the previous stage as a new feature and call the new classifier as SVMps.

RNN: Recurrent neural network (RNN) is a classifier of artificial neural network and the connections among units of RNN forming a directed cycle [30]. This property is equivalent to create an internal state of the network, which makes RNN describe dynamic temporal behavior, that is to say, RNN can use its internal memory to process arbitrary sequences of input, just like our time series with stage transition. From many kinds of RNN, Elman shows the ability of dynamic recurrent with varying ability, so in this paper, we apply Elman to train our RNN classifier, with one hidden layer, sigmoid function as the kernel, and sum of squares of errors as the evaluation function.

3.8   Personal Model and the Self-independent Model

For the practicability and reliability of the classifiers, different scenarios should be considered:

1. If the subject has historical recordings of BCG signal and the corresponding ECG and EEG for visual scoring of stages, the data can be used for constructing a personal model. The personal model inheres the subject's own characteristics, such as his sleep rhythm, activities pattern at daytime, and they will be totally reflected in the model, leading to a self-adaptive model, which shows excellent performance when his newly generated BCG data appended to the model.

2. The self-independent model seems more practical in real time applications, especially when the subject unwilling to wear any electrodes for ECG, EEG recording. They think the electrodes not only disturb their natural sleep but also regard them as patients, thus, it's difficult to collect the labeled trusted stages for their personal models. To avoid the behavior interference and psychological conflict, the self-independent model is demanded to be built. On account of each person's characteristic different with others, if we randomly choose some users that have training data to establish the stage recognition model and apply to new user, the accuracy will greatly reduce. Considering the reliability and practicability, a compromise solution is to divide the users into many groups, the training data of each group are associated same characteristics and share with similar sleep pattern. Then for each group we can build a model with the training data in this group. For a new person who doesn't have training data, we just judge which group the new user will belong, and use that model to do stage recognition.

Diverse studies have shown sleep structure changing with age and gender, such as the major sleep of the infant is in deep stage; slow wave sleep decreases gradually when growing up, which reflects on the longer sleep in the daytime, circadian rhythms appear different about the stage-advanced for infant and the elderly, the latter show earlier both in falling sleep and waking up than they were young. Besides that, in senior community, female's sleep structure is more stable than male, and women generally have more slow-wave sleep, which means the deepest sleep. So in this paper, we use the existing subjects' data to build self-independent model according to age and gender for a new subject.

4   Experiment Evaluations

To evaluate the performance of our models, the data of 56 subjects has been recorded at least 3 nights for the experiment, and we randomly select 70% of the data as training data, and the remaining 30% is test data. For the personal model, we use ten folds cross validation to divide the 56 subjects into 6 groups randomly, with the first five group 10 subjects and the last group 6 subjects. For each group, the features of time-domain, frequency-domain and the DFA value are all extracted at first, although the golden standard PSG identifies stage by dividing sleep time in epochs with length of 30s, in fact, each stage usually sustain at least 5~10 minutes, so we also use several minutes as the segment for the stage identification. Then PCA is used to reduce the dimension and the new attributes can make contribution rate cumulatively to 95%. Finally, we apply SVM, SVMps, and RNN to the test data, the average accuracy of each group is worked out by different classifiers. In this paper, we repeat our experiments 3 times. The results are shown in the flowing tables.

Table 3. Accuracy of SVM in personal model

Accuracy	(Training set)/ (Test set)					
(%)	10/56	10/56	10/56	10/56	10/56	6/56
Experiment 1	64.0000	71.4912	70.1571	58.7940	71.2389	70.1087
Experiment 2	69.6682	72.7273	67.7596	70.0000	72.0430	74.2857
Experiment 3	76.1658	57.9487	75.3695	56.4767	64.9289	76.5306
Average	69.9447	67.3891	71.0954	61.7569	69.4036	73.6417

Table 4. Accuracy of SVMps in personal model

Accuracy	(Training set)/ (Test set)					
(%)	10/56	10/56	10/56	10/56	10/56	6/56
Experiment 1	71.7822	74.0741	84.5771	78.7330	79.6117	76.7544
Experiment 2	73.5931	74.8744	79.6209	86.8182	72.1053	81.6038
Experiment 3	82.9016	71.5026	82.6733	79.3722	74.0884	76.3033
Average	75.4887	73.2169	83.9425	78.9461	74.4373	76.6040

Table 5. Accuracy of RNN in personal model

Accuracy	(Training set)/ (Test set)					
(%)	10/56	10/56	10/56	10/56	10/56	6/56
Experiment 1	64.5455	72.2222	68.4211	64.8649	72.2222	66.6667
Experiment 2	78.7234	68.5714	79.1667	79.7436	63.1250	73.3333
Experiment 3	76.1658	57.9487	75.3695	56.4767	64.9289	76.5306
Average	71.8750	67.0833	72.5000	68.2927	79.1667	80.9787

Table 3 shows the accuracy of SVM, whose features include time domain, frequency domain and the DFA value, the average of the three experiments on each group in range of [61.7569%,73.6417%]. While Table 4 shows the accuracy of SVMps, which has taken into account of the temporal transitions in different stages, the average accuracy is obviously improved to [73.2169%, 83.9425%] RNN automatically integrates transition behavior, which means RNN function should be better than others. However, compared with SVMps, each group's average accuracy generated by RNN decreased except the 5th as presented in fig 5.

We guess the reason why SVMps performs better than RNN is its intrinsic quality to deal with binary problem. Because the signal we wish to classify can be decompose to several binary classifications, as Fig.5 shown, the input features are distinguished into bed-away and on-the-bed state, then the latter can be subdivided into awake and sleep state which made up of REM and NREM, while NREM can be further refined by deep sleep and light sleep, these properties exactly match the SVMps's ability.

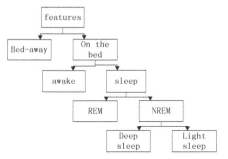

Fig. 5. Stage structure

In the evaluation of self-independent model, we group the subjects by gender and age, specifically, the age is divided into 16~35, 36~55, and 56~76, as shown in Table 6. However, it's inappropriate to use ten folds cross validation because the least number is only 5 in group of [male, 56~76] and [female, 16~35], so we use the leave on out method to train the self-independent models. Considering SVMps shows the highest accuracy in personnel model, we also use this algorithm in the self-independent model. The result (in table 6) shows that the age between 16~35 is more precise whether for male or for female, which reflects that the younger subjects may have more stable sleep stages than the older. Whatever, comparing the accuracy between male and female data set, more varieties is presumed to exist in the sleeping patterns of the female, resulting in lower accuracy than the male data set.

Table 6. Accuracy of SVMps in self-independent model

Gender	Age Group(year)	Number of Subjects	Maximum Accuracy (%)	Minimum Accuracy (%)	Average Accuracy (%)
Male	16~35	8	89.583	71.044	78.778
	35~55	18	82.758	66.667	76.536
	56~76	5	82.818	69.444	73.6111
Female	16~35	5	85.416	72.723	79.455
	35~55	14	83.333	65.278	75.395
	56~76	6	80.227	63.636	73.989

Moreover, in this paper, we take one minute as the short term features, and for the long term duration, different segment (from 1minute to 10minutes) have be applied for the accuracy evaluation. From Fig.6, different duration shows little variations on the accuracy, the 4 minutes and 6 minutes seem more precise than others, so in the following experiment, so 5 minutes has been our appropriate choice for the duration of long term.

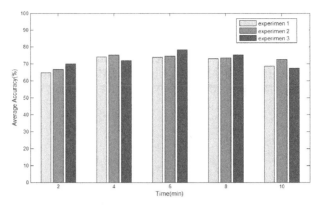

Fig. 6. Accuracy for different segment

5   Conclusion

This paper proposed systematic approach for sleep staging with BCG signal, acquiring from the continuous and non-invasive sensing platform. The contribution we made in this paper can be concluded: firstly, we extracted as complete as possible features for stage classification from short term to long term, from time domain to frequency domain; Secondly, SVM, SVMps and RNN were applied to train multiple classifiers, and the SVMps showed best performance, and it relied on that, one hand, it take into account of the inherent temporality in the REM-NREM cycle, on the other hand, its intrinsic quality just matches our classification problem; Thirdly, We designed personal model and self-independent model to adapt to different scenarios. Finally, according to relatively high accuracy of the experimental result, the work is effective for sleep staging. In the future work, we will encourage more subjects to participate in this work, and improve the accuracy of sleep staging.

Acknowledgments. We thank the reviewers for the valuable comments and for the time spent towards the improvement of the paper. This work is supported by the National Found of Science of China (61332013)and Scientific Program Grant of Xi'an (CXY1340-7).

References

[1] Feige, B., Al-Shajlawi, A., Nissen, C., et al.: Does REM sleep contribute to subjective wake time in primary insomnia? A comparison of polysomnographic and subjective sleep in 100 patients. Journal of sleep research **17**(2), 180–190 (2008)

[2] De Chazal, P., Heneghan, C., Sheridan, E., et al.: Automated processing of the single-lead electrocardiogram for the detection of obstructive sleep apnoea. IEEE Transactions on Biomedical Engineering **50**(6), 686–696 (2003)

[3] Kim, Y.E., Jeon, B.S., Yang, H.J., et al.: REM sleep behavior disorder: Association with motor complications and impulse control disorders in Parkinson's disease. Parkinsonism & Related Disorders (2014)

[4] Rechtschaffen, A., Kales, A.: A manual of standardized terminology, techniques and scoring system for sleep stages of human subjects (1968)

[5] Yılmaz, B., Asyalı, M.H., Arıkan, E., et al.: Sleep stage and obstructive apneaic epoch classification using single-lead ECG. Biomedical engineering online **9**, 39 (2010)

[6] Fell, J., Mann, K., Röschke, J., et al.: Nonlinear analysis of continuous ECG during sleep I. Reconstruction. Biological cybernetics **82**(6), 477–483 (2000)

[7] Ancoli-Israel, S., Cole, R., Alessi, C., et al.: The role of actigraphy in the study of sleep and circadian rhythms. American Academy of Sleep Medicine Review Paper. Sleep **26**(3), 342–392 (2003)

[8] Paradiso, R., Loriga, G., Taccini, N.: A wearable health care system based on knitted integrated sensors. IEEE Transactions on Information Technology in Biomedicine **9**(3), 337–344 (2005)

[9] Gu, W., Yang, Z., Shangguan, L., et al.: Intelligent sleep stage mining service with smartphones. In: Proceedings of the 2014 ACM International Joint Conference on Pervasive and Ubiquitous Computing, pp. 649-660. ACM (2014)

[10] Bruser, C., Stadlthanner, K., de Waele, S., et al.: Adaptive beat-to-beat heart rate estimation in ballistocardiograms. IEEE Transactions on Information Technology in Biomedicine **15**(5), 778–786 (2011)

[11] Cerutti, S., Bianchi, A.M., Mainardi, L.T.: Advanced spectral methods for detecting dynamic behaviour. Autonomic Neuroscience **90**(1), 3–12 (2001)

[12] Mendez, M.O., Matteucci, M., Castronovo, V., et al.: Sleep staging from Heart Rate Variability: time-varying spectral features and Hidden Markov Models. International Journal of Biomedical Engineering and Technology **3**(3), 246–263 (2010)

[13] Kortelainen, J.M., Mendez, M.O., Bianchi, A.M., et al.: Sleep staging based on signals acquired through bed sensor. IEEE Transactions on Information Technology in Biomedicine **14**(3), 776–785 (2010)

[14] Zeng, T., Mott, C., Mollicone, D., et al.: Automated determination of wakefulness and sleep in rats based on non-invasively acquired measures of movement and respiratory activity. Journal of neuroscience methods **204**(2), 276–287 (2012)

[15] Redmond, S.J., Heneghan, C.: Cardiorespiratory-based sleep staging in subjects with obstructive sleep apnea. IEEE Transactions on Biomedical Engineering **53**(3), 485–496 (2006)

[16] Unser, M., Aldroubi, A.: A review of wavelets in biomedical applications. Proceedings of the IEEE **84**(4), 626–638 (1996)

[17] Akay, M.: Time frequency and wavelets in biomedical signal processing (1998)

[18] Ashkenazy, Y., Lewkowicz, M., Levitan, J., et al.: Discrimination of the healthy and sick cardiac autonomic nervous system by a new wavelet analysis of heartbeat intervals. Fractals **6**(03), 197–203 (1998)

[19] Thurner, S., Feurstein, M.C., Teich, M.C.: Multiresolution wavelet analysis of heartbeat intervals discriminates healthy patients from those with cardiac pathology. Physical Review Letters **80**(7), 1544 (1998)

[20] Sprager, S., Zazula, D.: Heartbeat and respiration detection from optical interferometric signals by using a multimethod approach. IEEE Transactions on Biomedical Engineering **59**(10), 2922–2929 (2012)

[21] Malik, M., Bigger, J.T., Camm, A.J., et al.: Heart rate variability standards of measurement, physiological interpretation, and clinical use. European heart journal **17**(3), 354–381 (1996)

[22] Tarvainen, M.P., Niskanen, J.P., Lipponen, J.A., et al.: Kubios HRV—a software for advanced heart rate variability analysis. In: 4th European Conference of the International Federation for Medical and Biological Engineering, pp. 1022–1025. Springer, Heidelberg (2009)

[23] Clifforda, G.D., McSharryb, P.E.: A realistic coupled nonlinear artificial ECG, BP and respiratory signal generator for assessing noise performance of biomedical signal processing algorithms. In: Proc. of SPIE, vol. 5467, p. 291 (2004)

[24] Bianchi, A.M., Mainardi, L., Petrucci, E., et al.: Time-variant power spectrum analysis for the detection of transient episodes in HRV signal. IEEE Transactions on Biomedical Engineering **40**(2), 136–144 (1993)

[25] Arvind, R., Karthik, B., Sriraam, N., et al.: Automated detection of pd resting tremor using psd with recurrent neural network classifier. In: 2010 International Conference on Advances in Recent Technologies in Communication and Computing (ARTCom), pp. 414–417. IEEE (2010)

[26] Tarvainen, M.P., Ranta-aho, P.O., Karjalainen, P.A.: An advanced detrending method with application to HRV analysis. IEEE Transactions on Biomedical Engineering **49**(2), 172–175 (2002)

[27] Hu, K., Ivanov, P.C., Chen, Z., et al.: Effect of trends on detrended fluctuation analysis. Physical Review E **64**(1), 011114 (2001)

[28] Jolliffe, I.: Principal component analysis. John Wiley & Sons, Ltd (2005)

[29] Burges, C.J.C.: A tutorial on support vector machines for pattern recognition. Data mining and knowledge discovery **2**(2), 121–167 (1998)

[30] Graves, A., Liwicki, M., Fernández, S., et al.: A novel connectionist system for unconstrained handwriting recognition. IEEE Transactions on Pattern Analysis and Machine Intelligence **31**(5), 855–868 (2009)

Heart Rate Variability Biofeedback Treatment for Post-Stroke Depression Patients: A Pilot Study

Xin Li[1], Tong Zhang[1(✉)], Luping Song[1], Guigang Zhang[2], and Chunxiao Xing[2]

[1] Department of Comprehensive Rehabilitation, School of Rehabilitation Medicine,
China Rehabilitation Research Center, Capital Medical University, Bejing, China
horsebackdancing@sina.com, zt61611@sohu.com,
songluping882002@aliyun.com
[2] Tsinghua National Laboratory for Information Science and Technology,
Department of Computer Science and Technology,
Research Institute of Information Technology, Tsinghua University, Beijing, China
zhangguigang@163.com, xingcx@tsinghua.edu.cn

Abstract. Treatment for post-stroke depression (PSD) is a very complicated system engineering, and it need quite a long time to see the effect. In this paper, through clinical trials, we adopt the method of heart rate variability biofeedback treatment for PSD patients. Through analysis of clinical trials, we hope to improve the situation of emotion on patients, the autonomic nervous function and reduce the impact by the prognosis of heart rate variability biofeedback, with dynamic observation of indices of variation on heart rate variability biofeedback under pressure/non-pressure, and summary of training scheme for PSD patients. In our research, by activating and enhancing the Baroreceptor Reflex function, it can improve the HRV indices and make mood better. We focused on heart rate variability biofeedback influence on depression and anxiety in clinical trials of its impact and corresponding experimental results is obtained.

Keywords: Heart rate variability · Biofeedback · Stroke · Depression

1 Introduction

The post-stroke depression(PSD) [1][2] is a common complication of cerebral vascular disease, it refers to varying degrees of depression after cerebral apoplexy and symptoms persist for more than 2 weeks, often characterized by depression, slow thinking, anxiety, despair, irritability, sleep disorders, low self-assessment, lack of initiative and body fatigue and other symptoms. At present, most of PSD is diagnosed by symptoms and psychological assessment scale such as self-expression, which is lack of objectivity in diagnosis and evaluation of the quantitative basis. In recent years, heart rate variability (HRV) [3][4] research method has been greatly improved and extended. HRV is pulsing rhythm of heart rate that occurs over the changing time, with easy operation and testing of non-invasive, sensitive, intuitive and quantitative advantages. HRV is mainly influenced by sympathetic nerve and vagus nerve activity, and also the relative balance, reflecting the mutual restriction relations of autonomic nervous system activity and the

X. Yin et al. (Eds.): HIS 2015, LNCS 9085, pp. 69–78, 2015.
DOI: 10.1007/978-3-319-19156-0_8

cardiovascular system, therefore HRV may be considered to a convenient window for understanding the human body state of the autonomic nervous system function, which is the quantitative indicators of judgments, explanations and prediction on the autonomic nervous system activity. HRV has become the hotspot research frontier in the field of ECG (electrocardiogram) signal processing and methods.

Currently most of the clinical treatment of PSD with drug therapy and cognitive-behavioral therapy, although drug treatments have been affirmed by the clinical, it will not only improve the quality of life in patients with stroke, but also contribute to nerve function rehabilitation after stroke [5]. But there are still some patients treated with drugs that won't work, and some patients that relapse after discontinuation, in rare cases it is difficult to withstand adverse drug reactions. Cognitive behavioral therapy for depression in patients with psychotherapy, the focus should be on faith, changes in perception, thinking, thought, by correcting the irrational belief to change behavior, the goal of treatment is to establish new appropriate behavior. Cognitive-behavioral therapy aims to help patients recognize their own thinking and action on the negative attitudes, learn to control your emotions, to adapt to the environment, by correcting a patient's basic concept of preventing recurrence of depression. However, levels of HRV [6-10] in PSD patients is low, while sensitivity to stress and disease is improved, and PSD patients are difficult to adapt to the stress, chronically high levels of stress and more likely to suffer from cardiovascular disease, whose stroke recurrence rates are high. These patients tend to be poor psychological reaction of cognitive-behavioral therapy, medication and drug problems such as slow onset and a variety of side effects, so it is imminent to look for a more economical, simple and convenient needle for PSD patients, with no adverse effects of intervention.

Biofeedback therapy is a behavior treatment method of no trauma and almost no side effects, and with the help of the instruments it could enlarge the extremely weak physiological activity that can't be usually aware of and electrical activity of information inside the body, to become visible waveform and audible voice displayed out in instrument. Then individuals with visual, and hearing organ through feedback information can understanding their changes, and according to changes gradually in some degree learn to control and correct these activities of process. After training, the adjustment function eventually becomes a self-regulating mechanism, which is formed and maintained without the feedback instrument to control and adjust some of the psychological and physiological reaction skills. Through relaxation training, biofeedback reduces the level of muscle tension to eliminate patients with depression, anxiety and tension, enhance vagus nerve function, and reduce sympathetic tone, so as to achieve the goal of treatment. Biofeedback therapy is different from conventional drug therapy, and throughout the course of therapy patients are the active participants showing high enthusiasm combined with therapy, which making the curative effect is better.

HRV biofeedback [11-17] is a newly developed method of biofeedback therapy, which is used to treat those disease related with HRV decrease. Many experiments have found that HRV biofeedback can improve HRV indices and/or baroreceptor reflex function, thus affecting the clinical symptoms and prognosis.

2   Experiment Conditions Selection

In order to improve the accuracy of the research, in this paper, the experimental requirements on patient selection imposes certain conditions, mainly includes: the selected condition and the exclusions condition.

2.1   Selected Patients with the Following Conditions

① Ages 18 to 75, men and women not limited;
② Meet the diagnostic criteria of stroke according to the fourth national cerebrovascular disease academic conference in 1995, and the cranial CT or MRI confirmed, and accompanied by limb movement disorder at the first attack of stroke patients;
③ Meet the international classification of diseases coding (ICD-10) depression, without diagnostic criteria of psychotic symptoms, with or without anxiety, and the Hamilton depression rating scale (HAMD)-24, scores more than 20 points;
④ In the pathogenesis of stroke within 2 to 6 months after the test, the vital signs are stable;
⑤ Patients conscious, directional force intact, no significant disorder of memory, understanding and intelligence;
⑥ Primary school culture degree above;
⑦ To complete the testing and treatment, and signed informed consent.

2.2   Exclusion Standard Includes the Following Conditions

① Depressive state, with psychotic symptoms;
② Prior history of psychiatric disorders and mood disorders;
③ With serious pulmonary infection, central respiratory failure, electrolyte disorder, high fever disease that affects the heart activity;
④ With other organic diseases, history of arrhythmia (atrial fibrillation, frequent premature ventricular), hyperthyroidism, history of syncope and autonomic dysfunction, detection of drugs affecting the autonomic nervous system activity and substance;
⑤ Serious disturbance of consciousness, dementia and cognitive impairment and aphasia;
⑥ The brain stem infarction;
⑦ Severe dysarthria and swallowing disorders;
⑧ Recent home suddenly appeared accident or bad life stress incident (such as widowed, childless, laid-off etc.);
⑨ Fails to cooperate, not to follow treatment scheme, and patients after the Group 5 training Essentials still unable to master the essentials of breathing should be excluded.

3   Experiment Method

This experiment is the prospective randomized controlled research on the heart rate variability biofeedback treatment for PSD patients, it aims to understand the heart rate variability biofeedback emotional improvement in stroke patients, the autonomic nervous function and the influence of prognosis, with dynamic observation of indices of variation on heart rate variability biofeedback under pressure/non-pressure, and summary of training scheme for PSD patients.

This experiment provide a scientific experimental basis for the clinical application of HRV biofeedback therapy on PSD and evaluation on its efficacy, and also the application of objective methods for the future diagnosis and treatment of emotional and cognitive impairment after cerebral stroke and merged diseases related with HRV decrease, and improve their balance of autonomic nervous function, strengthen the baroreceptor reflex function and set up the experimental and theoretical basis. As a new treatment, HRV biofeedback has simple, safe and convenient operation, for clinical practice and accumulated valuable experience, become a useful supplement comprehensive rehabilitation.

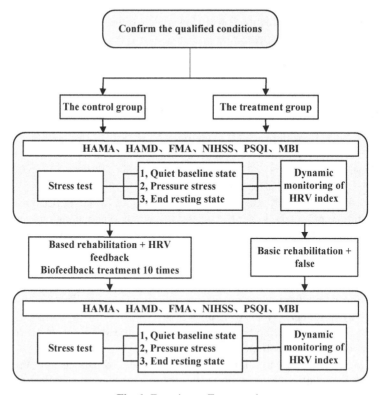

Fig. 1. Experiment Framework

With the development of the society, an aging society has arrived. Cerebrovascular disease, as a disease of the elderly, the incidence and morbidity in our country especially is higher than other diseases. The study opens up a new, scientific and effective method for the treatment of DSP, and in the domestic for a breakthrough, which will have significant improvement on relieving pain for patients at the same time and bring huge economic benefits and social benefits.

Figure1 shows the experiment framework which is our design process.

4   Experiment Results

We focused on heart rate variability biofeedback influence on depression and anxiety in clinical trials of its impact. Our experiment found that both the depressive symptoms and the anxiety symptoms were obviously improved.

4.1   The Influence of Heart rate Variability Biofeedback for Depression

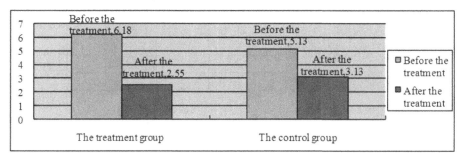

Fig. 2. HAMD anxiety somatization factor comparison between the two groups

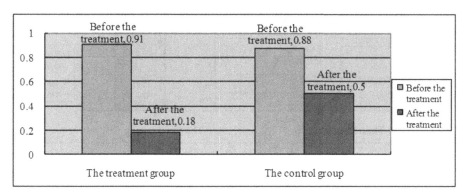

Fig. 3. HAMD weight factor comparison between the two group

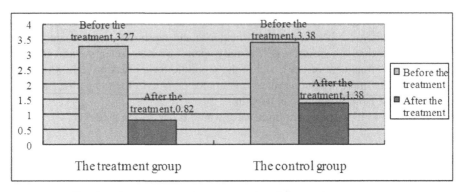

Fig. 4. HAMD cognitive factor comparison between the two groups

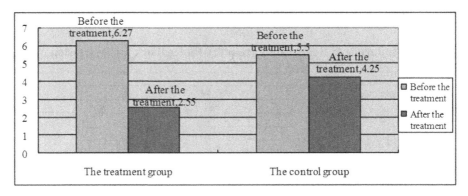

Fig. 5. HAMD block factor comparison between the two groups

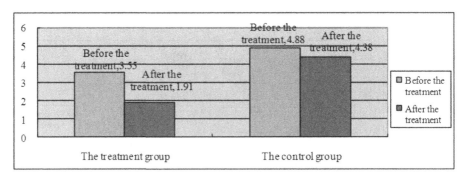

Fig. 6. HAMD sleep disorders factor comparison between the two groups

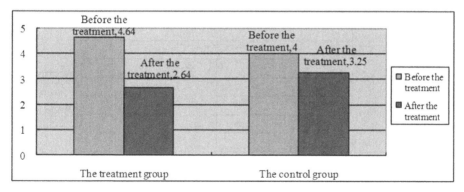

Fig. 7. HAMD despair factor comparison between the two groups

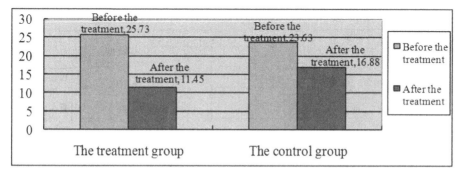

Fig. 8. HAMD depression scores comparison between the two groups

4.2   Experimental Results of Heart Rate Variability Biofeedback for Anxiety

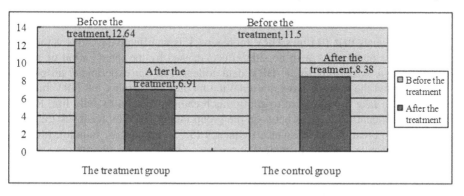

Fig. 9. HAMA spirit factor comparison between the two groups

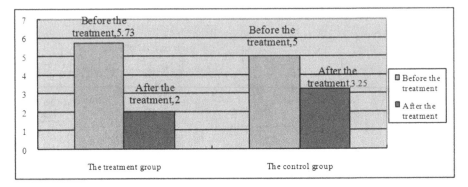

Fig. 10. HAMA body factor comparison between the two **groups**

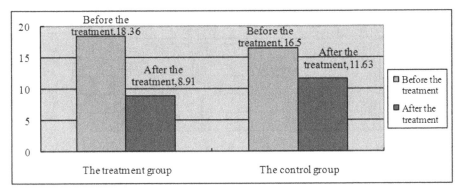

Fig. 11. HAMA anxiety scores comparison between the two groups

5   Discussion

This study reveals that 10 times HRV biofeedback is an effective treatment for post-stroke depression patients with no side effects caused by the intervention of antidepressant drugs. According to the HRV data collected in our experiment, all patients who completed the training have mastered the method of carrying out HRV biofeedback, and can take the initiative to apply this breathing method to daily life. Results showed significant differences between the group taking HRV biofeedback treatment and the group breathing at resonance frequency (5.5 to 6 times per minute). Mechanism for the change of HRV is unclear at present. After lots of authoritative research, Lehrer thought that the increase of HRV was caused by stimulation of baroreflex. And the baroreflex also plays an important role in achieving homeostatic state of autonomic function and the adaptability of entire cardiovascular system. Only when patients breathe at resonance frequency, baroreflex will be activated to the greatest extent. By behavioral therapy, patients strengthen the control of self-regulation on autonomic nervous function, which indicates the improvement of functional activity of vagus nerve.

Our experiment found that although the clinical symptoms, both the depressive symptoms were obviously decreased, unlike the Karavidas[3] results in significant improvement. I think the disease specificity of post-stroke depression disease may account for this. Most scholars favor the theory of "biological mechanism", which believes that the parts of the brain damaged and neurotransmitters are important factors in determining whether stroke patients suffer from depression. Although the observed indicators of the study did not involve the measure of various neurotransmitter and hormone levels, previous studies have showed that the depression combined stroke has a greater impact on HRV than mere stroke or simply depression, and its damage on autonomic nerve is more serious. Based on the above results, our experiment found that after 10 times HRV biofeedback, depression levels of patients were still in the recovery process, but they were not completely cured. There exists a need to increase the frequency and intensity of training to observe its long-term effect. The recovery mechanism of HRV biofeedback therapy for stroke patients with depression needs to be further studied.

6   Conclusion

In this paper, through clinical trials, we adopt the method of heart rate variability biofeedback treatment for PSD patients. We focused on heart rate variability biofeedback influence on depression and anxiety in clinical trials of its impact. We applied Heart Rate Variability (HRV) biofeedback to train PSD patients by a prospective randomized control study. This study reveals effectiveness of the HRV biofeedback on stroke patients' emotional improvement, autonomic nerve function and prognostic implications. HRV biofeedback is a beneficial adjuvant treatment for patients with post-stroke depression in rehabilitation training. Our findings suggest that 10 times HRV biofeedback is an effective treatment for post-stroke depression patients, especially on the improvement of depression levels and sleep disturbance.

In the future, we'll extend the follow-up time, add observed indicators of prognosis, and clarify their level of efficacy. Meantime, we will continue to deepen the HRV biofeedback and changes of individual psychological and physiological indexes in the treatment of pressure under stress, can also study HRV biofeedback index change on the level of consciousness, arousal, attention and other higher cognitive functions. There is no significant difference between the two groups. It is generally believed that depressed patients have memory and learning neural psychological defects, early research suggests depression in patients with nerve psychological defects could be secondary to depression, but recent studies have shown that psychological depression in patients with nerve defects can't explain completely by depression and other psychological factors. After treating depression improves, neuro-psychological defects still exist inside the patients. The next step could be a detailed observation of cognitive-related indicators. Correctly to handle the pressure stress, emotional stability, ease pain, improve sleep, enhance attention adaptability, and learning ability, which has important clinical significance for the prognosis of patients with cerebral stroke rehabilitation.

Acknowledgements. This study was supported by the National Basic Research Program of China (973 Program) No.2011CB302302. We would like to thank Dechun Sang, Songhuai Liu, Lin Wang, Shufeng Ji, from Bo Ai Hospital, Beijing. We also appreciate the research assistance provided by Yan Zhang MSc from Tsinghua University.

References

1. Ming-ming, Y.: Relationship among Depression, Anxiety and Possible Factors in Post-stroke Patients: 510 Cases Report. Chinese Journal of Rehabilitation Theory and Practice. **12**(6), 498–500 (2006)
2. Dai-qun, X., Rong, Y., Rong-mei, L., et al.: Analysis of Post-stroke Anxiety Disorders and the Related Factors. Huaxi Medicine **19**(1), 133 (2004)
3. Karavidas, M.K., Lehrer, P.M., Vaschillo, E.G., Vaschillo, B., Humberton, M., Buyske, S., et al.: Preliminary results of an open label study of heart rate variability biofeedback for the treatment of major depression. Applied Psychophysiology and Biofeedback **32**, 19–30 (2007)
4. Zucker, T.L., Samuelson, K.W., Muench, F., Greenberg, M.A., Gevirtz, R.N.: The effects of respiratory sinus arrhythmia biofeedback on heart rate variability and posttraumatic stress disorder symptoms, A pilot study. Applied Psychophysiology & Biofeedback **34**, 135–143 (2009)
5. National Conference on Cerebrovascular Disease Score Standards in Clinical Neurological Deficit for Stroke Patients (1995). Chinese Journal of Neurology, **29**(6), 381–383 (1996)
6. Lehrer, P.M.: Applied psychophysiology: Beyond the boundaries of biofeedback (mending a wall, a brief history of our field, and applications to control of the muscles and cardiorespiratory systems). Applied Psychophysiology and Biofeedback **28**(4), 291–304 (2003)
7. Kleiger, R.E., Miller, J.P., Bigger, J.T., et al.: Decreased heart rate Variability and its association with increased mortality after acute myocardial infarction. Am J Cardiol **59**, 256–262 (1987)
8. Carod Artal, F.J., Gonzalez Gutierrez, J.L., Egido Herrero, J.A., et al.: Post stroke depression: predictive factors at one year follow up. Rev Neurol, 16–31 (2002)
9. Hayee, M.A., Akhtar, N., Haque, A., et al.: Depression after stroke2analysis of 297 stroke patients. Bangladesh Med Res Counc Bull **27**(3), 96–102 (2001)
10. Nolan, R.P., Kamath, M.V., Floras, J.S., Stanley, J.: Heart rate variability biofeedback as a behavioral neurocardiac intervention to enhance vagal heart control. American Heart Journal **149**(6), 1137 (2005)
11. Dishman, R.K., Nakamura, Y., Garcia, M.E., et al.: Heart rate variability, trait anxiety, and perceived stress among physically fitmenand women. Int J Psychophysiol **37**(2), 121–133 (2000)
12. Monk, C., Kovelenko, P., Ellman, L.M., et al.: Enhanced stress reactivity in paediatric anxiety disorders, implications for future cardiovascular health. Int J Neumpsychopharmacol **4**(2), 199–206 (2001)
13. Slosh, R.P., Shapiro, P.A., Bagiella, E., et al.: Temporal stability of heart period variability during a resting baseline and in response to psychological challenge. Psyehophysiology **32**(2), 191–196 (1995)
14. Hayanao, J., Sakakibaba, Y., Yamada, A., et al.: Accuracy of assessmena of cardiac vagal tone by heart rate variability in normal subjects. Am J cardiol **67**, 199–204 (1991)
15. Hedman, A.E., Hartikainen, J.E.K., Tahvanainen, K.U.O., et al.: The high frequency component of hear rate variability reflects cardiac parasympathetic modulatin rather than parasympathetic 'tone'. Acta Physiol Scand **155**, 267–273 (1995)
16. Salahuddin, L., Cho, J., Jeong, M.G., et al.: Ultra short term analysis of heart rate variability for monitoring mental stress in mobile settings. In: Proceedings of the 29th Annual International Conference of the IEEE, pp. 4656–4659. IEEE EMBS, Lyon (2007)
17. David, W.W.: Physiological correlates of heart rate variability (HRV) and the subjective assessment of workload and fatigue in-flight crew: a practical study. In: People in Control. An International ConfeFence on Human Interfaces in Control Rooms, pp. 159–163. Cockpits and Command Centers, Manchester (2001)

A New Approach for Face Detection
Based on Photoplethysmographic Imaging

He Liu[1,2], Tao Chen[1], Qingna Zhang[1], and Lei Wang[1(✉)]

[1] Shenzhen Institutes of Advanced Technology,
Chinese Academy of Sciences, Shenzhen, China
{he.liu,wanglei}@siat.ac.cn
[2] Haerbin Institute of Technology, Harbin, China

Abstract. Face detection as a necessary first-step has been widely used in face recognition systems and many other applications. However, many effective face detection methods still stay in grayscale images. Nowadays, photoplethysmographic imaging (PPGi) for cardiovascular and hemodynamic analysis has become an attractive research area and pulsatile signal extracted from skin surface can be obtained using a digital camera under the condition of the ambient light. In this paper, we introduce a new approach of face detection based on the PPGi technology. First, a reference signal is required to calculate the standard value of the subject's heart rate. The frame images are sliced into many small regions and the frequency of every region is estimated, respectively. According to the predetermined threshold between the standard value and the calculated value, an index of the existence of the face region can be created. And then the binary image of the face region can be formed. Finally, an elliptical template can be formed using the edge information of the binary image. In the condition of different heart rate, we can obtain effective results.

Keywords: Face detection · Grayscale images · Photoplethysmographic imaging · Heart rate

1 Introduction

In the last decades, face detection is a rapidly growing research area. With the purpose of locating and extracting the face region from the backgrounds, many efficient face detection methods based on skin color characteristics have been proposed [1-4]. Face detection also has several applications in many areas such as video coding, video conferencing, content-based image retrieval, crowd surveillance and intelligent human-computer interfaces. The human face is a dynamic object and has a great variability in its appearance, which makes face detection become a difficult problem in computer vision and many other applications. In order to improve the accuracy of face detection, some efficient methods have been developed. Traditionally, methods that focus on facial landmarks (such as eyes, nose etc), that detect face-like colors in circular regions, or that use standard feature templates, were used to detect faces. However, these attempts don't improve the accuracy of face detection fundamentally. Face detection is still a challenge because of several difficulties, such as variable face

X. Yin et al. (Eds.): HIS 2015, LNCS 9085, pp. 79–91, 2015.
DOI: 10.1007/978-3-319-19156-0_9

orientations, different face sizes, partial occlusions of faces in an image, and changeable lighting conditions.

Photoplethysmography imaging (PPGi) as a new research field is used to extract physiological information in recent years. As a fact that volume of the blood in the blood vessels is constantly changing during the cardiac circulation system and human face is a part of a living body, we can learn that there is a constant blood flow in the subject's face region. Photoplethysmography (PPG) corresponds to the variations in reflected light due to cardiovascular blood volume pulse [5]. Nowadays, it has been shown that heart rate (HR) could be measured from human face with a simple consumer level digital camera under ambient light [6]. The noncontact methods to estimate HR can obtain very high accuracy.

In this paper, we propose a new methodology of face detection based on PPGi technology. The pulsatile signal extracted from face as a unique feature may be used to improve the robustness of noncontact face detection. The frame images obtained from the recorded video stream are sliced equally into many small regions. Then the frequency of every region is estimated, respectively. According to the predetermined threshold between the standard value and the calculated value, an index of the existence of the face region can be created. Because the human face can be approximate to an elliptical area, we use the edge information of the binary image of the subject's face region to fit out an accurate face region.

2   Method

2.1   Experimental Setup

We use a digital camera to record the videos of the subjects of our research team for analysis the information of the physiological signals. All videos were recorded in color (24-bit RGB with 3 channels × 8 bit/channel) at 30 frames per second (fps) with pixel resolution of 640 × 480 and saved in AVI format on the laptop. A total of ten healthy volunteers (eight males, aged from 24 to 35 with a mean age of 28.6 years; two females, both aged 25 years old), recruited from the Shenzhen Institutes of Advanced Technology, Chinese Academy of Sciences, were enrolled in this study.

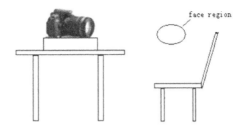

Fig. 1. Specific experimental environment when recording the subject's videos

Fig. 1 shows the experimental setup. Our experiments were conducted indoors and with the ambient light as the only source of illumination. The subjects were asked to seat at a desk in front of a digital camera at a distance of approximately 0.4 m from the camera lens and to keep normal breathing. The experiment procedure has three sessions for all subjects. In session 1, the subject is the state of rest. In session 2, the subject is the state after gentle exercise. In session 3, the third one is the state after intense exercise.

2.2   Frame Image Acquisition and Processing

In order to detect the subject's face region in our experiments, we use the technology of division the video streaming to obtain the single frame image sequence at 30 Hz. And then each image was equally divided into many small regions. The size of these small regions is 40×30 pixels. Image processing was performed with custom software written in Matlab, Mathworks. The result of the divided small region can be seen in Fig. 2. According to established theoretical model [7], physiological processes of heart pulsation lead to modulation in time of fractional blood volume at the heart-beat rate. Modulation of the blood volume results in the absorption modulation of the light penetrated in the skin, which leads to the intensity modulation of light reflected in vivo from the subject's skin. Therefore, the value of pixels with the same spatial coordinates (x, y) in series of recorded frames is also modulated in time with the heart-beat rate. This fact was confirmed in numerous experiments including those carried out recently with digital cameras in the reflection mode [8].

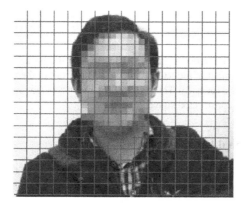

Fig. 2. The result of the divided small region

By recording a video of the facial region with a digital camera, the RGB channels pick up a mixture of the reflected pulsatile signal along with other sources of fluctuations in light due to motion artifacts. So each color sensor records a mixture of the original source signals with slightly different weight. For each frame image, the total number of the small regions is 16×16. Then the R、 G、 B channel of each small region of the images will be extracted. After these processing steps, all pixel values within each small region were spatially averaged to form a red, green and blue measurement point. After the spatial averaging operation, we can obtain the raw signal $x(t)$ of the G channel within the duration of the recorded video. In the previous literatures [6, 9], it is demonstrated that the result of G channel is better than the result of R channel and B channel when calculating the subject's HR. For the sake of simplicity, we always selected the G channel as the desired signal for further analysis.

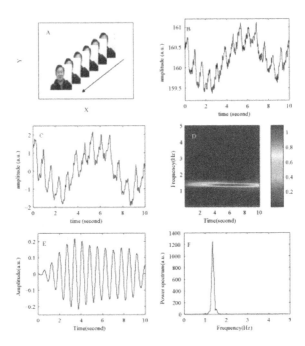

Fig. 3. The result of the reference signal. (a) The result of the frame images. (b) The result of the raw trace of the G channel of the RGB image. (c) The result of the processed signal. (d) The result of the Wavelet Transform. (e) The result of the reconstructed signal. (f) The result of the power spectrum of the reconstructed signal.

2.3   Reference Signal Formation

In order to analysis the characteristic of the pulsatile signal of the subjects, we firstly process the recorded video frames to generate a reference signal. We select the forehead area of the subjects as the region of interest (ROI) in our research to generate a reference signal. And then, the bounding box containing the forehead regions of the subjects were selected at the first frame of the recorded video. Coordinates of the selected forehead region remained the same for the whole sequence of the frame images in Fig. 3a. All pixel values within the selected ROI were spatially averaged resulting in a single mean value of each recorded frame. Time-trace of this mean value during the whole recorded video is shown in Fig. 3b. In Fig. 3b, we can see that the signal is a kind of time-varying signal. We want to obtain the frequency spectral characteristic of the time-varying signal, so we should transform the time-varying signal from time domain to frequency domain. As we can see from Fig. 3d, it was obtained by applying wavelet transform to the signal shown in Fig. 3c. Fig. 3e shows the reconstructed signal using the coefficients of the wave transform. Typical power spectrum curve of wavelet transform coefficients of the mean-pixel value of the located ROI is shown in Fig. 3f.

2.4   Signal Processing

In this study, interest of the underlying signal is the pulse wave of the cardiovascular. Signal processing is a key step for extracting the human body's physiological parameters. In our research, we use continuous wavelet transform (CWT) to filter the pulse signal. The CWT constructs a time-frequency representation of a signal and has been used to denoise or refine peaks [10] and significant points [11] in PPG signals. Inner product was used in continuous wavelet transform to measure the similarity between an analyzing function and a signal. Due to the width of the window is constantly changing when calculating the wavelet transform coefficients, so the continuous wavelet transform can detect the rapid changes in both time domain and frequency domain. This is the most significant advantage of wavelet transform when comparing to the Fourier transform and the short time Fourier transform. Many advantages have resulted in CWT being increasingly used for biological signals analysis [12, 13]. The non-stationary PPG signal is convolved with a child wavelet $\psi_{\tau,s}$, representing a scaled and shifted version of a mother wavelet ψ :

$$CWT_x^{\psi}(\tau,s) = \int_{-\infty}^{\infty} x(t)\psi_{\tau,s}(t)dt \tag{1}$$

$$\psi_{\tau,s}(t) = \frac{1}{\sqrt{|s|}}\psi(\frac{t-\tau}{s}) \tag{2}$$

where $\psi_{\tau,s}$ is the child wavelet, scaled by s and dilated by τ. ψ is the alleged mother wavelet. There is a relationship between analyzed frequencies and the scale parameter when we use wavelet transform to process signal problem. Decreasing s and shrinking the wavelet size results to cover a smaller signal in the time domain, leading to analyze higher frequencies and vice versa. According to the input signal properties and different application scope, we can choose different wavelet functions from a large set of standard mother wavelets for further analysis. The cmor3-3 wavelet has already been used to analyze PPG signals [14] and was employed in this study. The original signal can be reconstructed from the wavelet transform via the following inverse equation:

$$x(t) = \frac{1}{C_\psi}\int_0^{\infty}\int_{-\infty}^{\infty}\frac{1}{s^2}CWT_x^{\psi}(\tau,s)\frac{1}{\sqrt{|s|}}\psi(\frac{t-\tau}{s})d\tau ds \tag{3}$$

$$C_\psi = \int_0^{\infty}\frac{\left|\psi^{'(\xi)}\right|}{|\xi|}d\xi < \infty \tag{4}$$

where C_ψ is the admissibility condition and $\psi^{'}$ is the Fourier transform of ψ. The DC component is removed to reveal detailed information [15] on lower scales prior to performing the CWT. The equation as follows:

$$X_{AC}(t) = \frac{x(t) - \mu}{\sigma} \tag{5}$$

where μ and σ represent the mean value and standard deviation of the raw PPG signal $x(t)$. The waveform of the reference signal $X_{AC}(t)$ is shown in Fig. 3c. The CWT is then computed within an operational frequency band, set to [0.8, 2.0] Hz corresponding to 48-120 beat per minute.

The wavelet energy curve can be used to filter the wavelet transform coefficients, its maximum value in the frequency axis corresponding to the averaged HR. The pulse wave presents stronger amplitudes than those generated by noise and trends. A weighted product is applied between the energy curve and the CWT coefficients. And then, we use the inverse wavelet transform represented as Eq. 4 to reconstruct a denoised version of the raw signal. The cascade of these two operations-weighting the CWT and reconstructing the signal by inverse CWT - is employed to filter the PPG signal in the operational band [0.8, 2.0] Hz [16].

2.5   Define a 4-neighbourhood of the Divided Image Pixel Block

In image processing, 4-neighbourhood of the pixel as a basic concept has become one of the most common principles to determine whether the pixels are connected or not. In our research, we want to detect the appropriate regions to form a map of the subjects' HR. According to the concept of the 4-neighbourhood of the single pixel, we define a concept of the 4-neighbourhood of the divided small image pixel block. Accordingly, the custom 4-neighbourhood of the divided small image pixel block can be seen in Fig. 4.

	B1	
B2	B0	B4
	B3	

Fig. 4. The schematic plot of 4-neighbourhood. The function of the 4-neighbourhood is to detect the connectivity of the pixel block.

2.6   The Method of Obtaining the Proper Boundary of the Face Image

In order to obtain the useful information of each small image in our study, we applied fast Fourier transform to the reconstructed reference signal and the processed signal of each small region to obtain the frequency information. For the reference signal and the processed signal, the maximum value around 1.0 Hz can be read from the frequency-amplitude curve. After this step, a mathematical expression can be represented as Eq. 6 to calculate the result of the heart beats per minute. The specific mathematic expression as follows:

$$Value = f \times 60 \tag{6}$$

In Eq.6, the parameter *Value* represents the result of the heart beats per minute, and the parameter f represents the frequency of the reference signal and the processed signal.

Next, we calculate the result of each small image pixel block to preliminary locating the rough ROI. In this step, we define a threshold ξ ($\xi = 3$) to determine whether the detected area is appropriate or not. The specific mathematic expression as follows:

$$V_i = \begin{cases} fi, \|fi - std\| \le \xi \\ 0, \|fi - std\| \ge \xi \end{cases} i = 1,2,3,...,N \qquad (7)$$

for each i, we get a value of the subject's HR. The symbol f_i represents the value of the HR of each detected small region, parameter *std* represents the result of the subject's HR calculated by the reference signal and N represents the total number of the small image block. If the result of the heart-beat per minute of the subject meets the upper criteria of the Eq. 7, we will use the value as the effective heart-beat value of the subject. If not so, we will set the value to zero. This step can help us obtain the rough scope of the effective face region.

In order to further locating the ROI accurately, we use the function of the custom 4-neighbourhood to decide whether take the small region as an effective area or not. For each small image pixel block, the traversal algorithm of the 4-neighbourhood is used to obtain the most suitable regions of the frame image. And then, the values returned from the algorithm to form a map of detected regions of interest. After these processing steps, the results of the candidate region have been calculated.

Now, we introduce the judgment criterion of the connectivity of the divided small pixel block. As can be seen in Fig. 4, if the value of the image pixel block B0 meets the upper criteria of the mathematic Eq. 7, and there are at least two values of the image pixel block B1、 B2、 B3、 B4 meet the upper criteria of the mathematic Eq. 7, too. We will mark the area B0 as the regions of interest in our research. The rest results can be processed using the same method. If not so, we will delete the area and set the value to 0. Accordingly, the located rough scope of the subject's face region with different states can be seen in Fig. 5.

 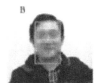

Fig. 5. The rough scope of the face region

2.7   The Method of Obtaining the Binary Image

After determining the value of the HR of each small area, the rough boundary of the face region can be obtained. In order to reach the goal that locating an elliptical face region, we should obtain the binary image. Next, we introduce the method to obtain the binary image. For each detected small area, we will set all pixels value to 1 if the value of the HR greater than zero. Accordingly, we will set all pixels value to 0 if the value of the HR equals to zero. The expression can be written as Eq. 8.

$$P_i = \begin{cases} 1, V_i > 0 \\ 0, Vi = 0 \end{cases} i = 1,2,3,...,N; j = 1,2,3,...,M.$$ (8)

For each i, the pixels value of the small region can be computed. The symbol V_i represents the value of each small detected area. The symbol P_i represents the pixel value of each small detected area. N and M represents the total number of the small image block and the total number of the pixels of each small image block respectively.

2.8   The Method of Ellipse Fitting

Robert operator is one of the most commonly used algorithms of the image edge detection. In this research, we use Robert operator to obtain the edge information of the binary image. After this step, the values of the edge of the binary image are equal to 1. According to the position of x-coordinate and y-coordinate of all the value 1, an optimal ellipse fitting function named fitellipse is used to calculate the parameters of the ellipse. These parameters can be marked as $A = (C_x, C_y, R_x, R_y, \theta)$. The parameters (C_x, C_y), (R_x, R_y), and θ represent the center coordinates, the length of the semi-major axis and short half shaft, and the rotation angle of the ellipse respectively. The input variables of the optimal ellipse fitting function are vector **x** and vector **y**. Vector **x** and vector **y** can be calculated by Eq. 9. The output results of the optimal ellipse fitting function are the parameters which meet the coordinate distribution of the vector **x** and vector **y**. The relationship between the coordinate position (x, y) and each parameter of A can be expressed as Eq. 9.

$$\begin{cases} x = R_x \times \cos\alpha \times \cos\theta - R_y \times \sin\alpha \times \sin\theta + C_x \\ y = R_y \times \cos\alpha \times \sin\theta - R_y \times \sin\alpha \times \cos\theta + C_{xy} \end{cases}, 0 \le \alpha \le 2\pi$$ (9)

According to the results returned from the function of fitellipse, an ellipse which is very similar to the shape of the face region can be drawn using a function written in ellipse.

2.9   Statistics

Box plot can be used to detect the outlier of the experimental results. In the process of slicing the video frame image into small regions, we are not able to determine the position of the eyebrows, beard and eyes precisely. So the map of detected face region could contain false values when comparing to the standard result of the subject's HR. In order to judge whether the detected face region is reasonable or not, we drawing the box plots to show the outlier of the proposed methodology which used to locate the rough scope of the face region.

3   Results

The key point of this paper is how to locate an accurate face region based on the result of the subject's HR. So calculating the HR of the subject is the most crucial step. In order to validate the correctness of the calculated result, a reference signal formed from the same frame images. Table 1 shows the calculated result of each small area. As can be seen from Table 1, the result contained two abnormal values (the number 0 lies in the row 5, column 7 and column 9 represent the abnormal result). But these error values are acceptable. The results of the subjects' HR of different state can be seen in Table 2.

Table 1. The map of the detected area. The light blue numbers represent the clustering characteristics of the face region, the numbers 0 lie in the row 5, column 7 and column 9 represent the abnormal result, the numbers 78 and 81 lie in the row 7, column 11 and row 13, column 9 respectively do not meet the definition of the 4-neighbourhood of the divided image pixel block.

0	0	0	0	0	0	0	0	0	0	0	0	0	0	0	0
0	0	0	0	0	0	0	0	0	0	0	0	0	0	0	0
0	0	0	0	0	0	78	81	81	78	0	0	0	0	0	0
0	0	0	0	0	78	81	81	81	81	0	0	0	0	0	0
0	0	0	0	0	78	0	81	0	84	0	0	0	0	0	0
0	0	0	0	0	78	84	84	81	78	0	0	0	0	0	0
0	0	0	0	0	81	81	81	84	84	78	0	0	0	0	0
0	0	0	0	0	81	84	81	81	84	0	0	0	0	0	0
0	0	0	0	0	0	84	81	81	81	0	0	0	0	0	0
0	0	0	0	0	0	81	81	78	84	0	0	0	0	0	0
0	0	0	0	0	0	78	81	84	78	0	0	0	0	0	0
0	0	0	0	0	0	0	81	84	0	0	0	0	0	0	0
0	0	0	0	0	0	0	0	81	0	0	0	0	0	0	0
0	0	0	0	0	0	0	0	0	0	0	0	0	0	0	0
0	0	0	0	0	0	0	0	0	0	0	0	0	0	0	0
0	0	0	0	0	0	0	0	0	0	0	0	0	0	0	0

Table 2. The results of the subjects' heart-beats with different states. State 1 represents the state of rest, state 2 represents the state after gentle exercise, and state 3 represents the state after intense exercise.

Subject number	State 1(bpm)	State 2(bpm)	State 3(bpm)
Subject 1	81±3	89±3	96±3
Subject 2	75±3	81±3	90±3
Subject 3	89±3	96±3	105±3
Subject 4	65±3	70±3	81±3
Subject 5	73±3	79±3	92±3
Subject 6	69±3	76±3	85±3
Subject 7	93±3	101±3	112±3
Subject 8	78±3	85±3	95±3
Subject 9	71±3	80±3	93±3
Subject 10	85±3	93±3	104±3

In order to obtain the binary image of the face region, the method described in the previous section (The method of obtaining the proper boundary of the face image) was used to calculate the position of up, down, left and right boundary scope of the face region. The result of the rough scope of the detected face region with different states can be seen in Fig. 5. In Fig. 6, we use the box plot to detect the outlier of the subject's HR. Fig. 6a represents the box plot of the HR with the state of rest. Fig. 6b represents the box plot of the HR with the state after gentle exercise. And Fig. 6c represents the box plot of the HR with the state after intense exercise. After this step, the outliers of the subject's HR can be detected. If the outliers are reasonable, the binary image of the face region with different state can be obtained. And then, the ellipse fitting function was applied on the edge image processed by the Robert operator to return the optimal elliptic parameters. Using these parameters returned from the ellipse fitting function, the result of the detected face region with different state can be seen in Fig. 7.

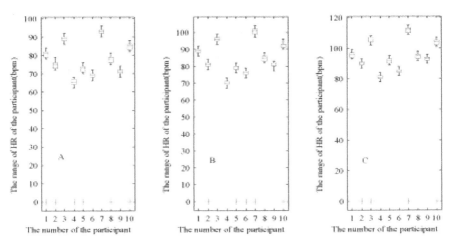

Fig. 6. The box plot of the heart rate with different states. (a) The box plot of the heart rate with the state of rest. (b) The box plot of the heart rate with the state after gentle exercise. (c) The box plot of the heart rate with the state after intense exercise.

4   Discussion

In this study, we detect the face region based on PPGi. Before recording the video, the subject was asked to find a comfortable position, and to breathe normally. In recent years, many scholars have proposed many efficient and robust face detection algorithm. However, these algorithms are based on color information. PPG is a non-invasive optical method to detect a cardiovascular pulse wave travelling through the human body. The basic form of PPG technology requires only two optoelectronic components: a light source to illuminate a part of the human body and a photo-detector to measure small variations in light intensity after light interaction with the illuminated part. The core of our method is based on the blood flow characteristic in a living body. As proposed in this research, in order to obtain an accurate signal to calculate the result of the subject's HR, we use the wavelet transform to remove noise from the raw photoplethysmographic signal of the G channel of the RGB image. This step is quite critical for subsequent processing. The result of the reference signal obtained from the same frame image can help us getting the correct calculated result for further analysis.

In Fig. 5, we can clearly see that the neck is also included in the detected face region. In our research, we found that we can detect the subject's HR in a small region. The size of the small region is width × height = 30 × 40 pixels. However, the size of the subject's neck is larger than the small region. So the detected region would contain the subject's neck. And the detected face with the ratio range between 0.7 and 2.1 is reasonable.

According to Eq. 6 and Eq. 7, a map of the detected area can be formed. Because of the influence of the eyes, beard and eyebrows, we can see a little abnormal result in Fig. 6 (the red + represents the abnormal number 0). In order to locate the face region accurately, we use the 4-neighbourhood of the divided small image pixel block to make a best decision. So the abnormal result would be contained in the map of the detected area. In order to obtain an accurate binary image, the morphological operation method and the hole filling method were adopted to process the area of the abnormal result. The method of obtaining the binary image proposed in this paper is different from the method of converting color space using the gray threshold. If the result of the subject's HR meets the upper criteria of the Eq. 7 and the connectivity of the 4-neighbourhood of the pixel block respectively, we will set all the pixel values of each small area to 1. So the result of our method would not contain many small holes phenomenon cause by the inconsistent color information.

After obtaining the edge information of the binary image, the coordinate position of the value 1 can be calculated in the rough scope of the image. Then we use the coordinate position as the input variable of the fitellipse function to calculate the parameters of the ellipse template. The result of the detected face region is effective with different states. After this research, we have found that the information of the subject's HR may be suit for emotion recognition and mental stress evaluation. For further study, we should research the potential value of the information of the HR in many other application fields.

5   Conclusions

In this paper, we have described and evaluated a novel methodology for face detection from video recordings of the human face and demonstrated an implementation using a digital camera with ambient daylight providing illumination. Wavelet transform plays an important role in removing noise and signal reconstruction. In order to locate the rough scope of the subject's face region, the custom 4-neighbourhood of the divided small image pixel block can help us to make a best decision. According to Eq. 8, we can obtain an accurate binary image. Obtaining the accurate binary image is a critical step for detecting the precise face region. We can draw a conclusion that our method based on the information of the HR has a very high precision.

Acknowledgment. This work was financed partially by the National 863 Program of China (Grant No. 2012AA02A604), the Next generation communication technology Major project of National S&T (Grant No. 2013ZX03005013), the Key Research Program of the Chinese Academy of Sciences.

References

1. Jesorsky, O., Kirchberg, K.J., Frischholz, R.W.: Robust face detection using the hausdorff distance. In: Bigun, J., Smeraldi, F. (eds.) AVBPA 2001. LNCS, vol. 2091, pp. 90–95. Springer, Heidelberg (2001)
2. Viola, P., Jones, M.J.: Robust real-time face detection. Computer vision 57(Suppl 2), 137–154 (2004)
3. Hu, W.C., Yang, C.Y., Huang, D.Y., Huang, C.H.: Feature-based face detection against skin-color like backgrounds with varying illumination. Information Hiding and Multimedia Signal Processing 2(Suppl 2), 123–132 (2011)
4. Chen, A.P., Pan, L., Tong, Y.B., Ning, N.: Face detection technology based on skin color segmentation and template matching. In: Second International Workshop on IEEE, Education Technology and Computer Science (ETCS), vol. 2, pp. 708–711 (2010)
5. Allen, J.: Photoplethysmography and its application in clinical physiological measurement. Physiological Measurement 28, R1–R39 (2007)
6. Verkruysse, W., Svaasand, L.O., Nelson, J.S.: Remote plethysmographic imaging using ambient light. Opt. Express 16(26), 21434–21445 (2008)
7. Cui, W.J., Ostrander, L.E., Lee, B.Y.: In vivo reflectance of blood and tissue as a function of light wavelength. IEEE Trans Biomed Eng 37(Suppl 6), 632–639 (1990)
8. Poh, M.Z., McDuff, D.J., Picard, R.W.: Non-contact, automated cardiac pulse measurements using video imaging and blind source separation. Opt. Express 18(10), 10 (2010)
9. Liu, H., Wang, Y., Wang, L.: The Effect of Light Conditions on Photoplethysmographic Image Acquisition Using a Commercial Camera. 2 (2014)
10. Soni, S., Namjoshi, Y.: Delineation of raw plethysmograph using wavelets for mobile based pulse oximeters. In: Proceedings of 5th Innovative Conference on Embedded Systems, Mobile Communication and Computing, pp. 74–84 (2010)
11. Peterek, T., Prauzek, M., Penhaker, M.: A new method for identification of the significant point in the plethysmografical record. In: Proc. 2nd International Conference on Signal Processing Systems, pp. 362–364 (2010)

12. Shastri, D., Merla, A., Tsiamyrtzis, P., Pavlidis, I.: Imaging facial signs of neurophysiological responses. IEEE Transactions on Biomedical Engineering **56**, 477–484 (2009)
13. Leonard, P., Beattie, T.F., Addison, P.S., Watson, J.N.: Standard pulse oximeters can be used to monitor respiratory rate. Emergency Medicine Journal **20**, 524–525 (2003)
14. Addison, P.S., Watson, J.N.: A novel time-frequency-based 3D Lissajous figure method and its application to the determination of oxygen saturation from the photoplethysmogram. Measurement Science and Technology **15**, 15–18 (2004)
15. Shastri, D., Merla, A., Tsiamyrtzis, P., Pavlidis, I.: Imaging facial signs of neurophysiological responses. IEEE Transactions on Biomedical Engineering **56**, 477–484 (2009)
16. Bousefsaf, F., Maaoui, C., Pruski, A.: Continuous wavelet filtering on webcam photoplethysmographic signals to remotely assess the instantaneous heart rate. Biomedical Signal Processing and Control **8**(Suppl 6), 568–574 (2013)

Biometrics Applications in e-Health Security: A Preliminary Survey

Ebenezer Okoh[1] and Ali Ismail Awad[1,2](✉)

[1] Department of Computer Science, Electrical and Space Engineering,
Luleå University of Technology, Luleå, Sweden
ebeoko-2@student.ltu.se, ali.awad@ltu.se
[2] Faculty of Engineering, Al Azhar University, Qena, Egypt

Abstract. Driven by the desires of healthcare authorities to offer better healthcare services at a low cost, electronic Health (e-Health) has revolutionized the healthcare industry. However, while e-Health comes with numerous advantages that improve health services, it still suffers from security and privacy issues in handling health information. E-Health security issues are mainly centered around user authentication, data integrity, data confidentiality, and patient privacy protection. Biometrics technology addresses the above security problems by providing reliable and secure user authentication compared to the traditional approaches. This study explores the security and privacy issues in e-Health, and offers a comprehensive overview of biometrics technology applications in addressing the e-Health security challenges. The paper concludes that biometrics technology has considerable opportunities for application in e-Health due to its ability to provide reliable security solutions. Although, additional issues like system complexity, processing time, and patient privacy related to the use of biometrics should be taken into consideration.

1 Introduction

The emergence of electronic health (e-Health) has proved to be very compelling for the health industry due to the many benefits it affords the industry. E-Health improves the quality of healthcare by making Patients Health Information (PHI) easily accessible, improving efficiency, and reducing the cost of health service delivery. Patients rarely get to spend much time with their physicians face-to-face. In spite of the benefits of e-Health, it still faces a number of security challenges that need to be addressed. E-Health data security and patient privacy stand out as top issues that health organizations implementing e-Health still grapple with, and to which they need solutions [1]. E-Health security requirements revolve around the basic principles of information security. E-Health security issues include the preservation of e-Health data confidentiality, data integrity, data availability, user authentication, and patient privacy protection [2].

Maintaining data security and user privacy in e-Health is therefore paramount. In order to ensure e-Health security from a technical point of view, it involves

X. Yin et al. (Eds.): HIS 2015, LNCS 9085, pp. 92–103, 2015.
DOI: 10.1007/978-3-319-19156-0_10

securing e-Health applications and their communication components. The underlying issue that is particularly important in relation to the security requirements of e-Health is the user authentication and authorization. In this context, achieving reliable user authentication forms the basis for all other measures to be achieved. Traditional authentication approaches such as user name, password, and access cards are not appropriate in the e-Health context due to the possibility of being lost, stolen, forgotten, or misplaced. In general, traditional authentication methods are not based on inherent individual attributes [3].

Biometrics is a fundamental security mechanism that assigns a unique identity to an individual according to some physiological (fingerprint or face) or behavioral characteristics (voice or signature) [4]. Therefore, biometrics is more reliable and capable than traditional authentication approaches of distinguishing between an authorized person and an imposter. Biometric traits cannot be lost or forgotten; they are difficult to duplicate, share, or distribute. Moreover, it requires the presence of the person being authenticated; it is difficult to forge, and unlikely for a user to repudiate [5]. Biometrics offers a sense of security and convenience both to patients and physicians alike. In order to stay ahead of the emerging security threats posed by e-Health, healthcare organizations are moving from traditional approaches to the utilization of biometrics technology.

This paper explores the security and privacy issues in e-Health as they continue to remain challenges for the healthcare industry. In addition, it seeks to embark on a review to highlight the applications of biometrics in addressing some of the e-Health security and privacy challenges. The research focus is on biometrics applications in user authentication and health data encryption. We believe that this study will provide a good foundation for further research in the area of healthcare data security and patient privacy protection.

The remainder part of this paper is structured as follows: Section 2 presents background on biometrics technology. Preliminary information about e-Health and its current security challenges is covered in Section 3. A detailed exploration of biometrics applications in e-Health security, and how they address e-Health security issues, is placed in Section 4. Section 5 presents a discussion on the current biometrics deployments in e-Health domain, and a discussion of future research directions. Finally, conclusions are documented in Section 6.

2 Biometrics Technology

Biometrics is the science of establishing the identity of an individual based on the physiological, chemical, or behavioral attributes of the individual [6]. In order to identify individuals based on their biometric traits, biometric systems need to go through two major phases, namely an enrollment phase and a recognition phase [7], [8]. Alternatively, biometric systems are regarded as pattern recognition systems consisting of four phases: sensor, feature extractor, database, and matcher [7]. Although, biometric systems support both identification (recognition) and verification (authentication) modes of operation, the appropriate mode is decided according the target application. Biometric identification refers to identifying an individual from a database of users based on his or her distinguishing biometric trait (unimodal) or traits (multimodal) [3]. However, verification mode ensures the authenticity of the identity claimed by an individual.

The requirements of biometrics deployment demand certain traits be used. Each biometric identifier has its own strength and weakness, and the choice of a certain biometric identifier is based on the systems needs [5]. Every biometric trait must fulfill, in different degrees, the following properties [7], [9]: universality (every person must possess the trait); uniqueness (the trait should be sufficiently distinct between persons); permanence (the trait should be invariant over time); measurability (the possibility of measuring the trait quantitatively); performance (achievable recognition accuracy); acceptability (the willingness of people to accept the system); and circumvention (the ability of the biometric system to defend against any system hacking operation). Table 1 shows a comparison of different biometric identifiers based on the aforementioned selection criteria. The the final score indicates the overall evaluation of the identifier.

In general, a similarity match score is used to measure the similarity between two feature sets from same or different biometric traits. A higher matching score provides a strong indication that the two biometric features originate from the same person. In practice, there are two basic techniques for measuring the accuracy of a biometric system; False Non- Match Rate (FNMR) and False Match Rate (FMR). These are also considered to be the two major errors made by a biometric system. FNMR refers to the probability that two samples of the same biometric trait from the same user are falsely declared as a non-match. Thus, the biometric system mistakenly rejects a genuine individual as an imposter. FMR refers to the probability that two samples from different biometric traits are mistakenly recognized as a match, and hence, the biometric system mistakenly accepts an imposter as a genuine individual [7].

There are other types of failures encountered by any biometric system. These are Failure to Capture (FTC), Failure to Acquire (FTA), and Failure to Enroll (FTE). FTA represents the proportion of times a biometric device fails to capture a sample when biometric characteristics are presented to it. FTE represents the proportion of users that cannot be successfully enrolled in a biometric system [6].

Table 1. A comparison between different biometric identifiers: 1 = High, 0.5 = Medium, and 0 = Low. The table is adapted from [4], [5], [9].

	Universality	Uniqueness	Performance	Acceptability	Circumvention	Score
Fingerprint	0.5	1.0	1.0	0.5	1.0	**4.0**
Face image	1.0	0.0	0.0	1.0	0.0	2.0
Iris pattern	1.0	1.0	1.0	0.0	1.0	**4.0**
DNA	1.0	1.0	1.0	0.0	0.0	**3.0**
EEG	1.0	0.0	0.0	0.0	0.0	1.0
Signature	0.0	0.0	0.0	1.0	0.0	1.0
Voice	0.5	0.0	0.0	1.0	0.0	1.5
Gait	0.5	0.0	0.0	1.0	0.5	2.0

There is a tradeoff between biometric systems FMR and FNMR which could be plotted on a Receiver Operating Characteristics (ROC) curve or Detection Error Tradeoff (DET) curve [3]. The ROC curve gives a measure of the system accuracy in a test environment [3]. The performance of a biometric system could also be determined by the Equal Error Rate (EER) of the system. The EER refers to the point in a DET curve where the FMR equals the FNMR. A lower value of EER indicates a better biometric system performance [6], [7].

3   Electronic Health (e-Health)

Recent advances in the field of telemedicine around the twentieth century paved the way for e-Health. Following that came developments in computerization, digitization of data, and digital networks which led to a multiplicity of e-Health applications [10]. Currently, e-Health comprises a whole range of services or systems at the edge of healthcare and information technology such as: telemedicine, which is defined as a remote healthcare delivery system using telecommunication and information technology; Electronic Health Records (EHR), which include electronic health information about a patient or individual; consumer health informatics, which is use of medical informatics to analyze consumer needs for information; health knowledge management, which aims to capture, describe, organize, share, and effectively use healthcare knowledge; medical decision support systems, which are interactive expert systems that assist health professionals with decision-making tasks; and mobile health (mHealth), which uses mobile devices for different applications in healthcare [10]. The underlying factor in all of these technologies is the digitization of data. In that regard, the term (e-Health) suggests digital health information in contrast to a paper-based system.

E-Health is an emerging field of medical informatics that refers to the organization and delivery of health services and information using the internet and related technologies [11]. In a broader sense, e-Health involves the application of information and communication technologies in healthcare. It involves all digital health-related information, encompassing products, systems, and services. The term health does not solely refer to medicine, disease, or healthcare but also comprises public health and healthcare.

The adoption of e-Health services achieves different goals including: increased efficiency in healthcare, enhanced quality care, evidence-based medicine, empowerment of consumers and patients by broadening the knowledge base of medicine, encouragement of new relationships between patients and health professionals, education of physicians and consumers, enabling information exchange and communication, extending the scope of healthcare; posing new ethical issues, and promoting equity in healthcare [11]. In concise terms, it promotes health information sharing, ensures effective healthcare, and empowers health consumers to manage their own health. It seeks to transform the healthcare system from a "provider-driven" model to a "patient-centric" paradigm [12].

Several studies that have been undertaken in the field of e-Health have demonstrated system architecture in order to represent a proposed e-Health system [12], [13], [14]. Several of these studies present a three-level system architecture of e-Health. For instance, in [12], the authors present an e-Health architecture consisting of three layers. The first layer consists of devices that help collect real-time data from patients. The second layer consists of the internet or interconnected devices that help transport the collected data from patients to third-party database servers or healthcare service providers. The third level is made up of intelligent systems to help in making health decisions. Similarly, in [13], the authors present a network layer architecture for an e-Health system.

3.1 Security Challenges in e-Health

There are, however, concerns about the security and privacy of patient health information. Privacy is considered one of the fundamental issues in e-Health. The electronic nature of health information introduces certain vulnerabilities that increase the possibility of security breaches occurring. E-health information can exist in three states: storage, transmission, and processing [15]. The threats associated with the different states are: threats to data confidentiality or privacy, threats to data integrity, threats to user authenticity, threats to availability, threats to storage, and threats to data transmission [15].

The confidentiality of patient data becomes a concern as healthcare professionals continue to transmit or share patient health information by relying on internet-based technologies. The privacy of the patient is always affected should such confidential information be disclosed. Effective access control is crucial in order to protect sensitive patient health information from unauthorized access. Established conventional authentication methods are known to have inherent vulnerabilities. Passwords, which can easily be compromised, thus making health data only as secure as the password is not a reliable security scheme. Password-based smart cards are a good example of that case.

In wireless healthcare, that is wireless sensor networks (WSN), it is essential to ensure secure communication among biosensors in order to protect the vital physiological data collected from patients. Communication within such an environment requires there to be confidentiality, integrity and authenticity of the data being communicated between the patient and the physician or medical center. Encryption helps to secure the transmitted data. However, there are some key factors that need to be considered such as encryption method, key generation, and key distribution, as the biosensors are resource constrained [16].

4   Biometrics in e-Health

Biometrics is increasingly gaining recognition within the healthcare environment as pressure increases on healthcare providers to reduce fraud, to provide secure access to medical records and facilities, to reduce costs, and to facilitate easier access to medical records [17]. The adoption of biometrics in healthcare goes along with the adoption of Electronic Health Record (EHR) systems as EHR makes the use of biometrics more efficient and effective [18]. As a consequence of

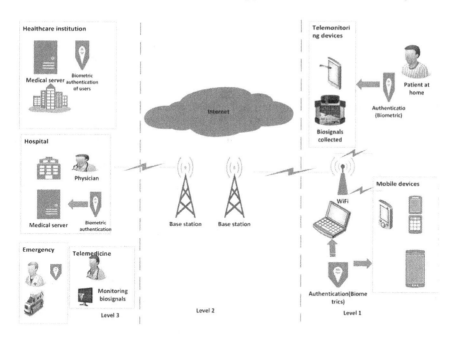

Fig. 1. System architecture of e-Health leveraging on biometric technology

the adoption of EHR, it is now easy for health professionals to view or tamper with patient records [19]. A secure authentication system in the form of biometric technologies, traits, or identifiers has been adopted by most healthcare organizations to meet the challenges for protecting patient privacy [19].

The current nature of biometrics technology adopted within the healthcare industry is based on physiological characteristics and multi-modal biometric systems, most of which are concerned with one-time verification [20]. Traditional biometric traits include fingerprints and iris patterns, which are considered to be static [21]. However, in recent times other potential biometric modalities have been studied within the healthcare industry based on biosignals [20]. The signal attributes of these modalities are time-varying, and thus dynamic. Within the medical setting, these biometric modalities, i.e. biosignals, are accessible and readily available as they have already been assessed as part of patient follow-up.

The biometric data of a patient or physician is used for authentication in order to access healthcare information. It provides a convenient authentication mechanism that removes the need to memorize long or complex passwords or PINs. As such, it is ideal for elderly people, especially those with mental disorders, and unconscious patients. In Fig. 1 level 1 is made up of all devices that form a network that helps to collect and transmit data from patients, or to gain access to health information by a consumer. The devices include medical sensors, mobile phones, and computers. Level 2 represents the main communication infrastructure that connects level 1 to level 3. Level 3 consists of those elements that deal with healthcare provision, the storage of health information, and telemedicine. In levels 1 and 3, patient or physician biometric data is used to provide authentication in order to gain access to health information.

Biosignals are ideal for a continuous biometric process, as they do not interfere with the regular tasks performed by the user [20]. Some of the biosignals that have received a lot of attention in terms of research are: electrocardiogram (ECG), electroencephalography (EEG), and photoplethysmography (PPG). An ECG is a diagnostic tool that measures and records the electrical activity of the heart in detail [22]. An EEG is a signal that represents the sum of the electrical activity of the functioning human brain [23]. PPG is a simple and low-cost optical technique that can be used to detect blood volume changes in the microvascular bed of tissue [24].

Other studies on ensuring e-Health security through the use of biometrics have been carried out in terms of authentication, data integrity, data confidentiality, and data authenticity. Data integrity, confidentiality, and authenticity may be achieved through biometric encryption. In a wireless Body Sensor Networks (BSN), sensors rely on biometric encryption for secure communication. BSNs consist of interconnected devices or sensors implanted in or worn on the human body in order to share information and resources. BSNs help provide healthcare services such as medical monitoring, memory enhancement, control of home appliances, medical data access, and communication in emergencies [32].

Through encryption, access to sensitive information is restricted, and thus protecting health information. An important aspect of biometrics cryptography is the use of biometrics to generate cryptographic keys. Biometrics are also used to generate authentication keys for data transmission in wireless communication [29]. The dynamic biometric traits are good for generating keys as a result of their randomness and time variance [29]. Several studies have proposed the use of dynamic biometric features such as ECG [25], [26], [27], [28], [29], and PPG [31] to generate keys for biometrics cryptosystems.

Specifically, in [29] the authors propose a biometric-based solution that combines encryption and authentication for wireless communication in BSNs. Similarly, the authors of [26] propose a biometric-based approach to ensuring secure communication in BSNs by employing biometrics to generate keys. The authors use physiological features such as ECG or PPG to generate cryptographic keys communicated within the network, thereby ensuring security. Usually, proposed methods extract features such as Interpulse Interval (IPI) from ECG or PPG in the time domain or in the frequency domain using Fast Fourier Transform (FFT). In order to provide a strong cryptosystems, the quality of the generated keys must be taken into consideration.

Two features are used to determine the quality of the generated keys: randomness and distinctiveness [33]. Distinctiveness determines if the keys generated can distinguish between different people. Metrics used to evaluate distinctiveness are FAR, FRR, and Hamming Distance(HD). Randomness ensures that the distinctive keys are unpredictable. Randomness is evaluated by computing the entropy of the keys generated. Table 2 shows a comparison in terms of distinctiveness

Table 2. A comparison of research contributions that use biometric traits (static or dynamic) to generate keys for authentication and encryption

Study	Data size	Biometric trait	Key length (bits)	Distinctiveness	Method of Distinctiveness	Randomness	Method of Randomness	Sampling rate (Hz)
[25]	84	ECG	128	Mean(HD)=64 when Threshold above 5; FRR almost zero(0) when Threshold <12	HD	Mean Entropy> 0.99	Entropy	250
[26]	79	ECG	128	Mean(HD)=64	HD	Mean Entropy> 0.99	Entropy	250
[27]	11	ECG	-	FAR almost zero(0)	FAR/FRR	FAR almost zero(0) when time variance >125	Time variance	125
[28]	-	ECG	128	FAR almost zero(0) when Threshold above 5; FRR zero(0) when Threshold <15	FAR/FRR	-	Time variance	-
[29]	9	ECG and PPG	64 and 128	-	HD	0.662 - 1	Entropy	1000
[29]	20	Fingerprint	64 and 128	-	HD	0.928 - 1	Entropy	-
[30]	31	ECG	128	Average(HD)=64	HD	0.996 - 1	Entropy	125
[31]	10	PPG	128	FRR almost zero (0) when Polinormal order(v) <4; FAR almost zero (0) when Polinormial order >11	FAR/FRR	-	-	60

and randomness of research contributions explored in this study. In Table 2, the "data size" represents the number of subjects from which the biometric features were generated, the key length represents the length of the generated keys in bits, and the sampling rate refers to the frequency (the number of times per second the biosignals are sampled).

5   Discussion and Future Vision

Biometrics technology has proven to provide a sure way of addressing the above e-Health security issues. In this context, the technology is used to provide identity verification, as well as encryption during exchange or transmission of health information. The use of biometrics encryption provides a secure means of protecting health information from attacks such as eavesdropping, data modification, and replay. It is evident that biometrics afford the healthcare industry several promising opportunities. As technology continues to advance, so do security and privacy issues that continue to be a major concern in the industry. To this end, biometrics have been shown to be efficient and robust in tackling security and privacy challenges in e-Health.

On the other hand, biometrics is not a silver bullet in that it cannot provide complete and enough reliable solutions to all security problems [34]. In spite of the robustness of biometrics, it still suffers from several attacks due to the inherent weaknesses that exist in a biometric-based authentication systems. Attacks on biometric templates could lead to vulnerabilities including the replacement of templates by an imposter to gain access, the spoofing of templates by an adversary to gain access, and the replay of attacks. Biometrics templates, when compromised, are impossible to replace as they are permanently linked to an individual. Therefore, the cancelable biometrics concept should be considered.

The total processing time (identification or verification time) is a crucial issue in any biometric system [35]. Biometric-based systems include many subprocesses such as enhancement or noise removal, feature extraction, feature matching, and classification. Attention should be given to the system's time consumed, feature extraction operations, and the large database classification, should be considered [36], [37].

Data encryption has received a lot of attention in healthcare. This is due to the fact that e-Health is pushing the frontiers of healthcare from health institutions to the home (mobile health, telemedicine, etc.), leveraging wireless communication. In any cryptographic system, key generation is vital for secure communication. In this, biometrics is increasingly proving to be very efficient and effective in cryptosystems in encrypting and decrypting sensitive information. Dynamic biometric features such as ECG, PPG, and EEG are useful in generating keys for encryption due to their randomness and time-variance [29]. This has resulted a number of research proposals regarding these aspects.

Future research may take many promising directions. First of all, future research should explore the potential benefits and limitations associated with the use of biometrics in cryptosystems in e-Health, such as, for instance, the constraints encountered in the generation and distribution of keys in wireless communication networks, or the strengths and weaknesses of the various biometric traits in key generation. Secondly, future research should continue to investigate how to provide robust authentication mechanisms in e-Health applications or systems using biometrics without undermining user access. Furthermore, there is a high demand for research on the adoption of biometric identification and verification systems for elderly people. The factors that influence the adoption of specific forms of authentication mechanisms in e-Health, as well as the implications of authentication mechanisms on the entire e-Health system, are interesting future research directions.

6 Conclusions

This paper has explored various literatures to determine the impact of using e-Health on the healthcare industry in terms of the benefits it affords to the industry as well as the challenges it poses. Patient e-Health data security and patient privacy are of the utmost concern in the domain of e-Health. Traditional authentication mechanisms, such as passwords and access cards, are not appropriate for addressing the current e-Health security and privacy issues due to their susceptibility to be lost, duplicated, or forgotten. Biometrics technology has proven to effectively address e-Health security and privacy challenges. Various forms of biometrics technology have been proposed in e-Health applications or systems ranging from unimodal to multimodal biometrics, continuous and unobtrusive authentication approaches, and in wireless sensor networks to secure communication channels. In addition, unconventional biometrics biosignals such as electrocardiogram (ECG), photoplethysmography (PPG), and electroencephalography (EEG) open new horizons for biometrics technology deployments in e-Health domain. In spite of all the benefits of using biometrics in e-Health, additional issues such as processing time, patient privacy related to using biometric traits, and biometric database protection should be taken into consideration.

References

1. Sharma, S.K., Xu, H., Wickramasinghe, N., Ahmed, N.: Electronic healthcare: issues and challenges. International Journal of Electronic Healthcare **2**(1), 50–65 (2006)
2. Katsikas, S., Lopez, J., Pernul, G.: The challenge for security and privacy services in distributed health settings. Studies in health technology and informatics **134**, 113–125 (2007)
3. Jain, A., Hong, L., Pankanti, S.: Biometric identification. Communications of the ACM **43**(2), 90–98 (2000)
4. Pratama, S.F., Pratiwi, L., Abraham, A., Muda, A.K.: Computational intelligence in digital forensics. In: Muda, A.K., Choo, Y.-H., Abraham, A., N. Srihari, S. (eds.) Computational Intelligence in Digital Forensics. SCI, vol. 555, pp. 1–16. Springer, Heidelberg (2014)

5. Jain, A., Ross, A., Pankanti, S.: Biometrics: A tool for information security. IEEE Transactions on Information Forensics and Security **1**(2), 125–143 (2006)
6. Jain, A.K., Flynn, P.J., Ross, A.A.: Handbook of biometrics. Springer (2007)
7. Jain, A.K., Ross, A.A.A., Nandakumar, K.: Introduction to biometrics. Springer (2011)
8. Egawa, S., Awad, A.I., Baba, K.: Evaluation of acceleration algorithm for biometric identification. In: Benlamri, R. (ed.) NDT 2012, Part II. CCIS, vol. 294, pp. 231–242. Springer, Heidelberg (2012)
9. Jain, A.K., Bolle, R., Pankanti, S.: Biometrics: Personal Identification in Networked Society. Springer (1999)
10. Sadr, S.M.H.: Consideration the relationship between ICT and ehealth. Journal of Biology, Agriculture and Healthcare **2**(8), 49–59 (2012)
11. Eysenbach, G.: What is e-health. Journal of Medical Internet Research **3**(2) (2001)
12. Bai, G., Guo, Y.: A general architecture for developing a sustainable elderly care e-health system. In: 8th International Conference on Service Systems and Service Management (ICSSSM), pp. 1–6. IEEE (2011)
13. Ahmed, S., Raja, M.: Integration of wireless sensor network with medical service provider for ubiquitous e-healthcare. In: 9th International Conference on High Capacity Optical Networks and Enabling Technologies (HONET), pp. 120–126 (2012)
14. Mukherjee, S., Dolui, K., Datta, S.K.: Patient health management system using e-health monitoring architecture. In: IEEE International Advance Computing Conference (IACC), pp. 400–405. IEEE (2014)
15. Adibi, S., Agnew, G.B.: On the diversity of ehealth security systems and mechanisms. In: Annual International Conference of the IEEE Engineering in Medicine and Biology Society. IEEE Engineering in Medicine and Biology Society, vol. 2008, pp. 1478–1481 (2007)
16. Cherukuri, S., Venkatasubramanian, K., Gupta, S.K.S.: Biosec: a biometric based approach for securing communication in wireless networks of biosensors implanted in the human body. In: International Conference on Parallel Processing Workshops, pp. 432–439 (2003)
17. Marohn, D.: Biometrics in healthcare. Biometric Technology Today **14**(9), 9–11 (2006)
18. Chandra, A., Durand, R., Weaver, S.: The uses and potential of biometrics in health care. International Journal of Pharmaceutical and Healthcare Marketing **2**(1), 22–34 (2008)
19. Krawczyk, S., Jain, A.K.: Securing electronic medical records using biometric authentication. In: Kanade, T., Jain, A., Ratha, N.K. (eds.) AVBPA 2005. LNCS, vol. 3546, pp. 1110–1119. Springer, Heidelberg (2005)
20. Silva, H., Lourenço, A., Fred, A., Filipe, J.: Clinical data privacy and customization via biometrics based on ECG signals. In: Holzinger, A., Simonic, K.-M. (eds.) USAB 2011. LNCS, vol. 7058, pp. 121–132. Springer, Heidelberg (2011)
21. Awad, A.I., Baba, K.: Evaluation of a fingerprint identification algorithm with SIFT features. In: The 3rd 2012 IIAI International Conference on Advanced Applied Informatics. Fukuoka, Japan
22. Baig, M.M., Gholamhosseini, H., Connolly, M.J.: A comprehensive survey of wearable and wireless ECG monitoring systems for older adults. Medical & Biological Engineering & Computing **51**(5), 485–495 (2013)
23. Paranjape, R., Mahovsky, J., Benedicenti, L., Koles', Z.: The electroencephalogram as a biometric. In: Canadian Conference on Electrical and Computer Engineering, vol. 2, pp. 1363–1366. IEEE (2001)

24. Allen, J.: Photoplethysmography and its application in clinical physiological measurement. Physiological Measurement **28**(3), R1–R39 (2007)
25. Zhang, G.H., Poon, C.C., Zhang, Y.T.: Analysis of using interpulse intervals to generate 128-bit biometric random binary sequences for securing wireless body sensor networks. IEEE Transactions on Information Technology in Biomedicine **16**(1), 176–182 (2012)
26. Zhang, G., Poon, C.C.Y., Zhang, Y.: A fast key generation method based on dynamic biometrics to secure wireless body sensor networks for p-health. In: 2010 Annual International Conference of the IEEE Engineering in Medicine and Biology Society (EMBC), pp. 2034–2036 (2010)
27. Hu, C., Cheng, X., Zhang, F., Wu, D., Liao, X., Chen, D.: OPFKA: Secure and efficient ordered-physiological-feature-based key agreement for wireless body area networks. In: Proceedings of IEEE INFOCOM, pp. 2274–2282. IEEE (2013)
28. Zhou, J., Cao, Z., Dong, X.: BDK: secure and efficient biometric based deterministic key agreement in wireless body area networks. In: Proceedings of the 8th International Conference on Body Area Networks, pp. 488–494. ICST (Institute for Computer Sciences, Social-Informatics and Telecommunications Engineering) (2013)
29. Zhang, G., Poon, C.C.Y., Zhang, Y.: A biometrics based security solution for encryption and authentication in tele-healthcare systems. In: 2nd International Symposium on Applied Sciences in Biomedical and Communication Technologies ISABEL, pp. 1–4 (2009)
30. Venkatasubramanian, K.K., Banerjee, A., Gupta, S.K., et al.: Ekg-based key agreement in body sensor networks. In: INFOCOM Workshops, pp. 1–6. IEEE (2008)
31. Venkatasubramanian, K., Banerjee, A., Gupta, S.K.S.: Plethysmogram-based secure inter-sensor communication in body area networks. In: IEEE Military Communications Conference, MILCOM 2008, pp. 1–7 (2008)
32. Darwish, A., Hassanien, A.E.: Wearable and implantable wireless sensor network solutions for healthcare monitoring. Sensors **11**(6), 5561–5595 (2011)
33. Poon, C.C.Y., Zhang, Y.T., Bao, S.D.: A novel biometrics method to secure wireless body area sensor networks for telemedicine and m-health. IEEE Communications Magazine **44**(4), 73–81 (2006)
34. Modi, S.K.: Biometrics in identity management: Concepts to applications. Artech House (2011)
35. Awad, A.I., Baba, K.: Fingerprint singularity detection: a comparative study. In: Mohamad Zain, J., Wan Mohd, W.M., El-Qawasmeh, E. (eds.) ICSECS 2011, Part I. CCIS, vol. 179, pp. 122–132. Springer, Heidelberg (2011)
36. Awad, A.I., Baba, K.: Toward an efficient fingerprint classification. In: Biometrics - Unique and Diverse Applications in Nature, Science, and Technology, pp. 23–40. InTech (2011)
37. Awad, A.I., Baba, K.: Singular point detection for efficient fingerprint classification. International Journal on New Computer Architectures and Their Applications **2**(1), 1–7 (2012)

Developing a Health Information Systems Approach to a Novel Student Health Clinic: Meeting the Educational and Clinical Needs of an Interprofessional Health Service

James Browne[1], Aileen Escall[1], Andi Jones[1(✉)],
Maximilian de Courten[2], and Karen T. Hallam[2]

[1] IPEP Clinic, Victoria University, Melbourne, VIC, Australia
{james.browne,aileen.escall,andi.jones}@vu.edu.au
[2] Centre for Chronic Disease, Victoria University, Melbourne, VIC, Australia
{Maximilian.deCourten,Karen.Hallam}@vu.edu.au

Abstract. This paper addresses the use of information management systems and IT capability to design and manage a university student teaching clinic in the Western suburbs of Melbourne. The clinic technology team had three main briefs, to support student learning and professional development, to provide quality health care to the community and to develop systems and platforms that facilitate the ability of the clinic to meet National Safety and Quality Health Standards (NSQHS). This paper highlights the role of health information systems in delivering on a clinic capable of these goals.

Keywords: Interprofessional education and practice · University teaching clinic · Ethics · Health information systems

The provision of skilled and experience workers for health care systems is a core goal of University health sciences programs. Research into student led clinics indicates they provide an effective health delivery model and deliver strong satisfaction score with patients, positive health outcomes [1] and improved student learning [2]. Innovations in health policy and education over the past decade have swung the operation of student led clinics towards the newer approach to health care provision known as Interprofessional Practice (IPP). The World Health Organisation (WHO) has identified IPP as a focus for health education worldwide [3]. This model may be a particularly appropriate fit with the Australian health system and training clinics as rates of chronic illnesses such as heart disease, diabetes, cancer, arthritis and mental illness become our greatest health needs [4].

In meeting both educational needs of students and clinical care needs of the community, University training clinics exist in a space between educational and healthcare worlds. In a recent consultative enquiry of 20 Australian and New Zealand clinics, Allan and colleagues [5] identified the tension between meeting the academic needs of the students engaged in the clinical service and providing appropriate and professional services to the community. The students need to experience and learn is

© Springer International Publishing Switzerland 2015
X. Yin et al. (Eds.): HIS 2015, LNCS 9085, pp. 104–110, 2015.
DOI: 10.1007/978-3-319-19156-0_11

sometimes discordant from the patients need for care, thus raising ethical dilemmas [6]. To further complicate these management issues, the regulatory environment in Australian health care system has changed significantly over the last decade in response to a new Health Records Act [7], the Information Privacy Act [8] and movement towards accreditation of health services through national and state level health service accreditation and recording requirements. A survey of the university sector indicates that most institutions are erring on the side of being student clinics that serve the public as their emphasis, with no University based student training clinic in Australia currently holding accreditation such as the National Safety and Quality Health Care Standards that are considered best practice standards for use in health services [9]. The purpose built VU IPEP clinic structure supports both clinical and student needs where small interview rooms or treatment spaces are linked technologically to assessment pods where as many as ten students engage in healthcare planning and learning activities. This new style of clinic and clinical practice is an example of a best practice health service and health education innovation.

1   Design of the Health Information System for an IPEP Task

Health information systems are viewed as central to improving the overall quality, safety and efficacy of health systems [10]. It is evident that as health care systems manage more complex and chronic illnesses that require multiple health fields to collaborate that information management systems plays a hidden but fundamental role in the ability to provide quality and safe health care for patients. In the VU IPEP clinic, the further addition of teaching and educational needs complicates the functionality requirements of the technology used in a typical clinic, therefore requiring tailoring of information management systems that move beyond specifically addressing clinical needs to incorporate educational solutions.

The IPE Clinic was designed and built to incorporate modern features found within ambulatory care centres, super clinics, hospitals and community health centres. The design aims to facilitate the professional learning continuum, enabling students to communicate interprofessionally in engaging in shared care and providing more coordinated services to clients. In designing the information technology systems, initial requirements were captured from the academic team and refined as clinical staff joined the project. Finally, consultation was sought from legal and accreditation bodies to validate and refine final requirements. These consultations led to two parallel themes regarding the clinic information management systems. The first requirement was to develop the technology to support the clinical practice. This included AV streaming for collaborative and remote consultation/supervision and securing a client management system which would support student led client sessions by including an approval mechanism for progress notes and which would incorporate the Service Coordination Tool Templates (SCTT) from the Victorian Department of Health [11]. The SCTT is a standardized package of assessments recommended for use in health care contexts by the Victorian Department of Health. They provide both the foundation information required by the clinical service but also information on disability and recovery that are equally important for provisional health staff to familiarize with best practice standards of reporting.

The second requirement of the information management systems was to support student learning, including the ability to record client sessions and to securely manage and control access to the recordings. This required a balancing of the needs between educational with the ethical and privacy needs of a clinic that is using national accreditation with the NSQHS as a benchmark for professional practice. The discussion of the needs analysis for both these issues and the solutions built into the health information systems policies and structure highlight the challenges of structuring the information management systems of a complex service in a way that maximizes usability and outcomes and protects valuable data.

2   AV Streaming and Recording

2.1   Learning and Teaching Capability via AV Streaming

To support learning and teaching, active collaboration, and connectivity between non-clinic locations (e.g. classrooms and offsite supervisors), all treatment and assessment rooms within the clinic are fitted with Audio-Visual (AV) conferencing systems. This technology allows practitioners in assessment rooms to conference in practitioners from other disciplines located in workrooms within the clinic. The nature of IPE means that up to 10 practitioners could be involved in an initial consultation (at the same time) or ongoing client treatment – rather than have all 10 present in the one room, streaming (aka video conferencing) is used to link multiple rooms. Building on from this, the scenario may arise where consultation with a supervisor external to the clinic may be required. This raises the need for AV streaming between health and University settings as well as within the clinic itself. Table 1 presents the needs analysis conducted across different stakeholder groups to develop an AV system that worked for multiple parties whilst maintaining privacy and health record management standards.

Although streaming from treatment rooms will primarily need to be controlled by policy and process and through education of students and supervisors, a number of technical safeguards have been put in place to support this. Video conferencing can only take place between VU conference rooms and/or VU users using Microsoft Office Communicator (this will enable staff to connect from remote sites via the VU VPN service). Where the call is initiated externally to the treatment room, the caller ID of the room/person dialing in will be displayed on the control panel in the treatment room and a ringtone will be audible – this will alert both practitioner and client to the incoming call and the practitioner will have the ability to accept or reject the call. This assists with maintaining the presence of informed consent as the client can observe the clinician or as treatment team provide access to the streaming.

Table 1. Needs Analysis: AV Streaming

Student learning	Clinic management	Patients/Carers	Privacy/regulatory
Ability to view high quality streaming video content, with permission, of assessment and treatment sessions in progress from locations within the clinic	Provide high quality and consistency of data streaming	Ensure Patients/ Carers provide informed consent to having their image and audio transmitted to other clinic rooms	Compliance with the Privacy and Data Protection Act [12]. Health Records Management Act (2002) in relation to sharing information protocols.
Ensure informed Consent is evident from Client / Student/ Supervisor	Ability to provide streaming from assessment pods, treatment and consultation rooms	Ensure that patients can request streaming of their session to be suspended or stopped	NSQHCS accreditation compliance. Focus on standard 1, 2 and 5.
	Incorporation of patient consent procedures into streaming access	Ensure informed consent is evident from carers, family, health workers included in assessments and treatment.	

2.2 Digital Asset Management System (DAMS) Capability

As well as allowing for live streaming of sessions to other rooms/sites, capability to record sessions has also been enabled allowing the use of recorded materials in classroom and teaching contexts at the University. The DAMS ~~system~~ allows for the distribution of high quality and editable clinical recordings of assessment and treatment session recordings to authorized University teaching staff both within the clinic and in the wider University setting. In addition, within the clinic these recordings provide a component of the client's clinical file (and are stored alongside consent documents), thus requiring secure storage and future accessibility based on freedom of information requests.

To maintain confidentiality and ensure informed consent, sessions are only recorded when written informed consent has been provided. In addition, patients and families may remove consent for recording during the course of a session or following a recording process. In order to comply with legislative [12] and accreditation guidelines regarding privacy obligations and compliance [11], the procedure for access and approval for use of recorded data is tightly monitored and controlled using information technology infrastructure and clinical policy documents.

The process of recording sessions begins with a student or clinician having to enter an authorization and password in order to record sessions. The system design also requires patient identification number for data management purposes and identification of the session as clinically or research based. As a final acknowledgement of importance of informed consent, students and clinicians are required to check this box on the room AV Touch Panel. Recorded sessions are securely encrypted and transferred from local storage in the clinic to the VU data centre and into VU's Enterprise Content Management system (Oracle Webcenter Content). File access is through the ECM environment when a senior authorized clinical staff member will ensure ethical fidelity through inspecting the informed consent for the recording, assessing if consent was removed and ensuring there were no other circumstances present that would indicate the file should not be viewed by clinical, research and academic staff. Clinical and research records are segregated to ensure confidentiality and the academic and research staff are responsible for the use of this data in accordance with the University teaching and research guidelines. At no time are these recordings released directly to students for use without a thorough review and authorization beforehand from clinical and academic staff.

Recorded content is maintained within the ECM platform in accordance with policies governing patient records and information. For legal and regulatory compliance reasons, academic staff will not have the ability to delete content from ECM. If content is no longer required it will be marked for archiving or disposal. Archived content will not be searchable or viewable by academic or clinical staff who are not authorised.

3   Practice Management and Clinic Health Information's Systems

Best practice health services are engaged in constantly improving practice to provide better patient care and health service practice. This focus on excellence in health care practice has rarely been discussed in relation to university based training clinics. In order to provide appropriate and timely patient clinical data, a practice management software package was selected from a variety used in medical practices across Australia. The health client management system eAlth (eAlth.net) was selected as the vendor showed a commitment to work with Victoria University to enhance their software to meet the specific needs of the IPEP Clinic. The software was specifically selected as it has the capacity to include clinical notes approval, multiple practitioner booking for appointments and the capability to incorporate the Victorian Government Service Co-Ordination Tool Templates [11]. The SCTT is a suite of standardized templates designed to facilitate service co-ordination and facilitate shared care within and between service providers. This template package will be rolled out through the client management software as it provides the qualitative and quantitative data required to measure performance against six of the ten NSQHSS [9]. The provider meeting this need was a major determinant of selection as the SCTT provides a platform for accreditation and best practice and specifically requires users to embed the templates directly into the practice management software.

4   Network Segregation

University students have access and use an extensive array of information technology and social media. This raises unique concerns when considering patient privacy and confidentiality issues [13]. In response, the clinic is developing clinical practice guidelines for the appropriate use of social media in health services based on legal, ethical and professional implications. Based on these findings and with intensive stakeholder engagement within Victoria University academic, legal, information security and clinical staff, guidelines around privacy in general and access to clinical information have been developed.

In support of these guidelines, the IPE Technology team has developed a network segregation design to isolate clinical software systems and facilities from the wider University network as well as allowing the clinical team to restrict the level of internet access students have whilst on placement at the IPE clinic and to support and maintain the privacy of client records/client information. A whitelist only approach has been taken, where only an agreed upon list of categories of web content are allowed, supported by the clinical governance framework to review and amend the list as needed. Being mindful of the needs of the students to access other content whilst on placement, access to the general Victoria University network has also been enabled for students at hot desks or through their own personal devices in student common areas within the IPE clinic. All students on placement will be provided access to devices to enable them to carry out daily activities. This includes capture and review of patient documentation, accessing external content and resources (e.g. MIMS medicine information catalogue), capturing content via a touchscreen device (paperless clinic). These devices can only access the IPE clinic network and therefore while they can access the client management software, they will be subject to the restrictions put in place via the network segregation design.

5   Conclusion

This technology use and tailored client management software will ensure that students gain 'real world' experience of documenting information into practice management software and complying with the best practices associated with accredited services. In turn, patients will have less need to repeat their histories and medical issues as interprofessional assessments and the Service Coordination Tool Template information are at the student/clinicians disposal in real time. The move to an interprofessional service approach has meant developing an interprofessional clinic that provides students with a quality education in an emerging health care model. In addition, the clinic must act in accord with the highest ethical standards and professional practices. The management information systems used to assist in managing these competing demands provides a unique opportunity for the VU IPEP Clinic to be the 'best of both worlds'.

References

1. Ponto, M., Paloranta, H., Akroyd, K.: An evaluation of a student led health station in Finland. Progress in Health Science **1**(1), 5–13 (2011)
2. Meah, Y.S., Smith, E.L., Thomas, D.C.: Student-run health clinic: Novel arena to educate medical students on systems based practice. Mount Sinai Journal of Medicine **76**(4), 344–356 (2009)
3. Gilbert, H.V., Yan, J., Hoffman, S.J.: A WHO Report: Framework for Action on Interprofessional Education and Collaborative Practice. Journal of Allied Health **39**(S1), 196–197 (2010)
4. AIHW: Australia's Health, 13. Cat. no. AUS 156. AIHW, Canberra (2012)
5. Allan, J., O'Meara, P., Pope, R., Higgs, J., Kent, J.: The role of context in establishing university clinics. Health and Social Care in the Community **19**(2), 217–224 (2011)
6. Christakis, D.A., Feudtner, C.: Ethics in a short white coat: the ethical dilemma that medical students confront. Academic Medicine **68**(4), 249–254 (1993)
7. Health Records Act. Victoria Parliament, Australia (2001)
8. Information Privacy Act. Victoria Parliament, Australia (2000)
9. Australian Commission on Safety and Quality in Health Care: National Safety and Quality Healthcare Standards (2011). http://www.safetyandquality.gov.au
10. Chaudhry, B., Wang, J., Wu, S., Maglione, M., Mojica, W., Roth, E., Morton, S.C., Shekelle, P.G.: Systematic review: Impact of health information technology on quality, efficiency, and costs of medical care. Annals of Internal Medicine **144**, 742–752 (2006)
11. Victorian Department of Health: Service Coordination Tool Template (2012). http://www.health.vic.gov.au
12. Privacy and Data Protection Act. Victoria, Australia (2014)
13. Cronquist, R., Spector, N.: Nurses and social media: Regulatory concerns and guidelines. Journal of Nursing Regulation **2**(3), 37–40 (2011)

A Stable Gene Subset Selection Algorithm for Cancers

Juanying Xie[✉] and Hongchao Gao

School of Computer Science, Shaanxi Normal University,
Xi'an 710062, PR China
xiejuany@snnu.edu.cn

Abstract. In order to solve the problem that the selected genes are depend on the train subset in the gene subset selection algorithms, we propose an assemble method to select the discrimination genes for cancers, so that a stable gene subset can be obtained. We randomly extract some proportional samples from train subset and cluster the genes of these samples in K-means, then select a typical gene from each cluster according to its weight estimated in Pearson correlation coefficient between genes and labels. This process is repeated several times. Those genes with high frequencies in the processes are selected to construct the selected gene subset. The power of the proposed method is tested on three very popular gene datasets, and the experimental results demonstrate that the new algorithm proposed in this paper has found the most stable gene subset with the highest classification accuracy.

Keywords: Gene selection · Gene subsets · K-means · Assemble · Pearson correlation coefficient · Cancers

1 Introduction

With the development of DNA microarray technology, there are more and more gene expression datasets with tens of thousands of genes and small numbers of samples. To analyze this kind of dataset, the first important thing is to reduce the dimensionality of it, that is to search and find those genes which can distinguish samples from different classes [5, 7, 8]. Therefore there are more and more experts focus on this field, and there are lots of gene selection algorithms being emerged [2, 12, 15]. However, the available gene selection algorithms cannot guarantee that the gene subset they found is stable. Many of them have got the disadvantages that the gene subset is variant with the different train subset from the same gene expression dataset. The worst case is that there is no one common gene in any two gene subsets. However, in bioinformatics area, especially for the medical doctors they usually want to find the specific and stable genes in which they can tell patients from normal people. Therefore, to find the stable gene subset has become an urgent issue in gene selection area.

It is well know that K-means [13] is a very fast and simple clustering algorithm, and it can be used to cluster big data [11]. So we adopts K-means to

X. Yin et al. (Eds.): HIS 2015, LNCS 9085, pp. 111–122, 2015.
DOI: 10.1007/978-3-319-19156-0_12

cluster genes into clusters, where the genes in a same cluster are very similar, and the ones in different clusters are dissimilar to each other. Then we select one typical gene from one cluster to construct the gene subset. We have demonstrated the correctness of the clustering based gene selection idea in [17]. However, the clustering result of K-means is depend on the initial centers, which caused the unstable in the gene subset. Furthermore, the variance of train subset on which the K-means runs accelerates the unstable of the selected gene subset. How to find the stable gene subset with high classification accuracy is a challenging problem in gene selection study [10, 18, 19].

In order to solve the aforementioned problem, this paper proposes an assemble method for selecting the discrimination genes of cancers, so that a stable gene subset can be obtained. We run K-means several times to get several gene subsets, then we merge the gene subsets and select the genes with high frequencies. We test the power of the new gene subset selection algorithm on three popular gene datasets. The experimental results prove that the new gene subset selection algorithm can find the most stable gene subset with highest classification accuracy compared to the famous gene subset selection algorithms, such as MRMR and SVM-RFE.

The paper is organized as follows: Section 2 introduces our proposed new gene subset selection algorithm in detail. Section 3 tests our proposed gene selection algorithm on three popular gene datasets, and compares its performance with MRMR and SVM-RFE in terms of the classification accuracy, variance and gene iteration rate. Section 4 draws some conclusions.

2   The Proposed Gene Subset Selection Algorithm

We adopt K-means to cluster genes, so that the similar genes are grouped into same cluster and the dissimilar genes are in different clusters. Then a typical gene is selected from one cluster, and the genes from each cluster comprise a gene subset.

2.1   The Importance of Genes to Classification

There are many metrics to evaluate the importance of a gene to classification, such as Relief-F, information gain, t-test and Wilcoxon Signed-rank test *et al* [8, 17]. We use Pearson correlation coefficient in equation (1) to assess the importance of a gene to classification.

$$R(i) = \frac{\sum\limits_{k=1}^{n}(x_{k,i} - \bar{x}_i)(y_k - \bar{y})}{\sqrt{\sum\limits_{k=1}^{n}(x_{k,j} - \bar{x}_i)^2(y_k - \bar{y})^2}} \tag{1}$$

where n is the total number of samples in a gene dataset, $R(i)$ means the importance of the ith gene to the classification, $x_{k,i}$ is the value of the ith gene in the

kth sample, $\bar{x}_i$ is the mean value of the ith gene, y_k, $\bar{y}$ are respectively the label of the kth sample and the mean of the labels for all samples in a gene dataset.

It can be seen from the equation (1) that $R(i) \in [-1,1]$, where $R(i) = 1$ means the ith gene is positive correlation to the label, and $R(i) = -1$ means the negative correlation between the ith gene and the label. The value of $|R(i)|$ varies from 0 to 1, and the higher the value of $|R(i)|$, the more importance is the ith gene to classification. When $|R(i)| = 1$ holds, the ith gene can tell patients from normal people correctly.

2.2   The Way to Partition a Dataset and to Estimate the Power of a Gene Subset

It is known that the selected gene subset may vary with the partition of a gene dataset. In order to reduce the influence of a dataset partition on the selected gene subset, we adopt bootstrap [9] to partition a gene dataset into train subset and test subset.

The different train subset may lead to the different selected gene subset, so we repeat our algorithm 50 times to get the statistical result of it. We calculate the classification accuracy of the selected gene subset in equation (2) [9], where M is the classification model built on the selected gene subset. The average classification accuracy of 50 runs of each algorithm is compared in our experiments.

$$Acc = 0.632 \times Acc(M)_{test\_subset} + 0.368 \times Acc(M)_{train\_subset} \qquad (2)$$

2.3   The Description of Our Algorithm

We partition a gene dataset into train subset and test subset in bootstrap [9], then we randomly extract samples from the train subset in proportion of 80%, and run K-means algorithm on the extracted samples to group similar genes into same clusters and dissimilar genes into different clusters. Then choose one typical gene from each cluster to construct a gene subset. This process is repeated 20 times, so we get 20 gene subsets. We choose genes with high frequencies in the 20 gene subsets to comprise the selected gene subset, and evaluate the property of the selected gene subset to classification in equation (2).

Here are the detail steps of our algorithm.

Input: $Data = \{x_i\}_{i=1}^n$, cluster number K for K-means, parameter γ for K-means repeating times, parameter φ for the proportion to extract samples from train subset, parameter τ for the number of genes in the selected gene subset.

Output: the selected gene subset and its classification accuracy.

step 1: data preprocessing, fill the missing values and normalize data;

step 2: partition dataset into $train\_subset$ and $test\_subset$, let $|train\_subset| = T$ and $cr = 1$;

step 3: randomly extract samples from $train\_subset$ in proportion φ, that is $T' = \varphi T$, and use K-means to cluster genes of extracted samples into clusters, and calculate the importance of genes in equation (1) using the extracted samples;

step 4: select the most important gene from each cluster to comprise a gene subset S;

step 5: save S to TS, let $cr = cr + 1$, if $cr \prec \gamma$, then go to *step* 3;

step 6: select the top τ genes with high frequencies from TS to construct the selected gene subset, then build a classification model on the selected gene subset, and calculate its classification accuracy in equation (2).

3   Experimental Results and Their Analysis

Experiments are conducted on three popular gene datasets including Leukemia [6] and Colon [1] and Carcinoma [14]. Table 1 describes the datasets. All the data are normalized in equation (3).

Table 1. Description of gene datasets

Gene datasets	Source	Number of genes	Number of samples
Leukemia	Golub, *et al* [6]	7 129	72 (47+25)
Colon	Alon, *et al* [1]	2 000	62 (40+22)
Carcinoma	Notterman, *etal* [14]	7 458	36 (18+18)

$$g_{i,j} = \frac{g_{i,j} - min(g_j)}{max(g_j) - min(g_j)} \qquad (3)$$

where $g_{i,j}$ is the value of the gene j in sample i, and $min(g_j)$ is the minimum value of gene j , and $max(g_j)$ is the maximum value of gene j.

We respectively adopt KNN [4] and SVM [16] as classification tools. The power of our algorithm proposed in this paper is compared with that of the popular gene subset selection algorithms including MRMR (minimum redundancy maximum relevance) [5] and SVM-RFE [8]. As a comparison we compared the performance of our algorithm with that of which K-means is executed only once on the whole train subset to select the gene subset. We named our algorithm as *S-Weight* and the other one with only once K-means execution as *Weight*. All the algorithms are respectively repeated 50 times and their average classification accuracy, variance of the classification accuracy and the gene iteration rate [5] of the selected gene subsets are compared.

The gene iteration rate of two successive selected gene subsets is computed in equation (4), where τ is the size of the selected gene subset, that is, the number of genes in the selected gene subset, and T is the times of each algorithm being repeated. In our experiments the T equals 50. We calculate the gene iteration rate of the selected gene subsets in equation (5) to assess the stable of the selected gene sunsets by each algorithm.

$$IRate_i = \frac{Subset_i \cap Subset_{i+1}}{\tau}, \qquad i = 1, 2, \cdots, T-1 \qquad (4)$$

$$Iteration\_rat = \frac{1}{T-1} \sum_{i=1}^{T-1} IRate_i \qquad (5)$$

We use the SVM library in [3] to conduct our experiments, and let the penalize parameter C for the linear kernel of SVM be 20. KNN is that embedded in MATLAB. The parameter K for KNN is set to be 5. All the codes are developed in MATLAB (version R2012a), and run on an Intel(R) Core(TM)2 Quad CPU Q9500@2.83GHz 2.83GHz PC with 4GB memory using Windows 7 (32 bit) operating system.

3.1   The Experimental Results on Colon

Fig. 1-3 respectively display the experimental results of algorithms on Colon dataset in term of average classification accuracy of the classifiers built on the selected gene subsets, variance of the classification accuracy, and the average gene iteration rate of the selected gene subsets of 50 runs of the algorithms. Where the subfigures (a) and (b) in Fig. 1-2 respectively display the results of algorithms when the SVM and KNN classifiers are used.

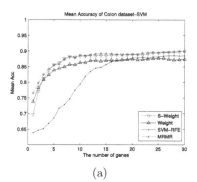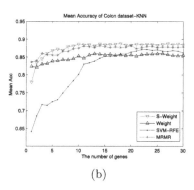

(a)   (b)

Fig. 1. The average classification accuracy of gene subsets by four algorithms on Colon dataset, (a) SVM, (b) KNN

The results in Fig. 1-(a) reveal that the performance of our proposed S-Weight is similar to that of MRMR, and both of the algorithms outperforms Weight and SVM-RFE. The results in Fig. 1-(b) reveal that our S-Weight algorithm has got the best performance when the KNN classifier is used, followed by MRMR. Both of the results in Fig.1-(a) and Fig. 1-(b) demonstrate that Weight outperformed SVM-RFE when the number of selected genes is less than 15, otherwise it was defeated by SVM-RFE in terms of mean accuracy no matter the classifier is SVM or KNN.

It can be seen from the results in Fig. 2-(a) and Fig. 2-(b) that the variance of the classification accuracy of selected gene subsets by our S-weight has got the

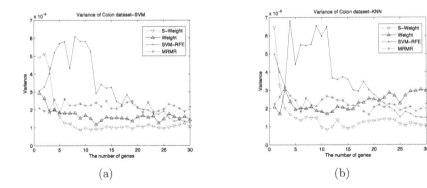

Fig. 2. The variance of classification accuracy of gene subsets by four algorithms on Colon dataset, (a) SVM, (b) KNN

minimum value, which means that our S-weight algorithm has found the gene subset with most stable property in classification accuracy. The performance of SVM-RFE in terms of variance is the worst one when the number of selected genes is less than 20. The performance of Weight and MRMR are in the middle place among the compared algorithms with a relative stable variance no matter how many genes are selected and which classifier is used.

The results in Fig. 3 reveal that there are more than 60% genes are same in the selected gene subsets by our S-Weight algorithm, followed by MRMR where there are more than 50% genes are duplicated in the selected gene subsets when the number of selected genes is greater or equal to 20. Weight has found genes with about 25% overlapping no matter how many genes are selected. The gene

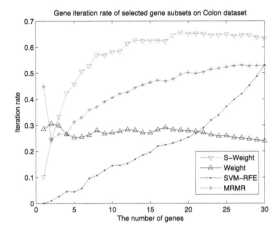

Fig. 3. The gene iteration rate of selected gene subsets by four algorithms of their 50 runs on Colon dataset

iteration rate of the selected gene subsets of SVM-RFE goes up with the number of selected genes.

The above analysis of four algorithms in terms of gene iteration rate and the variance of classification accuracy of selected gene subset on Colon dataset demonstrates that our S-Weight is the most stable gene subset selection algorithm among the popular gene selection algorithms including SVM-RFE and MRMR, and with the highest classification accuracy as well.

3.2 The Experimental Results on ALL/AML Leukemia

Fig. 4-6 display the experimental results of four algorithms on Leukemia dataset in terms of average classification accuracy, variance of the accuracy and the gene iteration rate of the selected gene subsets. Where the subfigures (a) and (b) of Fig. 4-5 respectively display the results of SVM and KNN classifiers are used.

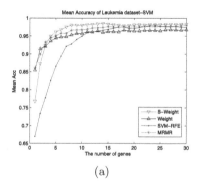
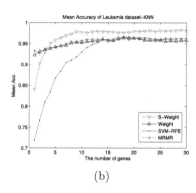

(a)   (b)

Fig. 4. The average classification accuracy of gene subsets by four algorithms on Leukemia dataset, (a) SVM, (b) KNN

From the results shown in Fig. 4-(a) and Fig. 4-(b), we can see that our proposed S-Weight algorithm has obtained the best classification accuracy, especially in Fig. 4-(b) where the KNN classifier is adopted, the performance of our S-Weight is much better than that of the other three algorithms. The results in Fig. 4-(b) still reveal that the Weight and MRMR have got the similar classification power no matter how many genes are there in the selected gene subset when KNN classifier is used. The SVM-RFE has obtained the similar performance with MRMR when there are more than 15 genes being selected, otherwise its performance is the worst when KNN classifier is used. The results in Fig. 4-(a) demonstrate that MRMR has got a little better performance than Weight does when the SVM classifier is used, and the SVM-RFE has obtained a little better performance than Weight when the size of the selected gene subset is greater than 10, otherwise it is the worst one among the four compared gene subset selection algorithms in terms of classification accuracy.

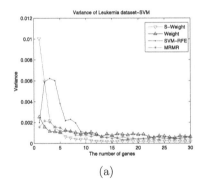 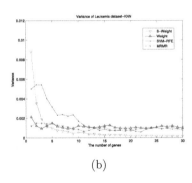

(a)   (b)

Fig. 5. The variance of classification accuracy of gene subsets by four algorithms on Leukemia dataset, (a) SVM, (b) KNN

The experimental results in Fig. 5 reveal that the proposed S-weight algorithm has found the gene subsets on which we can build a classifier with minimum variance of classification accuracy. The performance of SVM-RFE in terms of variance is the worst one when the number of selected genes is less than 10. The performance of Weight and MRMR are similar with a relative stable variance no matter how many genes are selected and which classifier is adopted.

The experimental results in Fig. 6 show that the gene iteration rate of the selected gene subsets by our S-Weight algorithm is up to 60% - 70%, which is much higher than that of other three gene selection algorithms. This means that S-Weight algorithm can find the most stable gene subset. The gene subset by SVM-RFE is the most unstable one whose gene iteration rate goes up with the

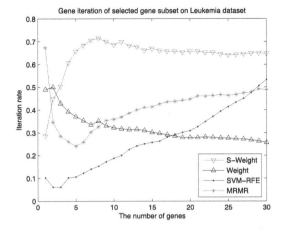

Fig. 6. The gene iteration rate of selected gene subsets by four algorithms on Leukemia dataset

number of genes in the gene subset. The gene iteration rate of selected gene subsets by MRMR is higher than that by Weight when the number of selected genes is more than 10.

3.3   The Experimental Results on Carcinoma

Fig. 7-9 display the experimental results of four algorithms on Carcinoma dataset respectively in term of mean classification accuracy of classifiers on corresponding gene subsets, and the variance of the classification accuracy, and the gene iteration rate of selected gene subsets when the algorithms are repeated 50 times.

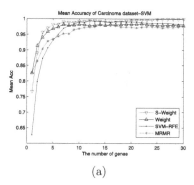 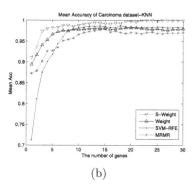

(a)   (b)

Fig. 7. The average classification accuracy of gene subsets by four algorithms on Carcinoma dataset, (a) SVM, (b) KNN

The experiments results in Fig. 7-(a) and Fig. 7-(b) reveal that S-Weight algorithm can found the gene subset with the highest classification accuracy, even up to 100% when the number of selected gens is up to 20. The other three algorithms have got very similar performance, especially when the number of selected genes is over 15. Although MRMR, SVM-RFE and Weight algorithms are not as good as S-Weight algorithm, they can find gene subsets whose classification accuracy is over 95% even up to 98%.

The comparison of variance of classification accuracy of selected gene subsets in Fig. 8-(a) and Fig. 8-(b) demonstrates that S-Weight algorithm can find the gene subsets with the lowest variance value. When the number of the selected genes is over 5, the variance of S-Weight reaches 0. Therefore, S-Weight is the best one among the four gene subset selection algorithms. From Fig. 8-(a), it can be seen that SVM-RFE, Weight and MRMR are very similar in terms of variance of the classification accuracy on the selected gene subsets when the SVM classifier is built. The results in Fig. 8-(b) reveal that MRMR is the worst one among the four gene subset selection algorithms when the KNN classifier is used, and SVM-RFE and Weight algorithms are similar to each other.

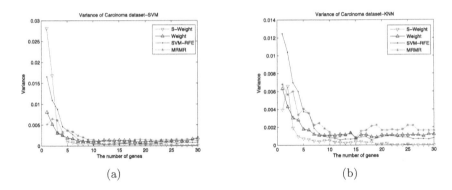

(a)   (b)

Fig. 8. The variance of classification accuracy of gene subsets by four algorithms on Carcinoma dataset, (a) SVM, (b) KNN

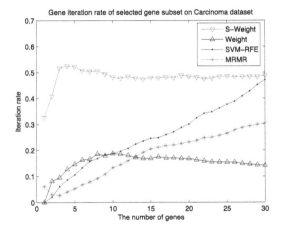

Fig. 9. The gene iteration rate of selected gene subsets by four algorithms on Carcinoma dataset

The experimental results in Fig. 9 show that our S-Weight is the most stable gene subset selection algorithm among the four compared algorithms. There are half genes are same in the selected gene subsets. The Weight algorithm is the worst one with the lowest gene iteration rate of no more than 20%. MRMR and SVM-RFE are not stable gene selection algorithms whose gene iteration rate goes up with the number of selected genes in the gene subset, but the upper bound of their gene iteration rate is no more than that of S-Weight.

4   Conclusions

This paper proposes a stable gene subset selection algorithm, named S-Weight. It randomly extracts samples from train subset and clusters the genes of the extracted samples in K-means, and estimates the importance of each gene of the extracted samples in Pearson correlation as well. Then it selects the most important gene from each cluster to construct the gene subset with K genes. This process is repeated several times, and the genes with high frequency will be selected to construct the selected gene subset.

The power of S-Weight is tested on three popular gene expression datasets, and compared with that of the famous gene selection algorithms including MRMR and SVM-RFE, and with that of Weigh algorithm which is the special case of S-weight where K-means is executed only once on the whole train subset to select the top K important genes to comprise the selected gene subset. The performances of the algorithms are compared in term of the classification accuracy of classifiers built on the selected gene subset, variance of the classification accuracy, and the gene iteration rate. All experimental results demonstrate that our proposed S-Weight algorithm can find the most stable gene subset with high classification accuracy. It outperforms MRMR and SVM-RFE and Weight.

It can be concluded that our S-weight to some extent has solved the exiting problem in gene selection area that the selected gene subset varies with the train subset.

Acknowledgments. We are much obliged to those who provide the public gene datasets for us to use. This work is supported in part by the National Natural Science Foundation of China under Grant No. 31372250, is also supported by the Key Science and Technology Program of Shaanxi Province of China under Grant No. 2013K12-03-24, and is at the same time supported by the Fundamental Research Funds for the Central Universities under Grant No. GK201503067.

References

1. Alon, U., Barkai, N., Notterman, D.A., Gish, K., Ybarra, S., Mack, D., Levine, A.J.: Broad patterns of gene expression revealed by clustering analysis of tumor and normal colon tissues probed by oligonucleotide arrays. Proceedings of the National Academy of Sciences 96(12), 6745–6750 (1999)
2. Bermejo, P., Gámez, J.A., Puerta, J.M.: A grasp algorithm for fast hybrid (filter-wrapper) feature subset selection in high-dimensional datasets. Pattern Recognition Letters 32(5), 701–711 (2011)
3. Chang, C.C., Lin, C.J.: Libsvm: a library for support vector machines. ACM Transactions on Intelligent Systems and Technology (TIST) 2(3), 27 (2011)
4. Cover, T., Hart, P.: Nearest neighbor pattern classification. IEEE Transactions on Information Theory 13(1), 21–27 (1967)
5. Ding, C., Peng, H.: Minimum redundancy feature selection from microarray gene expression data. Journal of bioinformatics and computational biology 3(02), 185–205 (2005)
6. Golub, T.R., Slonim, D.K., Tamayo, P., Huard, C., Gaasenbeek, M., Mesirov, J.P., Coller, H., Loh, M.L., Downing, J.R., Caligiuri, M.A., et al.: Molecular classification of cancer: class discovery and class prediction by gene expression monitoring. Science 286(5439), 531–537 (1999)
7. Guyon, I., Elisseeff, A.: An introduction to variable and feature selection. The Journal of Machine Learning Research 3, 1157–1182 (2003)

8. Guyon, I., Weston, J., Barnhill, S., Vapnik, V.: Gene selection for cancer classification using support vector machines. Machine learning **46**(1–3), 389–422 (2002)
9. Han, J., Kamber, M.: Data mining: Concepts and techniques. Morgan kaufmann (2006)
10. Han, Y., Yu, L.: A variance reduction framework for stable feature selection. Statistical Analysis and Data Mining: The ASA Data Science Journal **5**(5), 428–445 (2012)
11. Huang, Z.: Extensions to the k-means algorithm for clustering large data sets with categorical values. Data mining and knowledge discovery **2**(3), 283–304 (1998)
12. Lu, X., Peng, X., Liu, P., Deng, Y., Feng, B., Liao, B.: A novel feature selection method based on cfs in cancer recognition. In: 2012 IEEE 6th International Conference on Systems Biology (ISB), pp. 226–231. IEEE (2012)
13. MacQueen, J., et al.: Some methods for classification and analysis of multivariate observations. In: Proceedings of the Fifth Berkeley Symposium on Mathematical Statistics and Probability, vol. 1, pp. 281–297. Oakland, CA, USA (1967)
14. Notterman, D.A., Alon, U., Sierk, A.J., Levine, A.J.: Transcriptional gene expression profiles of colorectal adenoma, adenocarcinoma, and normal tissue examined by oligonucleotide arrays. Cancer Research **61**(7), 3124–3130 (2001)
15. Sasikala, S., Balamurugan, S.A., Geetha, S.: Multi filtration feature selection (mffs) to improve discriminatory ability in clinical data set. Applied Computing and Informatics (2014)
16. Vapnik, V.: The nature of statistical learning theory. Springer Science & Business Media (2000)
17. Xie, J., Gao, H.: Statistical correlation and k-means based distinguishable gene subset selection algorithms. Journal of Software **25**(9), 2050–2075 (2014)
18. Yu, L., Ding, C., Loscalzo, S.: Stable feature selection via dense feature groups. In: Proceedings of the 14th ACM SIGKDD international conference on Knowledge discovery and data mining, pp. 803–811. ACM (2008)
19. Yu, L., Han, Y., Berens, M.E.: Stable gene selection from microarray data via sample weighting. IEEE/ACM Transactions on Computational Biology and Bioinformatics (TCBB) **9**(1), 262–272 (2012)

Toward Establishing a Comprehensive Public Health Service Platform for Chronic Disease Management and Medication in China: A Practice in Building a Smart Hypertension Medical System

Yuncheng Hua[1], Jue Xie[2(✉)], Lei Liu[3], and Anjun Chen[1]

[1] 1j1 Intelligent Medical Technology, Suzhou Industrial Park, Suzhou, China
{hua.yuncheng,chen.anjun}@1j1ht.com
[2] Monash University–Southeast University Joint Research Institute, Suzhou, China
jue.xie@monash.edu
[3] Institute of Biomedical Sciences, Fudan University, Shanghai, China
liulei@fudan.edu.cn

Abstract. This research proposes a solution to establish an effective chronic disease prevention and control mechanism to strengthening public health management in China. This approach is to change from passive medication to active healthcare, which aims to prevent chronic diseases at early stage. The practice in developing one key subsystem of the proposed solution is demonstrated. It provides an intelligent medical platform that links hospitals, patients and community healthcare centers via the Internet to effectively achieve self-monitoring of health conditions and personalized medical treatment of hypertension.

Keywords: Chronic disease management · Blood pressure self-management · Remote health monitoring · Intelligent medical system · Health service platform

1 Introduction

With the dynamic development of China's social economy and rapid progress of technology, people's living standard has been constantly improved. While the average life span of Chinese residents is prolonged, the disease spectrum also experiences a major change. Chronic diseases, including cardiovascular disease, diabetes, chronic obstructive pulmonary disease, and chronic non-communicable cancer diseases, have occupied the first place in resident disease spectrum. According to statistics, in China the number of existing diagnosed patients with chronic diseases has reached 260 million. Annually, over 8 million people died from chronic diseases, which accounts for 85% of total death. The caused disease burden is 70% of the total measure, which already becomes a serious problem that hinders the social and economic development in China.

The occurrence of chronic diseases is closely related to various factors, such as dietary, lifestyle, sports, environment and heredity. Simply relying on existing healthcare system and medical model makes it hard to control and prevent chronic diseases

© Springer International Publishing Switzerland 2015
X. Yin et al. (Eds.): HIS 2015, LNCS 9085, pp. 123–132, 2015.
DOI: 10.1007/978-3-319-19156-0_13

effectively. By enhancing the management of public health, as well as providing Chinese residents with a comprehensive health management system that is based on modern science technology, it is able to change the care mode from passive medical treatment to active healthcare. The approach aims to prevent chronic diseases at early stage. It is essential to establish effective chronic disease prevention and controlling system, providing big data based, individualized treatment services that take each relevant factor into consideration. By this means, the effectiveness of disease treatment will be improved. It is imperative to build an integral public service platform, which is driven by residents' individual health needs, integrates contemporary scientific and technological achievements, and can provide residents comprehensive health management and personalized medical treatment.

The rapid and dynamic advance of contemporary science and technology, especially the network technology, cloud computing, big data, mobile Internet and wearable devices, has delivered fruitful outcomes in life science. Besides, the established regional medical information platform has provided a foundation for sharing medical treatment data. All these achievements make it technically possible to establish a comprehensive public health service platform, which can be employed to provide the public with synthetic health management information and personalized medical therapy based on big data applications.

This paper provides an overview of the comprehensive public health service platform, followed by an introduction of our first attempt of its implementation. The design and development of the 1j1 Smart Hypertension Medical System are presented with some preliminary results.

2   Overview of a Comprehensive Public Health Service Platform

It is perceived that a health service platform is an integral system of telemedicine, care management programs and e-health, which together would effectively prevent and control chronic diseases [1,2,3,4,5,6].

2.1   Telemedicine

Chronic disease therapy is over a long-term period, which needs continuous monitoring. The physiologic indexes of patients should be repeatedly observed in order to guide treatment or to promptly send interventions to patients. In traditional therapy methods, such as face-to-face patient-to-provider encounters, the medical instruments are devised to be operated by professional physicians in the clinical laboratory of hospitals. This leads to the instruments not practical for patients to be used at home for self-monitoring. Chronic disease patients have to take clinical examinations and therapies in hospitals or intensive care units, which would cost patients and physicians a great amount of time, money and energy. On a comprehensive health service platform, the functionality of telemedicine is designed to solve such a problem. By employing information and communication technologies, especially wearable devices together with Smartphone technologies, medical personnel could provide patients with professional healthcare remotely when such professional care services are not available face to face [7,8].

Telemedicine is designed to deliver healthcare and medical assistance from remote locations with help of latest telecommunication means. Wherever the health service is needed, professional medical care will be provided [9]. Presently, with the advance of telecommunication technology, the telemedicine can be implemented over ubiquitous wired or wireless communication methods, which makes it possible to employ tele-medicine in a health service platform [10,11]. As a result, highly expert-based medical care can be accessible to a wider range of patients, especially those who are in understaffed areas, such as rural health centers, vehicles, and airplanes, as well as for home monitoring [12]. In Europe, the telemedicine technology has been employed to manage heart failure, which is aimed to prevent crisis, treat heart disease and empower patients to manage their own health [13].

By integrating the telemedicine to the platform, the physiologic information that doctors receive will have a longer time span than it can be collected during the patients' normal hospitality stays [14]. On one hand, the information that collected by telemedicine is essential for treatment of chronic diseases and has good long-term effects on healthcare at home. On the other hand, based on the data derived from a considerable number of chronic disease sufferers, the experts have more information to study and research, thus more effective therapies can be provided to patients. The iterative process would also result in better health services. Patients therefore could save money, time and energy, as well as get better healthcare at home [15].

The monitoring over chronic diseases, for instance hypertension, is regarded as a complex process. Telemedicine in this case allows continuous monitoring of patients' physical index readings. In China, with rapid arise of obesity and ageing population, the risk of stroke, heart disease and kidney attack increases correspondingly. Although the primary cause of hypertension is yet unknown [14], the blood pressure of patients can be easily observed and controlled via various means. For example, many hypertension sufferers usually measure their blood pressure at home on a regular basis. The measured systolic and diastolic blood pressure can be used in the telemedicine function to determine whether an alert message needs to be sent, or the system should automatically request further actions. Once a patient connects to a telemedicine network, the blood pressure readings together with other relevant physiologic information will be transmitted to healthcare professionals or medical science web services. Feedback would then be returned to inform the patient about his/her physical condition.

Furthermore, on such a health service platform, challenges such as a lack of social care personnel and continuous healthcare are addressed. This patient-based approach is able to improve the existing chronic healthcare services. The approach integrates telemedicine with care management, which would promote data exchange between patients at homes, healthcare providers in hospitals, and clinical units [1]. It is aimed to use physiologic information to identify at-risk patients promptly and effectively. For instance, patients with hypertension could choose to upload physical condition changes onto a telemedicine program. The information can include the rise of blood pressure, adverse reactions, or behavior changes. The telemedicine program, which receives and analyses such information, will then send feedback to both patients and their care managers for taking further actions. By utilizing telemedicine tools, the care providers will gain more access to their patients, and therefore obtain more information from interactive communications.

2.2   Care management

Care management incorporates an exception handling approach, which would intervene in the occurrence of some exceptional cases. For instance, if some parameters exceed the pre-defined limits, the care management function would alert medical personnel to pay attention to a particular patient. The approach is designed to firstly identify the patient who appears to be at risk based on the analysis of patient's physical signs and symptoms. Second, care management program determines whether there is a need for care management interventions, and informs corresponding care managers [16]. At last, the care manager would contact the patients who are potentially at risk to ensure that they will receive in time and appropriate treatment. By this means, care managers will be able to intervene before their patients being sent to emergency units.

Another merit of integration of care management and telemedicine is to empower patients to be experts in managing their own health conditions through the provision of personalized health information and personal health records [17]. Interaction with the program would enable patients to obtain good knowledge of both their own health conditions and effective methods to better manage their own health. Patients thus are stimulated to participate in health management matters [18,19].

2.3   E-health

In addition to care management and telemedicine, the health service platform also incorporates e-health functionality. E-health is originally aimed at transforming medical records from paper to electronic format. By using well-designed computer systems, the billing and scheduling for patients can be automated, which would be cheaper, faster and more convenient than the manual approach. Such an EMR (Electronic Medical Record) or EHR (Electronic Health Record) system replaces handwritten medical notes to record patients' medical history [20,21]. Based on it, doctors are able to access and review patients' medical history conveniently, and to prescribe medicine or treatment more accurately and specifically. A few countries have adopted EMR/EHR systems, including U.S., Australia and China. In China, the government propels forward the EMR/EHR systems since 2005 [22,23,24].

Besides, e-health has a medical database foundation to support decision making on medication. Based on the customized information about a patient's medical problems, including physical data, symptoms, health complication, medical history of patients, allergy reaction and drug-drug interactions, an e-health system computes appropriate dosing and therapy for a particular patient [20]. By applying the best practice standards, an e-health system can also generate a list of patients who are identified to be at risk and need intervention. In addition, the data format of EMR/EHR in e-health system should be standardized to realize interoperability. The uniform data standard enables the EMR/EHR data to be shared and incorporated by different medical organizations or hospitals, and would help to overpass the obstacle of data transmitting in different units. The Ministry of Health (MOH) in China has ratified the study and research on the standards and specifications of EMR/EHR [22]. Using uniformed data standards makes it possible to gather patients' medical records from various sources. For instance, over 450 organizations have employed BlueButton+ API and promoted patients to access and download medical information, which would enable patients manage and improve their own health. In addition, the health information exchange could be promoted across different health organizations by using BlueButton [25,26]. The uniformed data standards would also help both the health service platform and various health organizations to share clinical information. All collected data would eventually be streamed to a data cloud managed by the health service platform for further research, analysis and reporting.

3   China National Health Big Data Framework and the 1j1 Practice

This research associates with a larger project "The development and application of a comprehensive health service platform based on big data applications" that is under the National Health Big Data Science and Technology Support Programme. In this framework, a "Learning Health System for Chronic Disease Management and Medication" is proposed and will be tested in heart health, specifically in monitoring and managing blood pressure of diagnosed patients. The final product will have three types of users, including patients, community practitioners, and medical specialists at hospitals. The collected data derived from patients would be assembled into a data cloud managed by the National Chronic Disease Centre for further study. The project aims at delivering an innovative and leading "self-Learning Healthcare System" (LHS). In LHS, the data cloud managed by the National Chronic Disease Centre would be designed to collect data routinely from patient care and clinical laboratories. The ever-growing data cloud is employed for LHS to "learn" iteratively via the following: (1) collecting and analyzing data; (2) studying existing data together with data from prospective studies to formulate updated treatment plans; (3) treating patients with new plan; (4) evaluating the treat outcomes from patients; and (5) putting forward new hypotheses for further research. Through such progress, LHS is able to provide quality and patient-centered health services as well as innovation continuity [27,28,29].

3.1   1j1 Smart Hypertension Medical System

The 1j1 Smart Hypertension Medical System aims at delivering a content service application, supported by China National Health Big Data Programme. The goal is to build a countrywide intelligent medical platform that links hospitals, patients and community healthcare centers via the Internet to effectively achieve self-monitoring of health conditions and personalized medical treatment of hypertension. At the stage of writing this paper, the development of intelligent medical software and hardware platforms will be soon released for clinical trial. Cooperations are carried out with the medical school at Shanghai Fudan University, where experienced clinical research professors are in charge of clinical trials designed for this research.

3.2   Conceptual Framework

The major architectural components of the proposed Smart Hypertension Medical System include a patient personalized service module, a care manager, a doctor module, and a central medical server, which are introduced below respectively:

The patient personalized service module is attached to monitoring devices, for instance a blood pressure monitor. It runs a monitoring application that receives patients' physiologic information, such as blood pressure systolic and diastolic values and heart rate. The patient frontend will activate alarms when interventions are received, and periodically exchange data with other modules, including the central monitoring server through the Internet. By this means, the patient service module is able to upload medical data onto the monitoring server and receive interventions from the care manager or the doctor module to alert corresponding patients.

Care manager is the module operates an observing application, which receives data transmitted from the patient service module, as well as feedback from the doctor module. The care manager sends interventions to the patient module when selected parameters exceed certain limits. It also notifies the doctor module to provide medical treatments to the patients that are at risk.

The doctor module receives messages from the care manager. It also refers to appropriate dosing and therapy generated by the central medical server. Within this module, doctors interact with patients directly, prescribing medicine or therapy with reference to clinical therapies retrieved from the central medical server. After applying medical treatment, doctors will assess the referral therapy based on the following factors: whether the therapy computed by the central medical server is useful to patients of a specific disease; how to improve the therapy; and how to alter the dosing in practical treatment. Such feedback will be sent to the central medical server.

A central medical server provides data persistence and management services, which store patient medical records, receive and persist updated medical information from the patient personalized service module and feedback from the doctor module. Its most important function is to compute appropriate dosing and therapy for a particular patient based on patient-specific information of a medical problem. The core of the central medical server is an ontology for the management of chronically ill patients together with the implementation of personalization. The ontology is consisted of medical management knowledge, including the knowledge of various diseases, corresponding signs and symptoms, as well as relevant interventions and treatments. When encountering with a patient, the personalization process is started. The medical information stored in patient's EHR system would be extracted and combined with the ontology. Based on pre-designed rules, the reasoning would be accomplished by a reasoner. By this means, the possible disease that the patient suffers, together with corresponding interventions and treatments, would be inferred and computed automatically. The personalized ontology that contains inferred knowledge will be relevant to a given patient and used for his/her treatment [30]. The foundation of such ontology is based on big data analysis. The medical data of patients diagnosed of the same disease are analyzed together with associated therapies. As a result, the most effective therapy will be recommended to the patient. Also based on doctor feedback, the therapy and intervention knowledge in ontology could be updated and adapted to different patients. This iterative process is employed to seek the most effective therapy for specific groups of patients, and to ensure the output can better facilitate doctors to make informed medical decisions.

The above four components interact with each other to accomplish the telemedicine, care management, and e-health functionalities that have been introduced in the previous section. The conceptual framework of this smart medical system is illustrated in Figure 1.

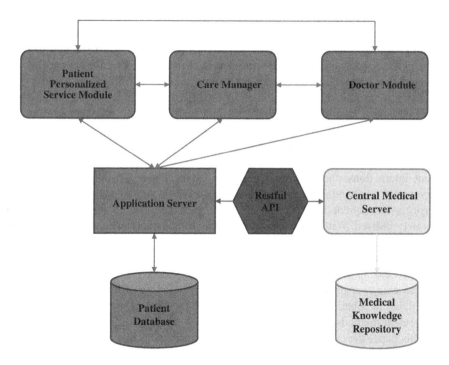

Fig. 1. Conceptual framework of the proposed Smart Hypertension Medical System

A patient's medical information is firstly transmitted and persisted into the patient database through an application server. The patient's information is subsequently conveyed to the central medical server. The central server will analyze the information to determine whether or not the patient is at risk. If so, the central server will send an alert to the care manager. Otherwise, the latest medical information of the patient will just be recorded in the patient database, and the patient's medical status will be updated accordingly. Doctors or care managers can access and enquiry the present and historical medical information of their patients.

After receiving an alert message about a particular patient, the care manager would choose an appropriate case doctor for the patient who has been identified at risk. It then will send a message to the doctor module in order to notify the case doctor that the patient needs to be treated immediately. The doctor will need to take immediate action to arrange medical treatment for the patient. Since the medical information of the patient is already transmitted to the central medical server, the server is able to suggest referral therapies based on the patient's medical data and relevant information retrieved from the medical knowledge repository. The doctor will then treat the patient accordingly with reference to suggested therapies. After the treatment is performed and completed, the doctor can send feedback on utilised therapies to the central medical server, which in turn will improve the service incrementally.

4   Conclusions

In China, chronic diseases, especially hypertension, have occupied the first place in public disease spectrum. The long-term treatment of chronic disease patients and the corresponding intensive expenses in both finance and time allocation impose great challenges. One innovative solution is to establish a comprehensive health service platform, which can diminish the geographical, financial, and temporal access problems faced by patients with chronic diseases. The philosophy behind this is the transition from passive medical treatment to active healthcare. By incorporating tele-medicine, care management, and e-health functionalities in medical data analysis and patient interactions, the platform is able to actively assist patients in performing interventions and sending emergency alerts. Moreover, via the analysis of big data of heterogeneous patient information, effective therapies can be quickly sought and accurately utilised. With reference to abundant clinical experience and feedback from experienced doctors, the reliability of the platform can be iteratively improved. The platform takes advantage of ubiquitous wired or wireless communication methods and online processing to enable active monitoring and modern healthcare. Also, the platform can empower patients to have in-depth understanding of their health conditions, as well as to obtain relevant knowledge on medical treatment and self-health management methods.

In this paper the conceptual framework of a smart medical system is presented for monitoring and medication of chronic diseases, the hypertension in particular. The system aims to meet the diverse needs of physician-diagnosed patients, minimizing cost and maximizing extensibility and reliability. Further research will be conducted to implement the proposed architectural components, and to test its usefulness and usability with patients and doctors through controlled clinical trials. The intelligent features of the system will be further investigated to enable automated learning from abundant patient information and effective treatments so as to generate useful therapy recommendations.

Acknowledgement. The Smart Hypertension Medical Systems project is part of an in-application larger project "The development and application of a comprehensive health service platform based on big data applications" under China National Health Big Data Science and Technology Support Programme. The project is going to be registered at the China National Chronic Disease Centre, and has already received strong support from Suzhou Development and Reform Commission in Jiangsu Province.

References

1. Laurence, C.B., Scott, J.J., Dendy, M., Howard, B.: Integrated Telehealth And Care Management Program For Medicare Beneficiaries With Chronic Disease Linked To Savings. Health Affairs **30**(9), 1689–1697 (2011)
2. Ekeland, A.G., Bowes, A., Flottorp, S.: Effectiveness of telemedicine: A systematic review of reviews. International Journal of Medical Informatics **79**(11), 736–771 (2010)
3. Young, L.B., Chan, P.S., Lu, X., Nallamothu, B.K., Sasson, C., Cram, P.M.: Impact of Telemedicine Intensive Care Unit Coverage on Patient Outcomes. ARCH. INTERN. MED. **171**(6), 498–506 (2011)
4. Lorig, K.R., Ritter, P., Stewart, A.L., Sobel, D.S., William, B.B., Bandura, A., Gonzalez, V.M., Laurent, D.D., Holman, H.R.: Chronic Disease Self-Management Program: 2-Year Health Status and Health Care Utilization Outcomes. Medical Care **39**(11), 1217–1223 (2001)
5. Lorig, K.R., Sobel, D.S., Stewart, A.L., Brown, B.W., Bandura, A., Ritter, P., Gonzalez, V.M., Laurent, D.D., Holman, H.R.: Evidence Suggesting That a Chronic Disease Self-Management Program Can Improve Health Status While Reducing Hospitalization: A Randomized Trial. Medical Care **37**(1), 5–14 (1999)
6. Blaya, J.A., Fraser, H.S.F., Holt, B.: E-Health Technologies Show Promise In Developing Countries. Health Affairs **29**(2), 244–251 (2010)
7. Amadi-Obi, A., Gilligan, P., Owens, N., O'Donnell, C.: Telemedicine in pre-hospital care: a review of telemedicine applications in the pre-hospital environment. International Journal of Emergency Medicine **7**(29), 1–11 (2014)
8. Gregoski, M.J., Mueller, M., Vertegel, A., Shaporev, A., Jackson, B.B., Frenzel, R.M., Sprehn, S.M., Treiber, F.A.: Development and validation of a smartphone heart rate acquisition application for health promotion and wellness telehealth applications. International Journal of Telemedicine and Applications **2012** (2012)
9. Pattichis, C.S., Kyriacou, E., Voskarides, S., Pattichis, M.S., Lstepanian, R., Schizas, C.N.: Wireless Telemedicine Systems: An Overview. IEEE Antenna's and Propagation Magazine **44**(2), 143–153 (2002)
10. Junnila, S., Kailanto, H., Merilahti, J., Vainio, A., Vehkaoja, A., Zakrzewski, M., Hyttinen, J.: Wireless, Multipurpose In-Home Health Monitoring Platform: Two Case Trials. IEEE Transactions on Information Technology in Biomedicine **14**(2), 447–455 (2010)
11. Ackerman, M.J., Filart, R., Burgess, L.P., Lee, I., Poropatich, R.K.: Developing Next-Generation Telehealth Tools and Technologies: Patients, Systems, and Data Perspectives. Telemedicine and e-Health **16**(1), 93–95 (2010)
12. Fortney, J.C., Burgess, J.F., Bosworth, H.B., Booth, B.M., Kaboli, P.J.: A Re-conceptualization of Access for 21st Century Healthcare. Journal of General Internal Medicine **26**(2), 639–647 (2011)
13. Anker, S.D., Koehler, F., Abraham, W.T.: Telemedicine and remote management of patients with heart failure. The Lancet **378**, 731–739 (2011)

14. Rotariu, C., Pasarica, A., Costin, H., Adochiei, F., Ciobotariu, R.: Telemedicine system for remote blood pressure and heart rate monitoring. In: Proceedings of the 3rd International Conference on E-Health and Bioengineering (2011)
15. de Toledo, P., Jimenez, S., del Pozo, F., Roca, J., Alonso, A., Hernandez, C.: Telemedicine Experience for Chronic Care in COPD. Information Technology in Biomedicine **10**(3), 567–573 (2006)
16. Morrison, L.G., Yardley, L., Powell, J., Michie, S.: What Design Features Are Used in Effective e-Health Interventions? A Review Using Techniques from Critical Interpretive Synthesis. Telemedicine and e-Health **18**(2), 137–144 (2012)
17. Wootton, R.: Twenty years of telemedicine in chronic disease management – an evidence synthesis. Journal of Telemedicine and Telecare **18**(4), 211–220 (2012)
18. Picard, R.W., Du, C.Q.: Monitoring Stress and Heart Health with a Phone and Wearable Computer. Offspring **1**(1), 14–22 (2002)
19. Hood, L., Friend, S.H.: Predictive, personalized, preventive, participatory (P4) cancer medicine. Nature Reviews Clinical Oncology **8**, 184–187 (2011)
20. James, B.: E-Health: Steps On The Road To Interoperability. Health Affairs (Millwood), 26–30 (2005)
21. Hess, R., Bryce, C.L., Paone, S., Fischer, G., McTigue, K.M., Olshansky, E., Zickmund, S., Fitzgerald, K., Siminerio, L.: Exploring Challenges and Potentials of Personal Health Records in Diabetes Self-Management: Implementation and Initial Assessment. Telemedicine and e-Health **13**(5), 509–518 (2007)
22. Gao, X., Xu, J., Sorwar, G., Croll, P.: Implementation of E-Health Record Systems and E-Medical Record Systems in China. The International Technology Management Review **3**(2), 127–139 (2013)
23. Jha, A.K., DesRoches, C.M., Campbell, E.G., Donelan, K., Rao, S.R., Ferris, T.G., Shields, A., Rosenbaum, S., Blumenthal, D.: Use of Electronic Health Records in U.S. Hospitals. The New England Journal of Medicine **360**, 1628–1638 (2009)
24. Xu, J., Gao, X.Z., Sorwar, G., Croll, P.: Current Status, Challenges, and Outlook of E-Health Record Systems in Australia. Springer, Heidelberg (2014)
25. Hogan, T.P., Nazi, K.M., Houston, T.K.: Technology-Assisted Patient Access to Clinical Information: An Evaluation Framework for Blue Button. JMIR Research Protocols **3**(1), e18 (2014)
26. Vogel, L.: "Blue button" access to medical records. CMAJ **182**(16), E746 (2010)
27. Abernethy, A.P., Etheredge, L.M., Ganz, P.A., Wallace, P., German, R.R., Neti, C., Bach, P.B., Murphy, S.B.: Rapid-Learning System for Cancer Care. Journal of Clinical Oncology **28**(27), 4268–4274 (2010)
28. Greene, S.M., Reid, R.J., Larson, E.B.: Implementing the Learning Health System: From Concept to Action. Annals of Internal Medicine **157**(3), 207–210 (2012)
29. Etheredge, L.M.: A Rapid-Learning Health System. Health Affairs **26**(2), 107–118 (2007)
30. Riaño, D., Real, F., López-Vallverdú, J.A., Campana, F., Ercolani, S., Ercolani, P., Annicchiarico, R., Caltagirone, C.: An ontology-based personalization of health-care knowledge to support clinical decisions for chronically ill patients. Journal of Biomedical Informatics **45**(3), 429–446 (2012)

TeenChat: A Chatterbot System for Sensing and Releasing Adolescents' Stress

Jing Huang[(⊠)], Qi Li, Yuanyuan Xue, Taoran Cheng, Shuangqing Xu,
Jia Jia, and Ling Feng

Deptartment of Computer Science and Technology,
Tsinghua University, Beijing, China
{j-huang14,liqi13,xue-yy12,ctr10,xsq10}@mails.tsinghua.edu.cn,
{jjia,fengling}@mail.tsinghua.edu.cn

Abstract. More and more adolescents today are suffering from various adolescent stress. Too much stress will bring a variety of physical and psychological problems including anxiety, depression, and even suicide to the growing youths, whose outlook on life and problem-solving ability are still immature enough. Traditional face-to-face stress detection and relief methods do not work, confronted with adolescents who are reluctant to express their negative emotions to the people in real life. In this paper, we present a adolescent-oriented intelligent chatting system called *TeenChat*, which acts as a virtual friend to listen, understand, comfort, encourage, and guide stressful adolescents to pour out their bad feelings, and thus releasing the stress. Our 1-month user study demonstrates *TeenChat* is effective on sensing and helping adolescents' stress.

Keywords: Adolescent · Stress sensing and easing · Chat

1 Introduction

With the rapid development of society and economy, more and more people live a stressful life. Too much stress threatens human's physical and psychological health [13,14]. Especially for the youth group, the threat is prone to such bad consequence as depression or even suicide due to their spiritual immaturity [4]. Hence, psychologists and educators have paid great attention to the adolescent stress issue [9,37]. Nevertheless, one big difficulty in reality is that most growing adolescents are not willing or hesitate to express their feelings to the people, but rather turn to the virtual world for stress release. Chatterbot (also known as chatbot or talkbot), as a virtual artificial conversation system, can function as a useful channel for cathartic stress relief, as it allows the conversational partner to finally get to say what s/he cannot say out loud in real life. Recently, [22] proposed a chatting robot PAL, which can answer non-obstructive psychological domain-specific questions. It collects numerous psychological Q&A pairs from the Q&A community into a local knowledge base, and selects a suitable answer to match the user's psychological question, taking personal information into

© Springer International Publishing Switzerland 2015
X. Yin et al. (Eds.): HIS 2015, LNCS 9085, pp. 133–145, 2015.
DOI: 10.1007/978-3-319-19156-0_14

consideration. However, in most situations, when users tell about their stress, they wouldn't only ask some psychological questions. Instead, they pour forth their woes sentence by sentence. and what the stressful people need is not only the solutions for their problems, but also the feeling of being listened, understood, and comforted. Comparatively, psychological domain-specific question-answer based chatting robots are rigid and insufficient in understanding and calming users' stressful emotions.

In this study, we aim to build a adolescent-oriented intelligent chatting system *TeenChat*, which can on one hand sense adolescents' stress throughout the whole conversation rather than based on a single question each time in [22], and on the other hand interact like a virtual friend to guide the stressful adolescents to gradually pour out their bad feelings by listening and comforting, and further encourage the adolescents by delivering positive messages and answers to their problems. To our knowledge, this is the first chatting system in the literature, designed specifically for sensing and helping release adolescents' stress in such stress categories as study, self-cognition, inter-personal, and affection during the virtual conversation. Our 1-month user study demonstrates that *TeenChat's* has achieves 78.34% precision and 76.12% recall rate in stress sensing and making the stressful users feel better.

The reminder of the paper is organized as follows. We review related work in Section 2, and outline our *TeenChat* framework in Section 3. Two core components for stress sensing and response generation are detailed in Section 4 and 5, respectively. Results of our user study are analyzed in Section 6. Section 7 concludes the paper and discusses future work.

2 Related Work

Chat Robots. Q&A systems respond to users by matching questions and question -answer pairs in knowledge bases [25,31], retrieving relevant documents and Web pages from local document collections and global Internet [17,24], or extracting answers from relevant documents or Web pages [15,21]. FAQ (Frequently Asked Questions) is a typical knowledge-based Q&A system, whose knowledge base accommodates frequently asked question-answer pairs. The main task of the system is to match users' questions to corresponding question-answer pairs [5].

As a special kind of Q&A system, chat robots (also called chatterbots, chatbots or artificial conversational systems) emphasize hominization, aiming to interact with users in a human-like friendly way. ELIZA [36] was the first chatbot, developed by Weizenbaum in 1960s. It acts like a psychotherapist to help speakers maintain the sense of being heard and understood. Inheriting the mechanism of ELIZA, another famous chatbot ALICE [34] engaged in a conversation with a human by applying some heuristical pattern matching rules to the human's inputs. ALICE won the Loebner Prize for the most human-like computer in 2000, 2001, and 2004. Since then, chat robots have found wide application areas. In education, they could help human users practice their conversational skills in foreign languages [29,41], act as virtual Confucius for promoting traditional Chinese culture[35] or build intelligent tutoring systems to tailor to individual needs [16,18]. In E-commerce, chat robots could help users find relevant products [6,12]. In medical health care, chat robots could give control/management advice to diabetes patients [23], impart knowledge about H5N1 pandemic crisis to community [12], answer adolescent sex, drug, and alcohol related questions [10] and general psychology specific questions [22]. Besides, recently developed chatbot systems [1,11,28] could recognize users' humoristic expressions and generate humorous sentences for time sharing and entertainment purpose.

Textual Emotion Recognition. Detection emotion through keywords is the most direct method [27,30]. [33] made use of lexical affinity to enhance the keyword-based detection accuracy. However, because of the existence of negation and various sentence structures, only considering keywords is not enough. [26,38] further applied natural language processing methods to parse sentences and proposed rules to reveal the relationships between a particular expression and emotion. [32,40] regarded emotion recognition as a classification problem, and used machine learning methods to classify a text into different emotions. [2,3] recognized emotion on the basis of some commonsense knowledge.

Stress Detection. Most existing stress detection methods rely on psychological scales and/or physiological devices, but in reality, people are not willing to go for a psychologist or take some contact sensors with them. Recently, researchers started to pay attention to the social media which also reveals users' stress signals. [39] proposed to detect adolescent stress from micro-blog. [20] investigated the correlations between users' stress and their tweeting contents, social engagement, and behavior patterns, and then built a deep neural network model to detect users' stress.

The *TeenChat* tool presented in this paper intends to serve adolescent chatters by sensing their possible stress in study, self-cognition, inter-personal, or affection throughout the conversation context, and encourage them to cope with the stress in a positive way.

3   System Framework

TeenChat works under the Browser/Server mode. Fig. 1 shows its framework. The user chats with *TeenChat* via an Internet browser. The *TeenChat* server is comprised of three major components, which cooperate as follows.

- **Chatting Manager**. After a user logins to the system, the *User Login&System Greeting* module sends a warm greeting to the user based on the historically detected stress result. If no historic stress is detected, *TeenChat* will send a greeting like a virtual friend *"Hello, hows doing?"*, or *"Is everything ok now?"*. if the user had some stress being detected through previous conversations, The *Feedback&Log Maintenance* module maintains and refreshes the detected stress result, and adjusts the response strategy based on feedback analysis (i.e., whether the chatting lasts long, whether the answers is effective to alleviate user's stress, etc.)

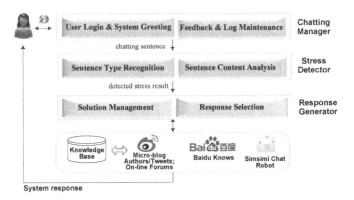

Fig. 1. *TeenChat* framework

- **Stress Detector**. To understand user's expected answer from the system, the *Sentence Type Recognition* module categorizes user's chatting sentence into *interrogative question, rhetorical question,* or *declarative sentence*. An interrogative question sentence like *"How to improve maths?"* or *What shall I do?"* may ask for objective or positive answers/suggestions, while a rhetorical question sentence like *"They should know me, shouldn't they?"* may reflect user's certain emotions to some extent. Furthermore, the *Sentence Content Analysis* module senses user's possible stress, including stress category and stress subcategory, based on the seven adolescent's stress-related lexicons. If the user's stress is sensed but no stress category/subcategory can be detected from the current chatting sentence, the previous or historic stress category/subcategory (if available) is assumed as the current stress category/subcategory. The working of the *Sentence Content Analysis* module is detailed in the next section.

- **Response Generation**. Based on the stress detection result as well as the chatting sentence type, the *Response Selection* module chooses an appropriate answer from the local Knowledge Base, Baidu Knows, or the existing chatting robot Simsimi Repository [28]. The aim is to help stressful users shift attention or express inner struggling, thus easing the pressure. The *Solution Management* module is responsible for setting up *TeenChat*'s response strategies during chatting, and pre-storing a large volume of positive answering sentences in a local knowledge base, to be managed and incrementally populated by crawling from on-line forums and influential micro-blog authors/tweets.

4   Stress Detection

From a user's input sentence c, *TeenChat* firstly tries to sense whether the user has some stress or not based on our stress-related emotion lexicon in Table 1. Meanwhile, it builds a linguistic dependency tree for c, whose root node is the core word of the sentence. *TeenChat* analyzes all possible linkage between the stress emotion word and stress category/sub-category words in the tree, and returns a set of triples of the form: (Stress, Category:l_c, SubCategory:l_s), where Stress takes value 0 (meaning no stress detected) or 1 (meaning stress detected), l_c is the path length between the negative emotional word and the category node, and l_s is the path length between the negative emotional word and the sub-category node. l_c/l_s can be null if there exists no path linking the negative emotion word and the category/sub-category word.

Table 1. Stress-Related Lexicons

I. Stress Emotion Lexicon		
Negative Emotion		*stress, stressful, pressure, nervous, unhappy, annoyed, annoying, bad, sad, etc.*
Positive Emotion		*happy, relaxed, good, fun, etc.*
Negation		*no, not, neither, etc.*
II. Stress Category/Sub-Category Lexicon		
STUDY	Homework	*homework, project, practice, assignment, etc.*
	Exam	*exam, grade, mark, rank, score, etc.*
	General	*history, math, physical, etc.*
SELF-COGNITION	Appearance	*ugly, fat, stout, etc.*
	Health	*sleepless, flustered, insomnia, fracture, stomachache, etc.*
	Inner-feeling	*foolish, stupid, awkward, incapable, self-distrust, etc.*
	General	*unconfident, inferior, abased, weak, etc.*
INTER-PERSONAL	Family	*father, mother, brother, sister, uncle, aunt, etc.*
	Teacher	*teacher, school, regulation, schoolmaster, etc.*
	Friend	*classmate, friendship, etc.*
	General	*quarrel, criticize, ridicule, etc.*
AFFECTION	Lover	*boyfriend, girlfriend etc.*
	Partner	*partner, etc.*
	General	*break-up, separate, secret-love, unrequited love, etc.*
GENERAL	(unknown category and sub-category)	

Example 1. Take sentence "*Always quarrelling with friends at school, so annoyed!*" for example. Fig. 3 gives its linguistic dependency tree, constructed by the linguistic analysis tool LTP [7]. The stress-related negative emotion word "*annoyed*" is linked to "*quarrel*" via a 1-length path, and to "*friend*" via a 3-length path. As "*quarrel*" belongs to stress category INTER-PERSONAL, and "*friend*" to its sub-category Friend, a user's stress in INTER-PERSONAL, in particular in the Friend aspect, is sensed from the sentence, denoted as (1, INTER-PERSONAL:1, Friend:3).

In case multiple stress categories/sub-categories are sensed, the one with the shortest path between the negative emotion word and the stress category or sub-category word is considered as the primary stress category/sub-category.

When the path length cannot help make distinction, the category similar to the historic stress category will be taken as the primary one. If the above also fails, the primary one is randomly determined. In this way, from each user's input sentence c, a detection result (`c.Stress`, `c.Category`, `c.SubCategory`) is returned, where `c.Stress=0` indicates no stress is discovered from the current sentence c, and `c.Category/c.SubCategory=null` indicates no category/sub-category word is found in c.

Considering user's short dialogue inputs, as well as the consecutiveness of stressful emotion remaining during conversation, we keep and refresh user's historic stress status, ((`h.Stress`, `h.Category`, `h.SubCategory`)) detected from the previous sentences as follows.

(1) When no stress is detected from the current sentence c, but detected from the history, if `h.Category==c.Category` and `h.SubCategory==c.SubCategory`, we mark `c.Stress=1`.

(2) When stress is detected from the current sentence c with a concrete category/ sub-category, which is/are missing from the history, we assign `h.Category=c.Category` and `h.SubCategory=c.SubCategory`.

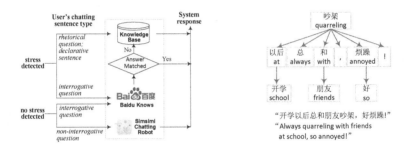

Fig. 2. *TeenChat* response strategies   **Fig. 3.** A dependence tree example

5   Response Generation Module

Fig. 2 gives *TeenChat*'s response strategies based on user's sentence type and the detected result (`c.Stress`,`c.Category`, `c.SubCategory`).

[**Case 1**] Stress being detected (`c.Stress==1`)

(1) For a user's **declarative sentence** or **rhetorical question**, *TeenChat* selects an answer from the *local knowledge base*, which accommodates abundant of positive response sentences in different categories/sub-categories to comfort, encourage, or guide stressful users.

(2) For a user's **interrogative question**, *TeenChat* goes to one of the largest Chinese Q&A community *Baidu Knows* to match the question with the given answer. Let Q_u be the user's input question, and Q_b be the closest question found in the Baidu Knows. If their matching degree $MatchDegree(Q_u, Q_b)$ is over a certain threshold θ, and meanwhile Q_b's corresponding answer has been adopted

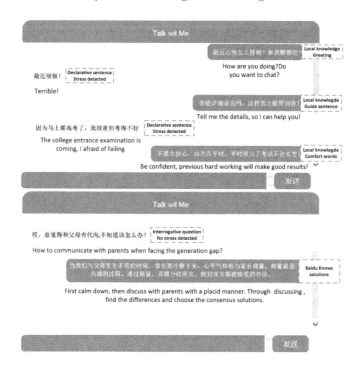

Fig. 4. *TeenChat* response examples of two topic categories

or agreed by at least one person, *TeenChat* will return Q_b's best answer to the user. Otherwise, *TeenChat* will search the *local knowledge base* and return a general positive answer, or just a joke to cheer up the user. The matching degree $MatchDegree(Q_u, Q_b)$ is computed based on the *effective node pairs* in the Q_u's and Q_b's linguistic dependence trees [19]. An *effective node pair* is a node pair (n_1, n_2), where n_1 is the core root node, n_2 is the direct child node of n_1, and n_2 represents a verb, noun, or adjective word. Given two effective node pairs $u = (u_1, u_2)$ and $b = (b_1, b_2)$, we define their similarity as:

$$sim(u,b) = sim((u_1, u_2), (b_1, b_2)) = \begin{cases} 1 & \text{if } (u_1 == b_1) \wedge (u_2 == b_2) \\ 0.5 & \text{else if } (u_1 == b_1) \wedge (u_2 \neq b_2) \\ 0 & \text{otherwise} \end{cases}$$

Let $E(Q_u)$ and $E(Q_b)$ denote the set of effective node pairs in the Q_u's and Q_b's linguistic dependence trees, respectively. Considering nodes' semantical equivalence, we replace any two nodes (one in $E(Q_u)$ and the other in $E(Q_b)$) with their sememe in Hownet (if existing) to ensure nodes' similarity as much as possible. The obtained equivalent effective node sets are denoted as $E^*(Q_u)$ and $E^*(Q_b)$, respectively. We have $MatchDegree(Q_u, Q_b) = \alpha \ SIM(E(Q_u), E(Q_b)) + (1 - \alpha) \ SIM(E^*(Q_u), E^*(Q_b))$, where $\alpha = 0.5$,

$$SIM(E(Q_u), E(Q_b)) = \frac{\sum_{u \in E(Q_u)} \sum_{b \in E(Q_b)} sim(u,b)}{Max\{|E(Q_u)|, |E(Q_b)|\}}, \text{ and}$$

$$SIM(E^*(Q_u), E^*(Q_b)) = \frac{\sum_{u^* \in E^*(Q_u)} \sum_{b^* \in E^*(Q_b)} sim(u^*,b^*)}{Max\{|E^*(Q_u)|, |E^*(Q_b)|\}}.$$

[**Case 2**] No stress being detected (`c.Stress==0`)

(1) For a user's `interrogative question`, the answering is the same as the one in *Case 1* (2).

(2) For a user's `non-interrogative question` input, *TeenChat* goes to the open Simsimi repository [28], which provides public API for developers to establish their own chatting robot.

Fig.4 shows some example responses about study and interpersonal skills.

6   User Study

6.1   Experimental Setup

We invited 10 students (aged between 15 and 22) from a high school and a university to participate in our 1-month study. We chose these students because the majority of the adolescent group are students and the selected students were suffering from more or less stress, as evidenced by their Cohen's Perceived Stress Scale (CPSS-14) results [8], which is commonly used to measure human stress level worldwide in psychology. To begin with, the users were told that *Teenchat* was a chatting system which could help them release stress and they could chat with *Teenchat* whenever necessary. During the experiment, we asked the users to do the following things: 1) Fill in the Chinese CPSS questionnaire every week to record the change of their stress status. 2) Evaluate the releasing effect of each conversation. 3) Give the ground truth to the stress status of each sentence in the conversation.

6.2   Experimental Results

After the 1-month user study, we obtained: 1) 62 conversations and 1063 chatting sentences in all, namely 6.2 conversations for each user and 17.2 utterances for each conversation in average. 2) 5 Chinese CPSS questionnaires for each user which record their change of stress status.

The accuracy of stress detection. For each conversation, we returned the stress detection result of each sentence to the user and ask the user to judge whether it is right or not. We used the *precision* and *recall* rate to evaluate the accuracy of stress detection. As Table 2 showed, the detection of stress existence has a good result with the precision rate of 78.34% and recall rate of 76.12%. For the detection of stress category, the recall rate of *affection* and *inter-personal* and the precision rate of *general* are lower than other categories, because some *affection* and *inter-personal* stress are denoted to the *general* stress. Apparently, the stress detection on study, the most common adolescent stress category, has the overall best result with the precision rate of 86.20% and the recall rate of 75.00%.

The effectiveness of stress release. We evaluated the effectiveness of stress release from three aspects:

The evaluation for the releasing effectiveness of each conversation. Users were asked to give a mark (1-5: represent feeling worse, not changed, a bit better, better and much better respectively) to evaluate the stress releasing effectiveness of each conversation. Fig. 5 shows that more than 60% conversations get a score higher than 2, namely, making the user feel better. And *Teenchat* is more effective in releasing study stress because detection result of study has higher accuracy.

The change mode of stressful sentence ratio in a conversation. For each conversation, we equally divided the whole chatting process into three stages (*early*, *middle* and *late*) according to time and computed the ratio of stressful sentences in each stage. Then we analyze the change $Change_n$ from one stage $Ratio_n$ to the next stage $Ratio_{n+1}$($Change_n = (Ratio_{n+1} - Ratio_n)/Ratio_{n+1}$). We consider $Change_n$ within ±10% as stable($\rightarrow$), $Change_n$ more than 10% as ascend($\uparrow$) and $Change_n$ less than −10% as descend($\downarrow$). The first four change modes of stressful sentence ratio in Table 3, denoted by column 2 and column3, mean that *TeenChat* is effective and the next five change modes mean that *TeenChat* is ineffective. As Table 3 showed, column 4 reports the frequency of conversations that satisfy the corresponding change mode and the percentage is shown in column 5. Column 6 and 7 report the sum of frequency and percentage of effective and ineffective conversations respectively.

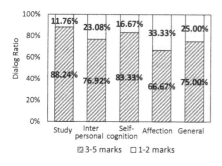

Fig. 5. 5 stress categories mark distribution

Table 2. Accuracy of stress detection

	Precision	Recall
Accuracy of stress existence detection		
Stress	73.15%	63.37%
No stress	83.53%	88.87%
Average	78.34%	76.12%
Accuracy of stress category detection		
Study	86.20%	75.00%
Self-Cognition	93.90%	46.27%
Inter-Personal	53.84%	76.56%
Affection	82.05%	42.60%
General	30.94%	76.92%
Average	69.39%	63.47%

The change of users stress status according to Chinese CPSS. For each user, we asked them to fill the Chinese CPSS questionnaire to record the evolving of their stress status. In the questionnaire, higher score represents heavier stress. We consider that score decreasing means the stress status has been improved, score increasing means the stress status has deteriorated. Table 4 shows that more and more users were feeling better as time goes by.

Table 3. Conversation distribution of the change mode about stressful sentence ratio

Change mode		Freq	Perc	Freq_sum	Perc_sum
Early-Middle	Middle-Late				
↓	↓	17	27.42%		
→	↓	7	11.29%		
↑	↓	8	12.90%	45	72.58%
↓	→	13	20.97%		
↓	↑	7	11.29%		
→	↑	0	0.00%		
→	→	6	9.68%	17	27.42%
↑	→	3	4.84%		
↑	↑	1	1.61%		

Row labels: Effective (first four rows), Ineffective (last five rows).

Table 4. Number of people of 3 kinds of stress status evolving type

	Improved	Not change	Deteriorated	Total
Week 1	2	0	8	10
Week 2	5	1	4	10
Week 3	5	1	4	10
Week 4	7	1	2	10

7   Conclusion

In this paper, we present an intelligent chatting system for sensing and releasing adolescents' stress. First, we built seven stress-related lexicons and used the natural language processing techniques to sense adolescents' stress. Then we designed the response strategies to act like a virtual friend to listen, comfort, encourage and understand the stressful adolescents to help release stress. Our user study showed a good result of *TeenChat* in stress detection and stress release. In our future work, we will make use of abundant resources in social network to improve the response effect, including collecting more answers with higher pertinency and efficiency. Then another direction we will consider is how to further solve the privacy problem of chatting processing.

Acknowledgments. The work is supported by National Natural Science Foundation of China (6137 3022, 61370023, 61073004), and Chinese Major State Basic Research Development 973 Program (2011CB302203-2).

References

1. Augello, A., Saccone, G., Gaglio, S., Pilato, G.: Humorist bot: bringing computational humour in a chat-bot system. In: International Conference on Complex, Intelligent and Software Intensive Systems. CISIS 2008, pp. 703–708. IEEE (2008)

2. Balahur, A., Hermida, J.M.: Affect detection from social contexts using common-sense knowledge representations. In: 2012 International Conference on Privacy, Security, Risk and Trust (PASSAT) and 2012 International Confernece on Social Computing (SocialCom), pp. 884–892. IEEE (2012)

3. Balahur, A., Hermida, J.M., Montoyo, A.: Detecting implicit expressions of sentiment in text based on commonsense knowledge. In: Proceedings of the 2nd Workshop on Computational Approaches to Subjectivity and Sentiment Analysis, pp. 53–60. Association for Computational Linguistics (2011)

4. Brain, S.: Statistic brain (2013). http://www.statisticbrain.com/teen-suicide-statistics/

5. Burke, R.D., Hammond, K.J., Kulyukin, V., Lytinen, S.L., Tomuro, N., Schoenberg, S.: Question answering from frequently asked question files: Experiences with the faq finder system. AI magazine **18**(2), 57 (1997)

6. Chai, J., Lin, J., Zadrozny, W., Ye, Y., Stys-Budzikowska, M., Horvath, V., Kambhatla, N., Wolf, C.: The role of a natural language conversational interface in online sales: A case study. International Journal of Speech Technology **4**(3–4), 285–295 (2001)

7. Che, W., Li, Z., Liu, T.: LTP: a chinese language technology platform. In: Proc. of Coling, pp. 13–16 (2010)

8. Cohen, S., Kamarck, T., Mermelstein, R.: A global measure of perceived stress. Journal of Health and Social Behavior, 385–396 (1983)

9. Colten, M.E., Gore, S.: Adolescent stress: Causes and consequences. Transaction Publishers (1991)

10. Crutzen, R., Peters, G.-J.Y., Portugal, S.D., Fisser, E.M., Grolleman, J.J.: An artificially intelligent chat agent that answers adolescents' questions related to sex, drugs, and alcohol: an exploratory study. Journal of Adolescent Health **48**(5), 514–519 (2011)

11. Fu, X.: xiaohuangji (2010). http://www.xiaohuangji.com/

12. Goh, O.S., Fung, C.C.: Intelligent agent technology in e-commerce. In: Liu, J., Cheung, Y., Yin, H. (eds.) IDEAL 2003. LNCS, vol. 2690, pp. 10–17. Springer, Heidelberg (2003)

13. Hammen, C.: Stress and depression. Annu. Rev. Clin. Psychol. **1**, 293–319 (2005)

14. Kasl, S.V.: Stress and health. Annual review of public health **5**(1), 319–341 (1984)

15. Katz, B., Lin, J.J., Loreto, D., Hildebrandt, W., Bilotti, M.W., Felshin, S., Fernandes, A., Marton, G., Mora, F.: Integrating web-based and corpus-based techniques for question answering. In: TREC, pp. 426–435 (2003)

16. Kerly, A., Hall, P., Bull, S.: Bringing chatbots into education: Towards natural language negotiation of open learner models. Knowledge-Based Systems **20**(2), 177–185 (2007)

17. Lab, M.A.: Start (2002). http://www.ai.mit.edu/projects/infolab/start.html

18. Latham, A., Crockett, K., McLean, D., Edmonds, B.: Adaptive tutoring in an intelligent conversational agent system. In: Nguyen, N.-T. (ed.) Transactions on Computational Collective Intelligence VIII. LNCS, vol. 7430, pp. 148–167. Springer, Heidelberg (2012)

19. Li, B., Liu, T., Qin, B., Li, S.: Chinese sentence similarity computing based on semantic dependency relationship analysis. Application Research of Computers **12**, 15–17 (2003)

20. Lin, H., Jia, J., Guo, Q., Xue, Y., Huang, J., Cai, L., Feng, L.: Psychological stress detection from cross-media microblog data using deep sparse neural network

21. Lin, J., Katz, B.: Question answering from the web using knowledge annotation and knowledge mining techniques. In: Proceedings of the twelfth international conference on Information and knowledge management, pp. 116–123. ACM (2003)
22. Liu, Y., Liu, M., Wang, X., Wang, L., Li, J.: Pal: a chatterbot system for answering domain-specific questions. In: ACL (Conference System Demonstrations), pp. 67–72. Citeseer (2013)
23. Lokman, A.S., Zain, J.M., Komputer, F.S., Perisian, K.: Designing a chatbot for diabetic patients. In: International Conference on Software Engineering & Computer Systems, ICSECS 2009
24. Microdoft: Encarta (2005). http://encarla.msn.com/
25. Moldovan, D.I., Rus, V.: Logic form transformation of wordnet and its applicability to question answering. In: Proceedings of the 39th Annual Meeting on Association for Computational Linguistics, pp. 402–409. Association for Computational Linguistics (2001)
26. Neviarouskaya, A., Prendinger, H., Ishizuka, M.: Textual affect sensing for sociable and expressive online communication. In: Paiva, A.C.R., Prada, R., Picard, R.W. (eds.) ACII 2007. LNCS, vol. 4738, pp. 218–229. Springer, Heidelberg (2007)
27. Olveres, J., Billinghurst, M., Savage, J., Holden, A.: Intelligent, expressive avatars. In: Proceedings of the First Workshop on Embodied Conversational Characters, pp. 47–55 (1998)
28. SIMSIMI: Simsimi (2009). http://www.simsimi.com/
29. Stewart, I.A., File, P.: Let's chat: A conversational dialogue system for second language practice. Computer Assisted Language Learning **20**(2), 97–116 (2007)
30. Subasic, P., Huettner, A.: Affect analysis of text using fuzzy semantic typing. IEEE Transactions on Fuzzy Systems **9**(4), 483–496 (2001)
31. Tapeh, A.G., Rahgozar, M.: A knowledge-based question answering system for b2c ecommerce. Knowledge-Based Systems **21**(8), 946–950 (2008)
32. Teng, Z., Ren, F., Kuroiwa, S.: Recognition of emotion with SVMs. In: Huang, D.-S., Li, K., Irwin, G.W. (eds.) ICIC 2006. LNCS (LNAI), vol. 4114, pp. 701–710. Springer, Heidelberg (2006)
33. Valitutti, A., Strapparava, C., Stock, O.: Developing affective lexical resources. PsychNology Journal **2**(1), 61–83 (2004)
34. Wallace, R.: Alice (2009). http://www.alicebot.org
35. Wang, X., Khoo, E.T., Fu, C.R., Cheok, A.D., Nakatsu, R.: Confucius chat: promoting traditional chinese culture and enhancing intergenerational communication through a chat system. In: 2013 International Conference on Culture and Computing (Culture Computing), pp. 123–128. IEEE (2013)
36. Weizenbaum, J.: Elizaa computer program for the study of natural language communication between man and machine. Communications of the ACM **9**(1), 36–45 (1966)
37. Wills, T.A., McNamara, G., Vaccaro, D.: Parental education related to adolescent stress-coping and substance use: development of a mediational model. Health Psychology **14**(5), 464 (1995)
38. Wu, C.-H., Chuang, Z.-J., Lin, Y.-C.: Emotion recognition from text using semantic labels and separable mixture models. ACM transactions on Asian language information processing (TALIP) **5**(2), 165–183 (2006)
39. Xue, Y., Li, Q., Jin, L., Feng, L., Clifton, D.A., Clifford, G.D.: Detecting adolescent psychological pressures from micro-blog. In: Zhang, Y., Yao, G., He, J., Wang, L., Smalheiser, N.R., Yin, X. (eds.) HIS 2014. LNCS, vol. 8423, pp. 83–94. Springer, Heidelberg (2014)

40. Yang, C., Lin, K.H., Chen, H.-H.: Emotion classification using web blog corpora. In: IEEE/WIC/ACM International Conference on Web Intelligence, pp. 275–278. IEEE (2007)
41. Zakos, J., Capper, L.: CLIVE – an artificially intelligent chat robot for conversational language practice. In: Darzentas, J., Vouros, G.A., Vosinakis, S., Arnellos, A. (eds.) SETN 2008. LNCS (LNAI), vol. 5138, pp. 437–442. Springer, Heidelberg (2008)

Ethical Quality in eHealth:
A Challenge with Many Facets

Marjo Rissanen[✉]

Aalto University School of Science, Espoo, Finland
`mkrissan@gmail.com`

Abstract. In eHealth, ethical quality refers to several other quality attributes. Understanding its versatile nature helps designers consider ethical requirements better in design processes. This can change the nature of a design process in a more pragmatic direction enhancing this way the total quality of products and services. The significance of ethical quality in eHealth increases also because the nature of given services changes rapidly. The growing number of distance-based services is one example. In the study, theoretical frames for design are considered in terms of ethical quality with a content analytical approach.

Keywords: eHealth · Ethical quality · Theoretical frames of design

1   Introduction

Ethical quality in eHealth projects has a significant role. There are many ethical codes for the eHealth area. These codes reflect different aspects of quality. Ethical quality attributes reflect customer, product, and process quality issues. In addition, ethical quality affects efficiency, image tasks, and broader societal issues. When the versatile essence of ethical quality is in focus more intensively, its control and management in eHealth projects may have a more pragmatic nature.

Many eHealth services are typical for applications of distance education and consumer support (e.g., applications for self-health management). Thus, e.g., many customer-targeted eHealth applications serve a venue for interactive knowledge processing between customers and health professionals without the need for clinic appointments. The question is not only about educational aspects but also about distance operational protocols. This fact also increases the demand level of many applications and not least in the ethical sense.

The study focused on the content and meaning of ethical quality in eHealth and its connection to other quality attributes. When ethical requirements are considered in the context of common quality facets, a wider perspective on ethical quality can be reached in the eHealth area. As well, aspects which are somehow hidden can be realized as ethical parameters more easily.

2   Methods

The theme area is examined by literature review which covered articles from areas of eHealth ethics, quality management, and eHealth design. Findings are considered with

© Springer International Publishing Switzerland 2015
X. Yin et al. (Eds.): HIS 2015, LNCS 9085, pp. 146–153, 2015.
DOI: 10.1007/978-3-319-19156-0_15

critical and content analytical approach. The study represents design science and concentrated on quality theoretical frames of design in eHealth. The role and meaning of ethical quality in eHealth in this frame combination formed the research focus. Quality theoretical considerations in general form an essential frame area of theoretical problem analysis in eHealth design.

3   eHealth Innovations and Ethics

Designing innovations in eHealth requires thinking about quality, which considers quality attributes and especially ethical aspects from view of versatile quality. Sophisticated evaluation is necessary for successful eHealth [1]. Ethical requirements must be considered when the first design ideas occur during the product planning phase [2]. Ethical acceptability of innovations means an always distinctive rule: If the idea in question is ethically acceptable and reasonable sustainability is predictable, then the continuous development and generation of the idea is meaningful. However, ethically non-acceptable ideas should be rejected during the idea phase or reconsidered and developed so they are ethically acceptable. This ethical evaluation is a process that might require a team with ethical expertise to define the potential of the presented product ideas even in the early developmental idea phase. If this early ethical evaluation is neglected, many resources are used perhaps in vain. Ethical quality today forms a more important aspect in eHealth design policy. When the product reflects innovation quality in eHealth area, its importance is understandable and its principle in balance with ethical requirements and therefore innovativeness and innovation quality are not equal concepts in this area [2]. However, ethical acceptability of eHealth products means in many cases maturation and validation iterations.

4   Ethical Codes and Emphasized Ethical Attributes

There are several ethical codes for eHealth. The foundation for ethical eHealth codes comes partially from the four principles approach for biomedical ethics [3]. The collection of ethical principles of the European Group on Ethics in Science and New Technologies (EGE) [4], [5] also forms the foundation for this theme area. This list contains the following aspects: respect for privacy and for the security of personal health data, confidentiality, trustworthiness, legitimacy, patient's informed consent for data use, transparency of standards, and patient access to electronic health records (EHRs). In principle, the same attributes get attention in most of the codes. However, some aspects are differently emphasized, and some aspects are unique. The Internet Healthcare Coalition (IHC) [6] emphasizes principles such as candor and trustworthiness, quality of the medical information content and services, informed consent, privacy and confidentiality, and high-quality commercial and professional practices. Quality, efficiency, education, and individualized care are the main ethical issues in the URAC Accreditation Guide (URAC) [7]. The HONcode covers authoritativeness, complementarity, privacy, attribution, justifiability, transparency, financial disclosure, and sponsorship [8] and was generated as an internal process in consultation with webmasters, information providers, and health consumers [9]. The principles of the Hi-Ethics Coalition contain the same attributes and also pay attention to consumer feedback (consumers' ability to evaluate the quality of the information), professionalism, data protection, and third party rating systems [9], [10]. eHealth Code of Ethics (eHealth) [6] emphasizes synergy creation among different entities, data quality and protection, self-evaluation, consumer and provider education [9]. Content, privacy, confidentiality, E-commerce, advertising, and sponsorship are underlined in the code of the American Medical Association (AMA) [9], [11], and broader consumer education and co-operative evaluation are mentioned in the European Union (EU) Action Plan (MedCERTAIN) [9], [10]. Anonymity requirement is emphasized in ISO/IEC (15408) [12] standard. There are also ethical issues addressing eHealth cloud management and computing.

Ethical attributes are also summarized and grouped into fewer categories. For example, Khoja et al. [13] collected and listed ethical and legal issues in their structured literature review. This list contains the following issues: management of health information on the Internet, health information privacy, consent for care in eHealth, medical malpractice liability, patient's right to access information, security of information during portability, control of malpractice, and cultural issues in communication. Miesperä et al. [14] collected features from this substance area in their literature review in six main areas: attributes of autonomy, privacy, confidentiality, consent, equality of service availability, and beneficence.

5   Ethical Quality and Its Reflect the Other Quality Dimensions

5.1   Pondering Ethics and Customer Quality

In general, customer quality refers to aspects that are important for consumers. Customer values also mean a more competitive advantage [15]. The recognized ethical dimensions refer in the first place to customer quality. The quality of the information content, accessibility, anonymity, respect for autonomy, discrimination, free and informed consent, justice, privacy and data protection, and safety represent all also customers' interests.

Customer activity and customer consideration form an area which is tried to support intensively with new eHealth innovations. In addition, customers' ideas may represent remarkable innovation [16], which may be valuable in new areas. The problem is that customers' opinions are heard typically when new products are at hand and when the first versions are tested or when the new products are in the market. When cost-intensive projects are planned which change service protocols in a remarkable way, it is reasonable to secure channels for the "customers' voice" and widen in this way also customers' rights. In this way, consumers have a greater role in evaluating new plans and ideas or give feedback when new products are planned for managing consumers' health, for example [2]. Consumers' role as an inspirational source for new products is therefore typically nowadays too limited. Often, there are not open and flexible channels where consumers can provide wishes and ideas freely to organizations and health policy designers or product designers. When the target is to reach the best professional practices, consumers' ideas about these processes should have a greater role. However, also customers' ideas and desires need their ethical evaluation iterations. Which ideas and desires are ethically acceptable, worthy, and possible to realize, and what are the wider reflections on society and the healthcare system?

Customers should also have rights in terms of options. Innovations in eHealth area change the healthcare system in many ways, but are all changes useful for or rewarding to all customers and aligned with their values? Acceptability must take place also at the individual level.

5.2   Ethics and Its Requirements for Product and Process Quality

All aspects that refer to customers' rights and requirements in the ethical sense are naturally challenges for production and product quality and form the essential focus when ethical principles are introduced into the design and design policy. In addition, the guidelines design and production line must develop self-evaluative protocols that guarantee that given requirements will be considered. In common quality terminology product quality refers to product features, performance, and perceived quality [17]. Production quality refers to design process and its evaluative protocols [18]. Beneficence and nonmaleficence means that "the eHealth tool should perform in a way that benefits the user" without causing harm [19]. This requirement refers to customer quality, but also represents challenges for production and process quality. This requires that production policy is controlled, and the quality of a product is evaluated in a versatile way. Product quality and ethical quality are not separate aspects. Content quality e.g., is also an ethical task. It is customers' right that the knowledge offered is trustable and right. Also, quality evaluation in this area is not a straightforward task; e.g., "quality remains an inherently subjective assessment, which depends on the type of information needed, the type of information searched for, and the particular qualities and prejudices of the consumer" [20].

Connected processes for system use must as well be carefully designed, controlled, followed, and evaluated. It is not enough that the product contains all given ethical requirements. The product must be evaluated in its use context, which includes connected processes. Thus, the purpose is to evaluate how well this product-process combination finally fulfills given ethical requirements and could serve customers' needs. The term dignity is often used when "the rights of elderly people" [19] are in question. Customer dignity is a principle which should be underlined in all design plans in this area. The product, connected processes, and customers form an entity and a chain that should be evaluated with deep enough sensitivity what comes to given ethical requirements. Beneficial products and services require attention to the process, product, and customer quality categories. Does the product deploy ethical principles, do the connected processes support these ideas, and are customers' reactions and ideas heard in a sensitive manner? Hence, novel products may be innovative in this area, but if they miss an ethical acceptability or when innovativeness is connected only with the technology change without real benefits, innovation quality is then questionable [2].

5.3   Ethics and Image Issues

Image is a product of communication, marketing, and production. Product image has a remarkable effect on consumer behavior [21] and innovation diffusion [22] and thus has an effect on a product's success in the market. The product image should be re-evaluated when allocation decisions are in question just to prevent too straightforward and unconsidered decisions in product procurement policy. Ethical quality in eHealth emphasizes "beneficence." However, "evidence for the beneficial impact of many eHealth technologies is still absent or at best only modest" [23]. Thus, image evaluation is a part of the ethical quality process. Evidence of trustworthiness does not mean only risk and performance of the system but also contains interactional and context-based information [24].

5.4   Ethical Issues and Efficiency

Resource allocation as an ethical task has also raised discussion in eHealth. Health consumers should have the opportunity to use online health services safely and effectively [25], and "public resources should be used fairly and efficiently" [26]. Public resources must be used in a way that produces a good return on investment (ROI). Thus, ethical considerations that are linked to cost intensity should take place when cost-intensive development projects are planned or when such allocations are funded with public resources. The question involves evaluation of alternative costs and fairness in prioritizing: How to allocate limited resources? Which development projects must be prioritized? In the health area, estimates and scenario planning that try to predict future trends in cost-intensive IT projects are usually demanding. Thus, eHealth technologies should be evaluated with a comprehensive set of measures [23]. These evaluations are part of the ethical quality process and its evaluation. Priority policy in health sector should be justified. Therefore, the questions of service intensity and option policy in healthcare are also questions of ethical nature. Which amount of service capacity will produce high-quality services in each area, and how can eHealth strategies help guarantee optimal care intensity?

5.5   Ethical Issues and Mission Fitness

Every eHealth project and product has an intended mission, and this mission must be transparent and obvious to the focus organization. Transparent and obvious mission means that mission clarity is acquired. If design ideology produces products that are aligned with the organization's values and mission statements, then mission fitness can be acquired [27]. However, this is not enough.

"Values have always implicitly driven the decisions of the organization" [28]. Mission statements for IT policy and IT products in eHealth must follow ethically acceptable values. This value filtering needs continuous evaluation; are these controlling values sustainable and acceptable? Thus, in this area mission formulation in organizations and in IT companies must recognize mission strategic considerations as tasks that are closely connected to ethical issues. In addition, this acceptability must be evaluated from the perspective of customers and their rights, by understanding the requirements of the product and process quality, and the economic consequences and societal impact. Only if mission statements are formulated by following truly ethical and quality requirements widely can we speak about acceptable mission quality. Table 1 shows the connection between quality areas and ethical principles.

Table 1. Quality Areas and Connected Ethical Principles in eHealth Area

Quality facet	Ethical core principles
Mission	Equality of availability, High-quality products and processes following ethical principles
Customer	Perceived: autonomy, privacy, confidentiality, service availability beneficence, consent
Product	High-quality products deploying given ethical requirements
Process	High-quality processes supporting given ethical requirements
Production	Production & maturation policy following given ethical guidelines
Efficiency	Cost-effective services and justified priority policy
Innovation	Innovation quality in balance with ethical requirements
Image	Trustworthiness in communication policy, image evaluation

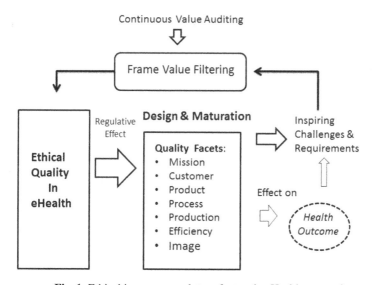

Fig. 1. Ethical issues as regulatory factors in eHealth maturation

6   Discussion and Conclusions

Ethical quality affects other quality attributes. However, this reflection means a two-way effect. As well, it is useful to concentrate on separate quality areas and to identify those requirements which are closely connected to ethical aspects. Usefulness and safety are attributes of product quality but as well challenges for ethical design. Service satisfaction refers to customer quality but is as well a challenge in ethical sense. Trust is associated as a product quality and an image quality factor but forms also an ethical requirement. In this way also separate quality areas form inspirational and iterative source for ethical considerations. New, identified requirements e.g., of customer quality need consideration of connected ethical aspects and in this way connect with ethical scheme (see Fig. 1). Understanding the versatile nature of ethical quality is essential. It helps designers understand and integrate ethical requirements better in a design process. This can change the nature of a design process in a more pragmatic direction. Evaluating also process outcome [29] is essential in eHealth. New innovations need evaluation in sense what are their social influence and reflections to the whole health care infrastructure. High value for patients should mean improved outcomes and good health [30]. Product maturation and validation means in eHealth area iterative production cycles. Development and research means typically continuous cycles of design, enactment, evaluation, and redesign [31] and this affects also maturation procedures which concern ethical acceptability of eHealth products.

The significance of ethical quality in eHealth grows all the time because eHealth innovations get more features and change their nature. For example, when eHealth services are distance based, issues of security play an important role. If the deep connection between ethical quality and other quality attributes is realized and considered in a design process, more quality for products and services can be embedded. One target of ethical quality is to produce the best professional practices. However, there is also evidence that in eHealth "best practice guidelines in effective development and deployment strategies are lacking" [23]. Consequently, if ethical quality requirements are approached by integrating ethical requirements and their reflections in all relevant quality areas and by understanding also the complexity of this challenging area, then more pragmatic design guidelines can be expected. Beside general guidelines also project based considerations are necessary.

References

1. Ammenwerth, E., Aarts, J., Berghold, A., Beuscart-Zephir, M.C., Brender, J., et al.: Declaration of Innsbruck. Results from the European Science Foundation Sponsored Workshop on Systematic Evaluation of Health Information Systems (HIS-EVAL). Methods Inf. Med. 1(45), 121–123 (2006). Supplement 1
2. Rissanen, M.: Prioritizing quality attributes in eHealth design. Leading transformation to sustainable excellence. 7th quality conference in the middle east. In: Proceedings of the Dubai 2014, pp. 133-142 (2014)
3. Beauchamp, T.L., Childress, J.F.: Principles of Biomedical Ethics, 5th edn. Oxford University Press, New York (2001)
4. European Commission. Opinion of the European Group on Ethics in Science and New Technologies. Ethical issues of healthcare in the information society, 13 (1999). http://ec.europa.eu/bepa/european-group-ethics/docs/avis13_en.pdf
5. European Commission. Press release of the European Commission Secretariat-General Directorate C, Secretariat of the European Group on Ethics in Science and New Technologies. http://ec.europa.eu/bepa/european-group-ethics/docs/cp13_en.pdf
6. California health care foundation. In: Proceed with Caution: A Report on the Quality of Health Information on the Internet Complete Study. http://www.chcf.org/~/media/MEDIA%20LIBRARY%20Files/PDF/P/PDF%20ProceedWithCautionCompleteStudy.pdf
7. Utilization Review Certification Commission. Health Web Site Accreditation Guide, Version 3.0. http://www.urac.org/docs/programs/URACHW2.1factsheet.pdf

8. Health On the Net Foundation. Certification Process. http://www.hon.ch/HONcode/Webmasters/StepByStep/StepByStep.html

9. Risk, A., Dzenowagis, J.: Review of Internet Health Information Quality Initiatives. J. Med. Int. Res. **3**(4), e28 (2001)

10. Coiera, E.: Information Epidemics, Economics, and Immunity on the Internet. We Still Know so Little about the Effect of Information on Public Health. Brit. Med. J. **317**, 1469 (1998)

11. Winker, M., Flanagin, A., Chi-Lum, B., White, J., Andrews, K., Kennett, R., DeAngelis, C., Musacchio, R.: Guideline for Medical and Health Information Sites on the Internet. J. Am. Med. Assoc. **283**(12), 1600–1606 (2000)

12. ISO/IEC Standard 15408 (2009)

13. Khoja, S., Durrani, H., Nayani, P., Fahim, A.: Scope of Policy Issues in eHealth: Results from a Structured Literature Review. J. Med. Internet Res. **14**(1), e34 (2012)

14. Miesperä, A., Ahonen, S.M., Reponen, J.: Ethical Aspects of eHealth- systematic Review of Open Access Articles. Fin. J. eHealth eWelfare. **5**(4), 165–171 (2013)

15. Poter, M.: Competitive Advantage. Huaxia, Beijing (1998)

16. Magnusson, P., Matthing, J., Kristensson, P.: Managing User Involvement in Service Innovation: Experiments with Innovating End Users. J. Serv. Res. **6**(2), 111–124 (2003)

17. Tenner, A., DeToro I.: Total Quality Management. Three Steps for Continuous Improvement. Addison-Wesley, Reading (1992)

18. ISO 9001: Quality Management Guidelines (2008)

19. Wadhwa, K., Wright, D.: eHealth: frameworks for assessing ethical impacts. In: George, C., Whitehouse, D., Duquenoy, P. (eds.) Legal, Ethical and Governance Challenges, pp. 183–201. Springer, Berlin (2013)

20. Wilson, P.: How to Find the Good and Avoid the Bad or Ugly: a Short Guide to Tools for Rating Quality of Health Information on the Internet. BMJ. **324**(9), 598–600 (2002)

21. Quester, P., Karunaratna, A., Goh, L.: Self-congruity and Product Evaluation: A Cross-cultural Study. J. Consumer Marketing. **17**(6), 525–535 (2000)

22. Moore, G., Benbasat, I.: Development of an Instrument to Measure the Perceptions of Adoption and Information Technology Innovation. Information Systems Research. **2**(3), 192–222 (1991)

23. Black, A., Car, J., Pagliari, C., Anandan, C., et al.: The Impact of eHealth on the Quality and Safety of Health Care: a Systematic Overview. PLOS Med. **8**, e1000387 (2011)

24. Nickel, P.: Ethics in e-Trust and e-Trustworthiness: The Case of Direct Computer-Patient Interfaces. Ethics Inf. Tech. **13**, 355–363 (2011)

25. Nuffield Council of Bioethics (2010)

26. Hood, C., Bougourd, S.: The Ethics of e-Health. Int. J. E-Health Med. Commun. **2**(2), 82–85 (2011)

27. Rissanen, M.: Machine Beauty – Should It Inspire eHealth Designers? In: Zhang, Y., Yao, G., He, J., Wang, L., Smalheiser, N.R., Yin, X. (eds.) HIS 2014. LNCS, vol. 8423, pp. 1–11. Springer, Heidelberg (2014)

28. Sapienza, A.: Creating Technology Strategies. How to Build Competitive Biomedical R&D. Wiley-Liss, New York (1997)

29. Donabedian, A.: An introduction to Quality Assurance in Health Care. Oxford University Press (2002)

30. Porter, M.: A strategy for health care reform- Toward a Value-based System. The New England Journal of Medicine. **361**, 109–112 (2009)

31. Design-Based Research Collective.: Design-based Research: An Emerging Paradigm for Educational Enquiry. Educational Researcher **32**(1), 5–8 (2003)

Experiences in Developing and Testing an Ambient Assisted Living Course for Further Education

Ilvio Bruder[1]([✉]), Andreas Heuer[1], Thomas Karopka[2], Juliane Schuldt[3], and Kerstin Kosche[3]

[1] Database Research Group, University of Rostock, Rostock, Germany
ilvio.bruder@uni-rostock.de
[2] BioCon Valley GmbH Greifswald, Greifswald, Germany
[3] Further Education, University of Rostock, Rostock, Germany

Abstract. There is a growing market for elderly care and assisted living. This trend is followed by a need for experts and professionals in health care and assistive technology. To target this need, the University of Rostock established a further education program for Ambient Assisted Living. The program consists of three courses and addresses the topics: 'information and communication technologies', 'ethics and law', 'consulting and communication' as well as 'assistive technology' in electronic health care. The courses are student-centered and especially designed for heterogeneous groups. The participants also get the opportunity to test currently available assisted living and e-health products.

This paper presents the concepts and experiences establishing these courses and focuses on technical aspects of the curriculum.

1 Introduction

The market of e-health solutions, e.g. fall detection and telemedicine, is growing and arouses more and more the interest of the mainstream society. However, complex concepts like Ambient Assisted Living (AAL) are discussed mainly among experts. For example, many people in health care do not know what e-health and AAL stands for. On the one hand, there are many interesting technical solutions (research prototypes as well as market-ready products). On the other hand, there are very few people who have an overview over the problems in e-health and who can apply an e-health solution for a given problem. The question is, how to apply the good solutions to the people who need those.

The University of Rostock established a further education program for AAL. In this course, managers in health care, caregivers, managers in the housing industry, decision makers, engineers and developers learn what the complex concept of AAL stands for. They discuss AAL as a socio-technical concept, which combines technical systems, social contact and service to support elderly people in their daily life at home. This further education program is composed of three extra-occupational certificate courses, each with a time frame of three months.

X. Yin et al. (Eds.): HIS 2015, LNCS 9085, pp. 154–164, 2015.
DOI: 10.1007/978-3-319-19156-0_16

The program was offered as a test for the first time in 2013. One year later the revised and optimized program took place. More than 40 people participated in the test program.

There are already graduate and postgraduate courses at universities: e.g. Assistive Technology MSc at the Coventry University or Ambient Assisted Living Courses at the Karlsruhe Institute of Technology and the University of Applied Sciences Krnten. These courses are integrated in regular master's degrees or in the context of education in the area of supporting people with disabilities. There are less initiatives trying to combine academic education and further education in the area of AAL.

First of all, the term Ambient Assisted Living (AAL) has to be defined. It is a term primarily used in Europe for initiatives for project funding in the European Union as well as national fundings in Germany and other european countries in the area of e-health, telemedicine, and elderly care (see also the web site of the EU AAL programme of the AAL Association [1]). Internationally, this topic is well known as assisted living and elderly care. Assistive technology is another term in this context. A possible taxonomy is declared in [2]. The classification of assistive technology in a broader sense is referred to [2]. AAL comprise not only technical but also medical, ethical and social, as well as legal aspects. Therefore, AAL projects are usually interdisciplinary. A good overview of the many aspects to be concerned is described in [4] with special attention on usability and psychological aspects.

With the project BAAL[1], funded by the German Federal Ministry of Education and Research, the University of Rostock extended their program of further education to the topic of Ambient Assisted Living. In this project an educational concept for an AAL program was developed. The program consists of three courses: (1) "Introduction to AAL", (2) "Ethics and Law in AAL", (3) "Consulting and Communication in AAL". There were two phases of course development in the project: a trial phase with a first time test of the courses and an evaluation phase with a second test of the courses using revised and restructured editions of curriculum and course material.

After the end of the BAAL project, the University of Rostock will offer these AAL courses regularly.

In the following, this paper presents the course concept and experiences. After a more detailed discussion of the target group (section 2), teaching approach and curriculum are presented in section 3. The realization of the trial phase is described in section 4.

2   Target Group and Educational Demand

The basis for participant-orientated educational offers is a profound identification of the educational demands of the target group.

Firstly, the target group has to be identified. At the beginning of the BAAL project, two main target groups were identified: on the one hand, managers in

---

[1] BAAL stands for Further Education in Ambient Assisted Living in German.

health care and caregivers; on the other hand engineers and technical staff who are involved in the development and distribution of AAL products. Later on, the course concept was opened for managers in the housing industry, designers and other professions which are involved in the development and implementation of AAL systems and concepts.

Secondly, the educational demands of the target group have to be analyzed and documented. Main results of this analysis were the need for a general overview over currently available AAL systems, the demand to gain insight into research in the field of AAL and to learn how to plan, implement and finance a complex AAL system.

Thirdly, educational objectives are determined. After finishing the program, participants should be able to plan and accompany the design and implementation of a complex AAL system for a specific demand, e.g. in private homes for elderly people or in residential care homes. Therefore, they need to understand the general technical functionality and the social dimension of an AAL system. They should be aware of ethical and legal aspects which come along with the implementation of AAL systems. And, not least, they should be able to find and discuss AAL solutions in interdisciplinary teams.

Fourthly, contents and didactic methods are chosen to meet the educational objectives. Didactic methods, used in the AAL program, supported the exchange of ideas between different professions and enable the participants to find multi-perspective solutions.

3   Teaching Approach

The AAL program is divided into three courses:

1. Course One: "Introduction to AAL"
   In this course, participants get an overview of AAL as a complex socio-technical concept to support mostly elderly people in their daily life at home. Participants learn how to plan, finance and implement AAL systems for special demands. They learn to understand the general technical functionality of AAL systems and get an insight into research and development of assistive technologies.
2. Course Two: "Ethics and Law in AAL"
   In this course, participants analyze and discuss the usage of assistive technologies from ethical and legal points of view. After finishing the course, they should be able to design projects regarding ethical and legal aspects and to advise users and organizations on ethical and legal aspects concerning AAL.
3. Course Three: "Consulting and Communication in AAL"
   In this course, participants learn how to communicate to different target groups of AAL, e.g. private customers and organizations in health care. They also learn how to advise on AAL in different situations and constellations. Participants practice their communicational skills and develop appropriate consulting schemes.

3.1 Teaching Technical Aspects for People Without a Technical Background

In the following, we want to focus on how technical aspects of assistive technologies are taught to people, who mostly have no technical background. The technical functionality of assistive technologies is part of the first course, "Introduction to AAL" [3]. This course is divided into a phase of self-study, two classroom seminars and exercises. The participants get learning material, consisting of didactically arranged texts, videos and internet resources.

In the first classroom seminar, concepts of technical systems are presented from an user's point of view as well as from a developer's point of view.

Initially, the participants are asked to complete the following sentence: "Technical products and systems disturb me if ...". No matter which professional background they have, all participants can answer this question. The answers are hints for attitudes and prejudices concerning assistive technologies. Later on, the participants are asked to describe, how technical products and systems have to be made to be really supportive. These thoughts are the basis for judging currently available products and systems in the field of AAL.

The participants do not only discuss these products, they can lay hands on them. In a so called show flat, they can see how fall detection works in a private setting and how smart a flat can be made today.

After visiting the show flat, they are invited into a smart laboratory at the University of Rostock, in which scientists and developers give an insight into research and new ideas of supporting people in their everyday life.

Having both experiences in mind, the visit of the show flat and the visit of the smart laboratory, the participants are divided into multi-professional groups. By using their individual professional perspective, they identify actual demands in supporting elderly people. They think about own designs and constellations for AAL systems, how to finance them and, finally, they reflect their solutions in terms of technical practicality and desirability. Some results of this group exercise are given in section 4.

The educational objectives of the course are:

- The participants know, which kind of products are currently available and which general ideas are matters of research.
- The participants understand, how assistive technology works in general.
- The Participants are able to judge, which kind of assistive technology is appropriate for which demand.
- The participants are able to use and consider different perspectives in planning an AAL concept.
- The participants are motivated to learn more about technical and social issues of assistive technologies and to join the public discourse on AAL.

After finishing the course, participants should be able to answer the following questions:

- *Question 1: What is assistive technology?*
  The term assistive technology is introduced from a technical point of view and is discussed in conjunction with the next question.
- *Question 2: What is "Ambient Assisted Living" (AAL)?*
  Ambient Assisted Living is assistive technology, which helps people managing their everyday life. The main objective is extending the time people can live in their preferred environment by increasing their autonomy, self-confidence and mobility. Examples for such supporting systems are fall detection systems, detection systems for water or fire damage, and cooperative devices like a doorbell which transmit the signal to the electric lighting or to the television.
- *Question 3: Which concepts are possible and reasonable realizing a fall detection?*
  Fall detection is used as an example for technical systems in health care with a couple of different solution approaches. Fall detection is possible using sensor technique on the body (e.g. acceleration sensors), using sensors integrated in the environment (e.g. intelligent carpet), and using a camera-based analysis.
- *Question 4: To what extent is there a Big Brother effect of sensor based assistive technology?*
  Sensor technology is always a kind of observation. Sensors are necessary for automatically recognizing situations, activities, and intentions. Sensor data are necessary to achieve the assistance objectives, but should be minimally used and stored (a.k.a. data avoidance or data minimization).
- *Question 5: Does a person using an electronic patient record become a transparent patient, i.e. someone who has lost his privacy? Which technical possibilities are available to avoid this?*
  There are other privacy compromising systems in daily life, for instance mobile phones or cars. An observation is possible much more extensively. However, assistive technology should be developed, that data is processed as near as possible at the person or sensor concerned. Only the bare minimum of data (the data needed to achieve the assistance objective) should leave the personal environment.

The course uses many examples in pictures and videos to describe assistance systems and their properties and capabilities. For explaining assistive technology to people without technical background, a layered architecture is used. The elementary architecture of an assistance system is described in Fig. 1. The five layers are from the bottom up:

1. Sensor technology and positioning
   There are many different and very small sensors which are integrated in many common devices, such as a positioning sensor in every smart phone.
2. Heterogeneous integration, spontaneous appliance cooperation
   Devices have to be connected for sharing their data and information. Most device cooperations are predefined today. In the future devices will be probably cooperated spontaneously.

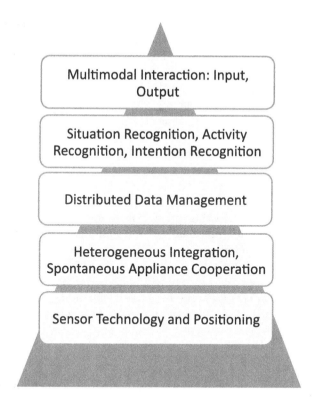

Fig. 1. Architecture Overview of an Assistance System

3. Distributed data management
   For an intelligent environment, it is necessary to join and manage data. Otherwise, data should be evaluated at the device where the data are collected. This is especially important for the protection of data privacy.
4. Situation recognition, activity recognition, intention recognition
   The recognition of situations, activities and user intentions is a difficult task for computers and works only in simple cases. This is currently a very active research area.
5. Multimodal interaction: input, output
   The output possibilities are very diverse. For user input, the recognition of speech, gestures, and facial expression may be important in the future.

For most of the participants in the AAL program, technical architectures like these are uncommon and not easy to understand. Therefore, everyday situations are used to illustrate the meaning behind the scheme.

One example to explain the architecture is a parking assistant. The positioning (lowermost layer in Fig. 1) is realized by distance sensors integrated in the bumper. Heterogeneous devices have to be interconnected (in the next layer): the sensors, the gear shift, the car radio and others. The data of these devices have to be integrated (in the distributed data management layer). Recognizing the situation and the driver's intention: the driver puts in the reverse gear, so the driver possibly wants to park back-in. The interaction with the user, i.e. driver (top layer in the architecture Fig. 1) is done using the car radio. The output is commonly a beep with changing intervals.

Another example is used for explaining the current limits of modern robotics. The limits of robotics in aiding humans can be demonstrated by comparing a human world championship football match and a robotic world championship football match using video recordings.

3.2   Special Issues

The special problem of protecting privacy is widely discussed in the course. Privacy and the right of informational self-determination are important aspects in data management in Germany and is legally protected. In the context of assisted living, there is a correlation between assistance functionality and privacy. In simple terms, the more assistance functionality is provided, the more privacy is lost. Privacy awareness is an absolute necessity for AAL experts.

The importance of privacy in designing AAL products arose in a usability test at the RWTH Aachen University [8], too.

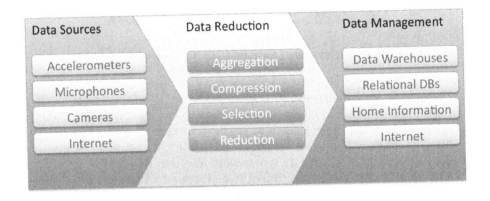

Fig. 2. Data Workflow in Assistance Systems

The possibilities designing AAL technology with decreased or minimized impact in losing privacy are explained using the data workflow in Fig. 2. On the left side, the data sources like sensors and cameras are depicted. On the right side, the handling, processing and analyzing as well as mining of interesting data using data warehouses, databases, and data mining tools are illustrated. Privacy-relevant data are collected at the sensors, cameras etc. and the loss of privacy happens during processing, analyzing and presentation of data at the latest. The collecting of data is possibly acceptable, if only the absolute relevant data is collected and data is immediately deleted after processing (also known as "process and forget"). The data should be processed and forgotten as fast as possible. The best approach would be if the data never leave the sensor. Shrinking the amount of data leaving the private environment, there are operations current systems can handle, such as selection and aggregation of data (the middle column of Fig. 2).

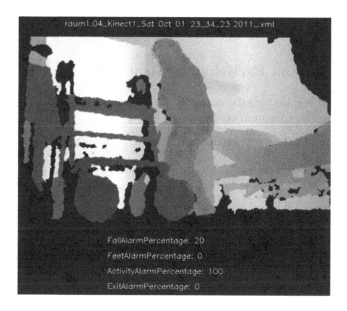

Fig. 3. How private is this data? Fall detection using depth maps colored from white (far) to black (near) with the person subsequently blue-colored

The question, which data are possibly privacy-relevant, leads usually to a controversial discussion. In the course, an example of an AAL project concerning fall detection is used to illustrate relevant questions. The project, which was realized by the University of Rostock and partners [5] uses a camera for fall detection. The participants are asked to discuss and evaluate the used technique. Fall detection is a good example to show problems in weighing up the advantages and disadvantages of an AAL solution. There are different solutions with different properties regarding limitations in user's mobility, privacy, user compliance, environment integration and reliability.

Participants usually discuss the following aspects:

– At which degree of fall endangering should the mobility of a person be observed or limited using an AAL solution?
– Is the fall detection suitable for a particular person? For instance, a wearable sensor may not be a good choice due to problems with compliance or unawares take off.

– Does the AAL solution provide the needed level of privacy? Especially, camera-based systems produce undesirable images and videos (e.g. depth maps in Fig. 3).

Fig. 3 shows an image of a depth map of an elderly resident

Exercising the exploration and evaluation of AAL technology, the participants should decide autonomous and independently: Is assisted living already reality or still vision from research. For this purpose, the participants have to develop an AAL solution for an own example mostly taken from their working environment.

4   Scenarios and Participants' Reactions

Before the first seminar starts, participants are asked about their expectations on an AAL course. Common answers are:

– Understanding the functionality of assistive technology and evaluating the benefits of such systems.
– Knowing what AAL costs and how to finance AAL systems
– Presentation, classification, and evaluation of systems regarding ethical aspects.
– Declarations on general legal conditions
– Information about available AAL solutions
– Learning how to develop concepts for AAL projects regarding own interests within the course.
– Exchanging experiences with other professions, learning more about other perspectives on AAL

After finishing the course, participants should be able to plan their own AAL concept. For deepening their understanding of technical principles, the participants were asked to develop AAL solutions in multi-professional groups. The participants have to develop the scenarios by describing the layers of the AAL reference architecture in Fig. 1. The scenarios are the results of brainstorming in the groups. Later on, they were discussed in terms of technical practicability, desirability, as well as ethical and legal aspects and user compliance. The following three examples illustrate what kind of systems they have in mind.

First idea of an AAL scenario is called "Communication against Isolation"
It is about a home information base for elderly with special needs, e.g. limited mobility.

System properties and developing thoughts are:

– Information should be viewable on television or on tablet computer
– using both devices as communication center and for video chats
– using speech interface for home control
– using always-on cameras and microphones in a Home Media Server environment
– charging the tablet computer by a cradle or a mat for induction charging

Second scenario idea: "Bedridden Person"
Bedridden persons often have decubitus problems. An automatic system of sensors and actuating elements integrated in a mattress or mattress cover should help to avoid decubitus.

System properties and developing thoughts are:

- Recognizing decubitus using pressure sensors in a mattress cover is better than using sensors for blood flow in the clothes is better than camera-based recognition of decubitus
- Actuating elements control the mattress achieving a pressure release
- Further procedures: Informing or alerting a care service
- Integration with vital signs using sensors in a bracelet or in clothes or in the mattress

Third scenario idea: "Shower Assistant"
Bathroom accidents and injuries are very common. A helping hand for washing and drying off someone is developed in this scenario.

System properties and developing thoughts are:

- Precondition: a seat in the shower
- Sensor system: camera, microphone for speech control, infrared sensors in shower
- Actuating elements: for controlling Water flow and temperature, automatic shower gel dispenser, handing towels, automatic hair blower, handing new clothes
- The shower assistant is not suitable for persons with a high care level. Otherwise, the system may be possible as a support for a nurse washing a patient, too.

The raised ethical aspects are further discussed in the next course "Ethics and Law in AAL".

After the courses, the participants were requested to answer questions about the courses, the lecturers, the organization, the material, and the personal conclusion. Positive aspects were the engagement of the lecturers and organizers and the outcome for the participants. After the first trial of the courses, the study material was evaluated negatively. The explanations in the study material were too technically-oriented for most of the participants. These parts of the study material have been revised for the second course.

5   Conclusions

This paper describes experiences in designing, realizing and establishing a further education course for Ambient Assisted Living. The course was developed within the project BAAL funded by an initiative of the German Federal Ministry of Education and Research for developing and establishing education concepts for AAL. The paper is focused on how technical aspects of AAL can be taught for a target group without a technical background. Basis for the development of such a course is a profound analysis of educational demands, which include the target groups ability to understand technical principles and connect them to their professional knowledge in fields like health care system and housing industry.

Lessons learned: People without a technical background want to connect new knowledge in technical fields to their everyday life experience and their professional knowledge. The participant?s different perspectives on technical issues can be precious. That is why such participants have to be encouraged to think about technical solutions in complex AAL concepts and to enhance the multi-professional AAL discourse.

In the future, an interesting test could be the evaluation of assistive technology in a virtual reality environment. In [7] an VR environment for AAL services for interacting and evaluating prototypes.

A look into the future of AAL job profiles has been done by [6]. These emerging job roles are described in detail and are related to existing professions. It will be interesting to see, if AAL experts becomes an accepted further education or if the AAL expert becomes a stand-alone profession.

References

1. AAL Association. Ambient Assisted Living Joint Programme – ICTfor ageing well. http://www.aal-europe.eu. (accessed: December 30, 2014)
2. Doughty, K., Monk, A. Bayliss, C., Brown, S., Dewsbury, L., Dunk, B., Gallagher, V., Grafham, K., Jones, M., Lowe, C., McAlister, L., McSorley, K., Mills, P., Skidmore, C., Stewart, A., Taylor, B., Ward, D.: Telecare, telehealth and assistive technologies do we know what were talking about?. Journal of Assistive Technologies **1**(2) (2007)
3. Heuer, A., Karopka, T., Geisler, E.: Introduction to AAL (Study Material of the BAAL project). University of Rostock, German (2014)
4. Leitner, G., Fercher, A.J.: AAL 4 ALL – A matter of user experience. In: Lee, Y., Bien, Z.Z., Mokhtari, M., Kim, J.T., Park, M., Kim, J., Lee, H., Khalil, I. (eds.) ICOST 2010. LNCS, vol. 6159, pp. 195–202. Springer, Heidelberg (2010)
5. Marzahl, C., Penndorf, P., Bruder, I., Staemmler, M.: Unobtrusive fall detection using 3d images of a gaming console: concept and first results. In: Wichert, R., Eberhardt, B. (eds.) Ambient Assisted Living. ATSC, vol. 2, pp. 135–146. Springer, Heidelberg (2012)
6. Panagiotakopoulos, T., Theodosiou, A., Kameas, A.: Exploring ambient assisted living job profiles. In: Proceedings of the 6th International Conference on PErvasive Technologies Related to Assistive Environments. ACM (2013)
7. Sala, P., Kamieth, F., Mocholi, J.B., Naranjo, J.C.: Virtual reality for aal services interaction design and evaluation. In: Stephanidis, C. (ed.) Universal Access in HCI, Part III, HCII 2011. LNCS, vol. 6767, pp. 220–229. Springer, Heidelberg (2011)
8. Ziefle, M., Wilkowska, W.: Why traditional usability criteria fall short in ambient assisted living environments. In: Proceedings of the 8th International Conference on Pervasive Computing Technologies for Healthcare. ICST, Brussels, Belgium (2014)

Prognostic Reporting of p53 Expression by Image Analysis in Glioblastoma Patients: Detection and Classification

Mohammad F. Ahmad Fauzi[1(✉)], Hamza N. Gokozan[2], Christopher R. Pierson[2,3],
Jose J. Otero[2], and Metin N. Gurcan[4]

[1] Faculty of Engineering, Multimedia University, Cyberjaya, Selangor, Malaysia
faizal1@mmu.edu.my

[2] Department of Pathology, The Ohio State University, Columbus, Ohio, USA
{Hamza.Gokozan,Jose.Otero}@osumc.edu

[3] Department of Pathology and Laboratory Medicine, Nationwide Children's Hospital,
Columbus, Ohio, USA
Christopher.Pierson@nationwidechildrens.org

[4] Department of Biomedical Informatics, The Ohio State University, Columbus, Ohio, USA
Metin.Gurcan@osumc.edu

Abstract. In this paper, we present a computer aided diagnosis system focusing on one important diagnostic branchpoint in clinical decision-making: prognostic reporting of p53 expression in glioblastoma patients. Studies in other tumor paradigms have shown that the staining intensity correlates with TP53 mutation status, and that gliomas show inter-tumoral heterogeneity in p53 mutation status. Increasing diagnostic accuracy by computer-aided image analysis algorithms would deliver an objective assessment of such prognostic biomarkers. We proposed a method for the detection and classification of positive and negative cells in digitized p53-stained images by means of a novel adaptive thresholding for the detection, and two-step rule based on weighted color and intensity for the classification. The proposed thresholding technique is able to correctly locate both positive and negative cells by effectively addressing the closely connected cells problem, and records a promising 85% average precision and 88% average recall rate. On the other hand, the proposed two-step rule achieves 81% classification accuracy, which is comparable with neuropathologists' markings.

Keywords: Cell detection · Cell classification · Digital pathology · p53 analysis

1 Introduction

In neurosurgery, if a decision is made to biopsy or excise an intracranial mass, the surgeon will often opt to submit a specimen to pathology for intraoperative consultation where a cytologic prep (smear) and/or frozen section is performed. Additional tissue is then submitted for formalin fixation and paraffin embedding (FFPE) where

© Springer International Publishing Switzerland 2015
X. Yin et al. (Eds.): HIS 2015, LNCS 9085, pp. 165–173, 2015.
DOI: 10.1007/978-3-319-19156-0_17

pathologists report the tumor type, WHO grade, and additional prognostic markers such as Ki67 labeling index and p53 expression status.

Tumor protein p53 in humans is encoded by the TP53 gene. The p53 protein is crucial in multicellular organisms, where it regulates the cell cycle and functions as a tumor suppressor, preventing cancer. Studies in other tumor paradigms have shown that the staining intensity correlates with TP53 mutation status [1]. Furthermore, gliomas show inter-tumoral heterogeneity in TP53 mutation status [2].

Reporting p53 expression as a proxy for TP53 mutation status is highly subjective. Therefore, our goal is to develop image analysis algorithms to accurately and objectively quantify immunohistochemical p53, hence improving diagnostic reporting as well as clinical decision-making. These algorithms will aid and supplement pathological interpretation.

In this paper, we report the results of our preliminary work in classifying positively and negatively-stained cells in p53 immunohistochemical staining. Histopathological analysis of tissues has been gaining a lot of interest and is being applied to many different diseases such as follicular lymphoma [3-11], neuroblastoma [11-18] and glioblastoma [19]. Nevertheless, to the best of our knowledge, there has been no previous work in analyzing negative and positive staining intensities for reporting p53 expression.

The paper is organized as follows. Section 2 describes the methodology of the work where the ground truth generation and the proposed cell detection and classification processes are described. Section 3 discusses experimental evaluations of the proposed system against the ground truth. Finally conclusion and future works are discussed in Section 4.

2   Methodology

For the analysis of p53 immunohistochemical staining, slides were scanned at 40x magnification using a high-resolution whole slide scanner Aperio (Vista, CA) ScanScope^{TM} at the resolution of 0.23 micrometer/pixel. The digitized slides were then transferred to a server where a web-based software is in place for the pathologists to independently mark the cells to determine the ground truth.

Retrospective cases were evaluated from the Pathology Tissue Archives of The Ohio State Unviersity Wexner Medical Center using an IRB approved protocol. Several cases of high grade glioma were procured. Inclusion criteria included the need for an unequivocal diagnosis and grade (confirmed by the neuropathologist) that had undergone p53 immunohistochemistry.

2.1   Ground Truth Generation

To determine the ground truth for p53 staining, two board-certified neuropathologists and one pathology research fellow reviewed several scanned/digitized slides immunostained with p53. First, to determine inter-observer variability, the three pathologists scored separately the status of each cell in a high-power field (HPF) --at 40x magnification-- as "negative stain," "weak intensity," "moderate intensity," or "strong intensity." Then, using a similar grading scheme, one of the pathologists proceeded to mark another five HPFs from five different cases. In this preliminary work, the objective is to classify the positively and negatively-stained cells, hence the "weak intensity", "moderate intensity" and "strong intensity" marked cells are grouped together as positively-stained cells.

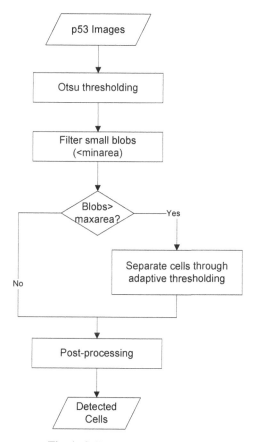

Fig. 1. Cells detection process

2.2   Cells Detection

Fig. 1 shows the flowchart of the proposed cell detection process. Given a digitized p53 stained image, we first convert the image into gray scale by only considering the luminance channel. Otsu thresholding is then applied to convert the luminance image into binary, separating the cells (blobs) from the background. The binary image is then cleaned by filtering very small and isolated blobs (blobs smaller than a certain minimum threshold, minarea). While Otsu thresholding is a very simple and straightforward technique in detecting dark objects from a light background, due to the lack of spatial information, it is prone to grouping closely connected cells together as a single cell, which will affect the cell counting process significantly.

To address this, we propose a novel adaptive thresholding scheme for any detected blobs with total area greater than a particular maximum threshold maxarea. The adaptive thresholding checks if a large detected blob consists of multiple cells by searching for potential valley within the blob, and proceeds to segment the blobs further if they do. For a 40x magnification image used in our experiment, a suitable minarea and maxarea threshold was found to be 300 and 1000 pixels (~70 and 230 µm2), respectively.

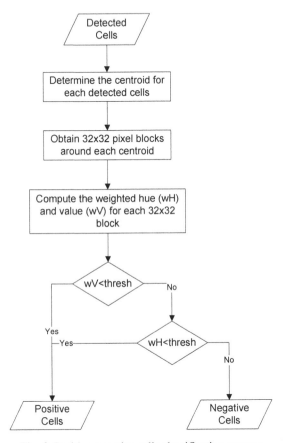

Fig. 2. Positive-negative cells classification process

2.3   Cells Classification

Fig. 2 shows the flowchart of the proposed positive-negative cell classification process. The classification of the cells into positive or negative will be based on the intensity and color of the cells, hence the image is first converted into HSV (Hue-Saturation-Value) color model. For each of the detected cells found in the previous section, their centroid is determined and 32x32 pixel blocks are extracted around each centroid. The weighted Hue and Value are calculated for each block and these values are used for classifying the cells. The weights used are inversely proportional to the pixels' distance to the centroid, with those closer to the center of the block receiving higher weight, and those further from the center receiving less weight.

Negative p53-stained cells tend to be blue (higher Hue) and less intense (higher Value), while positive p53-stained cells tend to be brown (lower Hue) with varying intensities. Based on these properties, we propose a two-step classification rule:

1. If the weighted Value (wV) for a block is less than a particular threshold (darker), the block will be classified as containing positive cell, regardless of its weighted Hue (wH).
2. Otherwise, the classification depends on weighted Hue, with wH less than a particular threshold means the block contains positive cells, and wH more than the threshold means it contains negative cells.

From experiment, suitable threshold value for both wH and wV is found to be 70.

3   Experimental Results

We first analyze the inter-observer variability during ground truth generation before discussing the performance of the proposed cell detection and classification methods against the ground truths.

3.1   Inter-observer Variability

Table 1 shows the summary of cell marking between the three pathologists. Overall the three pathologists are all able to detect more than 1000 cells within the image, although the classification into positive and negative cells differs quite significantly. Table 2 further examines the pathologist agreement by looking at their classification of each cell. Each column gives the number of cells where the pathologists are in agreement with each other. For example, in the first row, pathologists A and B gave the same classification for 966 cells (207 for positive cells, and 759 for negative cells), which is equivalent to 83.8% of the 1153 total cell marked. From the table, we can see that the agreements between any two pathologists are between 78.8% and

Table 1. Positive and Negative Cell Counts by Different Pathologists

	Positive	Negative	Total
Pathologist A	781	325	1106
Pathologist B	868	285	1153
Pathologist C	720	378	1098

Table 2. Marking Agreement Between Pathologists

	Positive	Negative	Total	Pctg
A&B	207	759	966	83.8
A&C	235	673	908	78.8
B&C	220	691	911	79.0
A&B&C	173	641	814	70.6

83.8%, which drops to 70.6% when all three pathologists are considered. This shows that even expert pathologists differs quite significantly in classifying positive and negative cells in digitized p53-stained images.

3.2   Cells Detection

Table 3 summarizes the performance of the proposed cells detection technique. 'Cases' refers to the different digitized tissue, 'GT' is the ground truth by pathologist A, B or C, 'TP' is the true positive (correctly detected cells), 'FP' is the false positive (incorrectly detected cells) and 'FN' is the false negative (missing or undetected cells). Precision and recall are defined by:

$$Recall = \frac{TP}{TP + FN}$$

$$Precision = \frac{TP}{TP + FP}$$

The proposed detection method recorded 85% precision and 88% recall rate. The recall rate in particular is very promising as all cases recorded more than 80% rate. This suggests that the proposed system is able to detect as much cells as identified by the pathologists. The precision rate on the other hand is slightly lower, suffering from slightly high false positive cases. Some of this is also caused by the pathologists missing some cells when marking the ground truth. Note that there could be more than 1000 cells in one viewed field causing the pathologists to unintentionally miss some of the cells.

Table 3. Performance of the Proposed Cell Detection Technique

Cases	GT	TP	FP	FN	Precision	Recall
1	A	844	188	32	0.96	0.82
1	B	878	200	49	0.95	0.81
1	C	852	187	49	0.95	0.82
2	A	420	77	43	0.91	0.85
3	A	221	12	73	0.75	0.95
4	A	257	15	30	0.90	0.94
5	A	185	9	82	0.69	0.95
6	A	172	23	69	0.71	0.88
		Average			**0.85**	**0.88**

3.3   Cells Classification

Table 4 shows the classification accuracy for the six images. The classification accuracy is defined by:

$$Accuracy = \frac{Correctly\ classified\ cells}{Total\ number\ of\ cells}$$

As seen from the table, the accuracy varies between 0.76 and 0.95, with an average of 0.81. Considering the agreement between any two pathologist is between 78.8% and 83.8%, and between all three pathologists is 70.6%, the results obtained is very promising, suggesting that the   proposed system measures up well with the given task.

Table 4. Summary of Classification Accuracy

Cases	GT	Correctly Classified	Incorrectly Classified	Accuracy
1	A	652	192	0.77
1	B	681	197	0.78
1	C	691	161	0.81
2	A	224	96	0.77
3	A	193	28	0.87
4	A	209	48	0.81
5	A	175	10	0.95
6	A	130	42	0.76
		Average		**0.81**

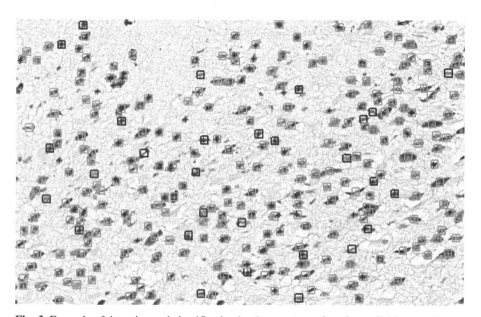

Fig. 3. Example of detection and classification by the system against the available ground truth (Case 4), where the positive and negative cells identified by the system are marked with green and blue squares respectively. The positive and negative cells identified by the pathologist are marked with green and blue asterisks respectively.

For case 1, we can also compare how the system measures against the different ground truth of the three pathologists, and in this particular case, it tends to agree more with pathologist C. Fig. 3 shows one example (Case 4) of the detection and classification against the available ground truth. The positive and negative cells identified by the system are marked with green and blue squares respectively. For reference purposes, the positive and negative cells identified by the pathologist are marked with green and blue asterisks respectively.

4   Conclusion

We have proposed a method for the detection and classification of positive and negative cells in digitized p53-stained images by means of Otsu and adaptive thresholding for the detection, and two-step rule based on weighted color and intensity for the classification. The proposed method is able to achieve 85% average precision and 88% average recall rate for cells detection, and 81% accuracy in classifying them into positively or negatively stained cells.

Considering the confusing nature of differentiating weakly stained positive cells from certain negative cells and even non-cells, and the fact that inter-observer variability is rather high (only 70% agreement among three pathologist), the proposed system provides promising results for detection and classification tasks. We are currently working on further classifying the positively-stained cells into different staining strength (weak, moderate, strong), which is even more challenging as the inter-observer variability is much higher.

References

1. Yemelyanova, A., Vang, R., Kshirsagar, M., Lu, D., Marks, M.A., Shih, I.M., Kurman, R.J.: Immunohistochemical staining patterns of p53 can serve as a surrogate marker for TP53 mutations in ovarian carcinoma: an immunohistochemical and nucleotide sequencing analysis. Mod Pathol **24**, 1248–1253 (2011)
2. Ren, Z.P., Olofsson, T., Qu, M., Hesselager, G., Soussi, T., Kalimo, H., Smits, A., Nister, M.: Molecular genetic analysis of p53 intratumoral heterogeneity in human astrocytic brain tumors. J. Neuropathol. Exp. Neurol. **66**, 944–954 (2007)
3. Sertel, O., Kong, J., Catalyurek, U., Lozanski, G., Saltz, J., Gurcan, M.: Histopathological Image Analysis using Model-based Intermediate Representations and Color Texture: Follicular Lymphoma Grading. Journal of Signal Processing Systems **55**, 169–183 (2009)
4. Sertel, O., Lozanski, G., Shana'ah, A., Gurcan, M.N.: Computer-aided detection of centroblasts for follicular lymphoma grading using adaptive likelihood-based cell segmentation. IEEE. Trans. Biomed. Eng. **57**(10), 2613–2616 (2010)
5. Sertel, O., Kong, J., Lozanski, G., Shanaah, A., Gewirtz, A., Racke, F., Zhao, J., Catalyurek, U., Saltz, J.H., Gurcan, M.: Computer-assisted grading of follicular lymphoma: High grade differentiation. Modern Pathology **21**, 371A–371A (2008)
6. Sertel, O., Kong, J., Lozanski, G., Catalyurek, U., Saltz, J.H., Gurcan, M.N.: Computerized microscopic image analysis of follicular lymphoma. Proceedings of SPIE Medical Imaging: Computer-Aided Diagnosis **6915**, 1–11 (2008)
7. Samsi, S.S., Krishnamurthy, A.K., Groseclose, M., Caprioli, R.M., Lozanski, G., Gurcan, M.N.: Imaging mass spectrometry analysis for follicular lymphoma grading. In: Proceedings of Annual Int Conf of the IEEE Engineering in Medicine and Biology Society, pp. 6969–6972 (2009)
8. Samsi, S., Lozanski, G., Shana'ah, A., Krishanmurthy, A.K., Gurcan, M.N.: Detection of follicles from IHC-stained slides of follicular lymphoma using iterative watershed. IEEE Trans. Biomed. Eng. **57**(10), 2609–2612 (2010)
9. Oger, M., Belhomme, P., Gurcan, M.N.: A general framework for the segmentation of follicular lymphoma virtual slides. Comput. Med. Imaging Graph. **36**(6), 442–451 (2012)

10. Belkacem-Boussaid, K., Sertel, O., Lozanski, G., Shana'aah, A., Gurcan, M.: Extraction of color features in the spectral domain to recognize centroblasts in histopathology. In: Proceedings of Annual Int. Conf. of the IEEE Engineering in Medicine and Biology Society, pp. 3685–3688 (2009)
11. Akakin, H.C., Gurcan, M.N.: Content-based microscopic image retrieval system for multi-image queries. IEEE Trans. Inf. Technol. Biomed. **16**(4), 758–769 (2012)
12. Teodoro, G., Sachetto, R., Sertel, O., Gurcan, M.N., Meira, W., Catalyurek, U., Ferreira, R.: Coordinating the use of GPU and CPU for improving performance of compute intensive applications. In: Proceedings of IEEE Int. Conf. on Cluster Computing and Workshops, pp. 437–446 (2009)
13. Sertel, O., Kong, J., Shimada, H., Catalyurek, U.V., Saltz, J.H., Gurcan, M.N.: Computer-aided Prognosis of Neuroblastoma on Whole-slide Images: Classification of Stromal Development. Pattern Recognition **42**(6), 1093–1103 (2009)
14. Ruiz, A., Sertel, O., Ujaldon, M., Catalyurek, U.V., Saltz, J., Gurcan, M.N.: Stroma classification for neuroblastoma on graphics processors. International Journal of Data Mining and Bioinformatics **3**(3), 280–298 (2009)
15. Ruiz, A., Kong, J., Ujaldon, M., Boyer, K., Saltz, J., Gurcan, M.N.: Pathological image segmentation for neuroblastoma using the GPU. In: Proceedings of 5th IEEE Int. Symp. on Biomedical Imaging: From Nano to Macro, pp. 296–299 (2008)
16. Gurcan, M., Pan, T., Shimada, H., Saltz, J.H.: Image analysis for neuroblastoma classification: hysteresis thresholding for cell segmentation. In: Proceedings of APIII, Vancouver, BC (2006)
17. Cambazoglu, B., Sertel, O., Kong, J., Saltz, J.H., Gurcan, M.N., Catalyurek, U.V.: Efficient processing of pathological images using the grid: computer-aided prognosis of neuroblastoma. In: Proceedings of Challenges of Large Scale Applications in Distributed Environments (CLADE), Monterey Bay, CA, pp. 35–41 (2007)
18. Sertel, O., Catalyurek, U.V., Shimada, H., Gurcan, M.N.: A combined computerized classification system for whole-slide neuroblastoma histology: model-based structural features. In: International Conference on Medical Image Computing and Computer Assisted Intervention, pp. 7–18 (2009)
19. Fauzi, M.F.A., Gokozan, H.N., Elder, B., Puduvalli, V.K., Otero, J.J., Gurcan, M.N.: Classification of glioblastoma and metastasis for neuropathology intraoperative diagnosis: a multi-resolution textural approach to model the background. In: Proceedings of SPIE Medical Imaging 2014: Digital Pathology (2014)

Identification of Schizophrenia-Associated Gene Polymorphisms Using Hybrid Filtering Feature Selection with Structural Information

Yingying Wang[1], Zichun Zeng[1,2], and Yunpeng Cai[1(✉)]

[1] Shenzhen Institutes of Advance Technology, Chinese Academy of Sciences,
Shenzhen, People's Republic of China
yp.cai@siat.ac.cn
[2] University of Science and Technology of China, Hefei, People's Republic of China

Abstract. Schizophrenia is a complex and severe neurological disorder that affects lots of people worldwide. Despite its strong evidence of heritability revealed by lots of genetic studies, research for locating of schizophrenia associated genes remains frustrating as numerous efforts had failed to identify biomarkers that could strongly impact the diagnosis and prognosis of schizophrenia. The major challenge lies in the weak discrimination of single gene marker and the enormous number of gene variants that exist in human genome. In this paper we propose a hybrid feature selection method that utilizes the biological structural information of the gene variants to tackle this problem. A set of statistical techniques are developed to encourage the clustering of multiple informative SNP variants on the same gene, which boost the probability of finding biologically meaningful features and suppresses false discoveries. As a result, the proposed method achieves significantly better performance on a published schizophrenia human genome data set compared with previous studies, with an area-under-ROC-curve of 65% and an odd ratio of 2.82 (95%CI: 1.80 – 4.40). 36 gene markers are discovered to be associated with the onset of schizophrenia with many of which verified directly or indirectly by previous literature. The method proposed in this paper can be also adopted for efficient control of false discoveries in finding biomarkers from genomic data.

Keywords: Schizophrenia · Biomarkers · SNP · Feature selection

1   Introduction

Schizophrenia is a heterogeneous and multi-factored disease that affects approximately 0.5-1.2% of individual worldwide [1]. Schizophrenia is very complex partly due to the complicating of brain and the enormous neuronal interconnections and permutations thereof in humans. It is thought to be caused by both genetic and environmental factors and the interactions between them [2]. Though genetic factors are considered to be the main issues since schizophrenia has a heritability of about 80%, the research based on genetics has been frustrating because numerous efforts had failed to identify biomarkers that could strongly impact the diagnosis and prognosis of schizophrenia. However, with the development of high-throughput genotyping technologies, many biomarkers especially single nucleotide polymorphisms (SNPs, also termed as

© Springer International Publishing Switzerland 2015
X. Yin et al. (Eds.): HIS 2015, LNCS 9085, pp. 174–184, 2015.
DOI: 10.1007/978-3-319-19156-0_18

common genetic variants) have been identified to be associated with schizophrenia as some studies shown [3-6].

Considering the major goal of schizophrenia genetic research is to choose a list of genetic loci with significant biomarkers, machine learning methods become good choices since they have been applied in many biological-related researches successfully such as microarray analyses, etc. In the field of schizophrenia, few studies had adopted machine learning methods from different aspects. One study identified 36 SNPs related to schizophrenia using logit linear models to represent the relationship between genotype and risk of schizophrenia. Results indicated that a Bayesian approach could identify genes possibly involved in the etiology of schizophrenia [7]. To identify relationships between brain structure volumes and cognitive performance, and the differences of these relationships between control and schizophrenia patients, a study used a Bayesian decision-theoretic method to find morphological biomarker features that best explained neuropsychological test scores in the context of a multivariate response linear model with interactions [8]. A study paid attention to the brain cortical thickness in order to investigate possible subtypes of schizophrenia patients using Lloyd's k-means cluster analysis and found no subtypes specific to patients [9]. Another study used a hybrid machine learning method for fusing fMRI and SNP data to classify schizophrenia patients and healthy controls [10]. These studies showed that machine learning methods can identify biomarkers (such as SNPs) with biological significance for the deep researching of schizophrenia.

Nevertheless, despite these attempts, the genetic origin of schizophrenia remains almost unrevealed. Specifically, most of the above works merely discovers a set of weak associated biomarkers (most of which have statistical significance $p > 0.001$), without giving a complete prediction model. Most of them are not cross-validated or have only marginal separation on the validation data. Although in [10] the authors claimed to achieve 87% accuracy in leave-one-out cross validation of a small data set, they actually used the information of the validation sample (with label information) during the feature selection phase, hence the result is not a real cross-validation accuracy, but should be regarded as a training accuracy which is not externally validated and the replicability is questionable. Hence, finding a discriminative model for separating schizophrenia vs. normal genotypes will still be a milestone in the research of schizophrenia genomics.

The major challenge in finding replicable schizophrenia gene markers is that this disease is likely caused by a collection of genetic factors but no gene is discovered to be strongly informative. Due to the large number of human gene variation factors (for example, there are approximately 10 million SNPs on the human genome) and the restricted number of samples under study, a large number of false-positive biomarkers will be selected which seems to be informative on the training data but will fail in the validation data. Most existing feature selection methods are not powerful enough to control the false-positive rate in such a high dimension and weak indicator case.

In this paper we propose a feature selection strategy to tackle this problem by taking into account the distribution information of the selected factors on the genomic structure. Specifically, the clustering of multiple informative features on the same gene or chromosome will provide an additional indication that these features are not likely random. For example, some previous works have found a set of schizophrenia-associated SNPs clustered on the same gene [6] or a set of genes on the same chromosome [11]. By exploiting this character and favor clustered features, we are able to select features that are more reliable and control the false positive rate. A crucial issue is to quantitatively describe the degree of enrichment for features on a gene or a chromosome. We employ the idea of multi-dimensional chi-square test and design a hybrid pipeline to pick out a set of gene variants that are enriched on a few genes. As a result, we derive a prediction model that achieves a C-statistics accuracy of 0.65 on a ten-fold cross-validation test, which is significantly higher than previous results. A set of schizophrenia-associated genes, and SNPs on them, are identified, which are proved to be with rational biology interpretation.

2   Material and Methods

2.1   Dataset

We downloaded SNP array data GSE27923 [11] from NCBI GEO [12, 13]. The dataset contained 120 schizophrenia patient-parents trio samples. In all the 360 persons detected, 128 were schizophrenia patients (including 120 schizophrenia patients, 6 of these patients' father and 2 of these patients' mother were also schizophrenia patients) and 232 were healthy controls. Four SNP array platforms were used for each person: Affymetrix Human Mapping 50K Hind240 SNP Array, Affymetrix Human Mapping 50K Xba240 SNP Array, Affymetrix Human CentHindAv2 SNP Array and Affymetrix Human CentXbaAv2 SNP Array. The SNP probes could be mapped to 115,117 NCBI dbSNP [14] entries altogether, which scatter on all 22 human chromosomes and each SNP entry contains three sub-genotypes.

2.2   Overall Framework

Fig.1 demonstrates the framework of the overall procedure in this paper. We split the original data in to ten folds randomly. In each iteration, 9 folds of the data are used for

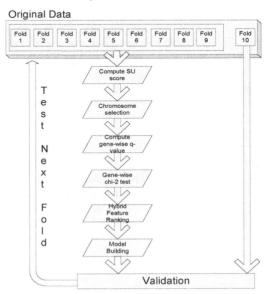

Fig. 1. Framework of the feature selection and validation procedure

model building and one fold for model validation. The procedure is iterated until all folds are used for validation. The compound result of all validations is used to evaluate the performance of the model. In order to deal with the high dimensional nature of the data and the small sample size, we propose a hybrid feature selection scheme combining multiple steps, which will be introduced in the next section.

2.3   Feature Selection

2.3.1   Symmetric Uncertainty

Because the gene SNP features are expressed in categorical variables, traditional filtering methods for continuous variables such as Student's t-test are not able to apply to the data directly. Although one can convert categorical variables into continuous one using encoding techniques, due to the small number of samples and imbalance distribution of attribute values, traditional filtering methods usually have poor performance after conversion. On the other hand, chi-square test is often used for detecting the statistical significance between groups of categorical attributes but is known to be too sensitive to the variance of the data, hence is not suitable for feature selection. In this paper we use the symmetric uncertainty (SU) [15] as the metric for filtering feature selection, which is expressed by the following equation:

$$SU(X, Y) = \frac{2I(X,Y)}{H(X)+H(Y)} \tag{1}$$

Where X is the values of samples on the studied variable and Y is the class labels of sample, I is the mutual information between X and Y, $H(X)$ and $H(Y)$ are the entropy of X and Y, respectively. A higher SU score indicates a higher distinction between different classes of samples on feature X.

Symmetric uncertainty has been previously employed in some feature selection methods (e.g., FCBF [16]) but in our experiment we found that these methods perform poorly on the   schizophrenia data, because by using the symmetric uncertainty as the only metric for selection, many false positive features are included in the model. In this paper, we propose multiple statistical technologies to tackle this problem and avert the short-coming of previous approaches.

2.3.2   Chromosome Ranking and Selection

The high dimensional nature of the gene SNP array and the limited number of samples poses a severe challenge to feature selection. In order to pick out reliable features, a trade-off should be considered between the completeness of the feature set and the control of false discoveries. In this paper we apply a conservative strategy that we only consider genes on a chromosome with a significant number of informative features.   Although some informative features will be lost by using this strategy, it is discovered that the false discovery rate is efficiently lowered. The detailed procedure of chromosome selection is described below:

1. Compute the SU score of each SNP variable;
2. Sort all variables by their SU score in descending order;
3. For a given variable i, suppose r_i is the rank order of the variable, the rank score for the variable is given by $rs_i = \max(100-r_i,0)$;
4. The rank score for a chromosome is calculated as:

$$S_{chr} = \frac{\sum_{v_i \in \Xi} rs_{v_i}}{|\Xi|} \qquad (2)$$

where Ξ is the set of all SNP variables located on the chromosome chr and $|\Xi|$ is the number of SNP varialbles on that chromosome

5. Chromosomes with rank score >0.1 are selected and the SNP variables located on the chromosomes are all included for next feature selection steps.

2.3.3   Gene-Wise Benjamini–Hochberg Correction

The Benjamini–Hochberg procedure [17] is a technique for false discovery rate control which take into account the total number of variables under consideration. A larger number of variables considered will increase the risk of false discovery and thus more stringent criteria should be applied to control the risk. On the other hand, a larger number of informative features will imply more chance of finding true positive. The BH procedure applied a balancing strategy by re-calculating the measurement of significance as:

$$q_k = \min\left(\frac{m}{k} p_k, q_{k+1}\right), \quad k = m - 1 \dots 1, \quad q_m = p_m \qquad (3)$$

where $\{p_k\}$ is the ordered set of the p-values for all variables derived from a normal statistical test (such as Student's t-test or chi-square test), satisfying $p_1 \le p_2 \le \dots \le p_m$, and m is the total number of variables in a given data set.

One thing to address is that unlike Student's t-test or chi-square test, there is no traditional measurement of significance for symmetric uncertainty. Nevertheless, we empirically observe that the distribution of SU score approximates the chi-square distribution. Hence we used the following method to calculate the significance (p-value) of SU score for each variable:

$$p_{SU}(X_k) = 1 - F\left(\frac{SU(X_k,Y)}{mean_{i \in \Omega}(SU(X_i,Y))}, 1\right) \qquad (4)$$

where $F(x,1)$ is the cumulative distribution function for the chi-square distribution with degree of freedom 1, Ω is the entire set of all variables and X_k is the variable under investigation.

It should be noted that the calculation of p-value is uniform for all variables, while the calculation of the q-value is applied on SNPs located on each gene separately. By this means, genes with a large number of SNP mutations are filtered with a more strict criteria and the overall chance of false discovery is suppressed, leading the selected features to be more stable.

2.3.4   Gene-Wise Chi-square Test

The BH procedure is powerful in reducing the number of false features. However, it does not provide a mechanism to boost informative genes. In biology, the phenomenon that a significant number of disease-associated SNPs clustering on the same gene provide a strong indicator that the gene should play an important role on the development of the disease. To quantitatively measure this phenomenon and enough clustered feature, we apply a multi-dimensional chi-square model:

$$p(G) = \min_{j=1..|G|} \left(1 - F\left(\frac{\sum_{k=1..j} SU(X_k, Y)}{mean_{i \in \Omega}(SU(X_i, Y))}, j\right)\right) \tag{5}$$

where $G = \{X_1, X_2, ..., X_{|G|}\}$ is a set of SNP variables on the same gene which are sorted in increasing values of their single-SNP significance $p_{SU}(X_k)$. Eq. 5 seeks for an optimal number of variables which maximizes the statistical significance of the model, and use it as the significance of the gene. In this manner the clustering effect of informative variables on the same gene is encouraged.

2.3.5   Hybrid Feature Selection Scheme

With the above procedure we got three kinds of evaluation scores for each SNP variable: SU score, the q-value of the SNP with the gene, and the chi-square p-value of the gene that the SNP belongs to (SNPs belonging to the same gene are all assigned the same p-value). We then rank each score individually for all variables selected in section 2.3.3, with SU score in descending order and p-value or q-value in ascending order. The largest rank of the three ranks is used as the rank of the variable. After that, the 30 top-ranked variables in each fold of training dataset are selected for model building.

2.4   Model Building

The Naïve Bayes Classifier

$$P(Y = y_0|X) = P(Y = y_0) \prod_{i=1}^{m} P(x_i | Y = y_0) \tag{6}$$

is adopted as the prediction model for clinical outcomes of gene variables. Here $y_0=0$ indicates a healthy outcome and $y_0=1$ indicates a disease outcome. $X = \{x_1, ..., x_m\}$ is a test sample with m feature variables selected on the above steps. The prior probability $P(Y)$ and conditional probabilities $P(x_i|Y)$ are computed from the training data set with Laplace smoothing applied [18].

In each round of cross-validation test, each validation test sample is assigned a predicted probability. After the entire ten-fold cross-validation is finished, the prediction results are merged together using the predicted probability as the unified outcome. The probability P=0.5 is then used as a cut-off to separate the samples into high risk (P>=0.5) and low risk (P<0.5) groups. The odds ratio between the two groups is computed, and a receiver operating characteristic (ROC) curve [19] is plotted based on the data to evaluate the performance of the derived models.

3   Results

Fig.2 depicts the odds ratio obtained by the models created in this paper and its comparison to previous results. With the probability cut-off P=0.5, our model achieves an odds ratio of 2.82 (95% CI: 1.80 – 4.40) which is significantly better than previous reported results on cross-validation data. The odds ratio results of Purcell [3] and Shi [6] are taken directly from the original report of their papers, with ratios converted to be always larger than 1. The result of Yamada [11] is computed using their published data (which is also the material used in this paper) using the best result of the selected biomarkers reported in their paper. Among twenty SNP variables reported in [11], only two variables have the 95% CI of the odds ratios completely larger than 1 (1.98 [CI: 1.22-3.21] for SNP rs10496761, and 1.89 [CI: 1.18-3.04] for SNP rs1048076, respectively). Hence, although the calculated odds ratio of [11] is relatively high, it is not obtained on a validation set and hence the comparison is biased to their results. Even so, they are still surpassed by our results. Moreover, these two SNPs only identify 24% and 35% of the patients, respectively. When combining them together, the number of false positive patients grows a lot and the odds ratio drop to near 1. Thus the gene markers reported in previous study [11] is not capable of making accurate prediction.

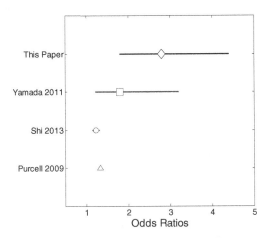

Fig. 2. Comparison of the odd ratios obtained by the result of this paper and previous studies in Purcell [3], Shi [6], Yamada [11], respectively. The markers show the positions of the mean odds ratio and the lines show the positions of the 95% confidence intervals (CI). The CI of the Purcell marker was not reported.

Fig.3 depicts the obtained ROC curve following the ten-fold cross validation pro-cedure, the area under ROC curve (AUC) is 0.65. As a comparison, using traditional filter selection methods such as t-test or chi-square test achieved a poor AUC of near 0.5. By carrying out a permutation test using 1000 permuted datasets, we further con-firmed that the result obtained on real dataset is superior to those on permuted data (p<0.001) and thus the discovered model is not likely a false discovery. Although the discrimination is not very strong for the patient and healthy group, the result already outperforms previous ones where only marginal separations were obtained.

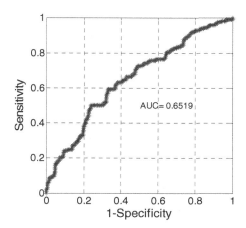

Fig. 3. The receiver operating characteristic (ROC) curve obtained from ten-fold cross valida-tion results on the studied dataset using the proposed method

In ten-fold cross-validation, altogether 74 SNP variables are selected for model building in different folds. Genes with at least 10 hits in total during the ten rounds are chosen for biological analysis. Table 1 listed the 36 SNP variables selected and their biological literature previously reported. We see that most SNP variables are located on the X chromosome and autosome No.1, despite that usually 6-8 chromo-somes will be considered after the chromosome selection step 2.3.3, and many SNPs are clustered on the same gene, which exactly as the algorithm expected. Through literature search, we found that 6 out of the 16 total genes have been known to be biomarkers for schizophrenia, and an additional 3 genes are linked with the gene regulation or metabolic functions regarding brain functions, which all persuades that our method is powerful of discovering biological relevant gene variants. Moreover, our study also discovered some new informative genes that help to predict the onset of the disease. The biological meaning of these genes will be further validated through further external validations with more data.

Table 1. List of selected gene biomarkers selected by the methods proposed in this paper. The symbol * denotes that the gene is known to be directly connected with schoziphrenia in literature, and + denotes that it is involved in some processes related to the disease or brain function disorders.

Chromosome	SNP ID	Gene Name	Gene Function	Literature
X	rs996106	PPP1R2P9	protein phosphatase 1, regulatory (inhibitor) subunit 2 pseudogene 9	[20]+
	rs723028			
	rs205869			
	rs205870			
	rs4986541			
	rs2410977			
X	rs2285634		intron variant TRAPPC2/OFD1	[21]*
X	rs5980419	IDS	iduronate 2-sulfatase	
	rs6540313			
	rs7065976			
X	rs431207	DMD	dystrophin	[25]*
	rs725979			
	rs1921386			
	rs1921395			
	rs436628			
X	rs6522686	NAP1L3	nucleosome assembly protein 1-like 3	
1	rs2282729	TNR	tenascin R	[23][24]*
	rs10489316			
	rs10492392			
	rs1385540			
	rs3766680			
	rs4570382			
	rs10489311			
1	rs10493026	RUNX3	runt-related transcription factor 3	
1	rs10489202	MPC2/BRP44	mitochondrial pyruvate carrier 2	[10]*
1	rs149912	DCAF6	DDB1 and CUL4 associated factor 6	[10]*
3	rs1348990		no info	
3	rs879161	PHC3	polyhomeotic homolog 3	
	rs7638400			
3	rs7619166	ACTRT3	actin-related protein T3	
3	rs10510897	CADPS	Ca++-dependent secretion activator	[27]+
17	rs3815341	CCL11	chemokine (C-C motif) ligand 11	[22]*
17	rs10515122	ANKFN1	ankyrin-repeat and fibronectin type III domain containing 1	
	rs7207271			
19	rs3810137	ZNF225	zinc finger protein 225	[26]+
	rs9304639			

4   Conclusion

The enormous number of gene variants that exist in human genome poses a major challenge to genomics studies and the discovery of disease-related gene biomarkers, especially when in the situations where no single strong correlated genes exist. In this paper we proposed a hybrid feature selection method that utilizes the biological structural information of the gene variants, and adopted a set of statistical techniques to make use of the clustering feature of multiple informative SNP variants on the same gene, thus boost the probability of finding biologically meaningful against false discoveries. Our study showed that the proposed method achieved significantly better performance on the discovery of schizophrenia associated gene markers. In the future, the proposed method will be also applied in other types of genomic data mining for efficient control of false discoveries in biomarkers discoveries.

Acknowlegements. This work was supported by Shenzhen Municipal Science and Technology Research Development and Funds and Platform Construction Plan Key Laboratory Program (CXB201111250113A), Shenzhen Basic Research Fund (JCYJ2013-0329155553732), the Promotion Funds for Key Laboratory in Shenzhen (ZDSY-20120617113021359) and Shenzhen Innovation Funding for Advanced Talents (KQCX20130628112914291).

References

1. Takahashi, S.: Heterogeneity of schizophrenia: Genetic and symptomatic factors. Am. J. Med. Genet. B Neuropsychiatr. Genet. **162B**, 648–652 (2013)
2. Rethelyi, J.M., Benkovits, J., Bitter, I.: Genes and environments in schizophrenia: The different pieces of a manifold puzzle. Neurosci. Biobehav. Rev. **37**, 2424–2437 (2013)
3. Purcell, S.M., Wray, N.R., Stone, J.L., Visscher, P.M., O'Donovan, M.C., Sullivan, P.F., Sklar, P.: Common polygenic variation contributes to risk of schizophrenia and bipolar disorder. Nature. **460**, 748–752 (2009)
4. Shatz, C.J.: MHC class I: an unexpected role in neuronal plasticity. Neuron. **64**, 40–45 (2009)
5. Kwon, E., Wang, W., Tsai, L.H.: Validation of schizophrenia-associated genes CSMD1, C10orf26, CACNA1C and TCF4 as miR-137 targets. Mol. Psychiatry **18**, 11–12 (2013)
6. Shi, Y.Y., Li, Z.Q., Xu, Q., Wang, T., Li, T., et al.: Common variants on 8p12 and 1q24.2 confer risk of schizophrenia. Nature Genetics **43**, 1224–1227 (2011)
7. Hall, H., Lawyer, G., Sillen, A., Jonsson, E.G., Agartz, I., Terenius, L., Arnborg, S.: Potential genetic variants in schizophrenia: a Bayesian analysis. World J. Biol. Psychiatry **8**, 12–22 (2007)
8. Laywer, G., Nyman, H., Agartz, I., Arnborg, S., Jonsson, E.G., Sedvall, G.C., Hall, H.: Morphological correlates to cognitive dysfunction in schizophrenia as studied with Bayesian regression. BMC Psychiatry **6**, 31 (2006)
9. Lawyer, G., Nesvag, R., Varnas, K., Frigessi, A., Agartz, I.: Investigating possible subtypes of schizophrenia patients and controls based on brain cortical thickness. Psychiatry Res. **164**, 254–264 (2008)
10. Yang, H., Liu, J., Sui, J., Pearlson, G., Calhoun, V.D.: A Hybrid Machine Learning Method for Fusing fMRI and Genetic Data: Combining both Improves Classification of Schizophrenia. Front. Hum. Neurosci. **4**, 192 (2010)
11. Yamada, K., Iwayama, Y., Hattori, E., Iwamoto, K., Toyota, T., Ohnishi, T., Ohba, H., Maekawa, M., Kato, T., Yoshikawa, T.: Genome-wide association study of schizophrenia in Japanese population. PLoS One **6**, e20468 (2011)

12. Edgar, R., Domrachev, M., Lash, A.E.: Gene Expression Omnibus: NCBI gene expression and hybridization array data repository. Nucleic Acids Res. **30**, 207–210 (2002)
13. Barrett, T., Wilhite, S.E., Ledoux, P., Evangelista, C., Kim, I.F., Tomashevsky, M., Marshall, K.A., Phillippy, K.H., Sherman, P.M., Holko, M., et al.: NCBI GEO: archive for functional genomics data sets–update. Nucleic Acids Res. **41**, D991–995 (2013)
14. Sherry, S.T., Ward, M.H., Kholodov, M., Baker, J., Phan, L., Smigielski, E.M., Sirotkin, K.: dbSNP: the NCBI database of genetic variation. Nucleic Acids Res. **29**, 308–311 (2001)
15. Witten, I.H., Frank, E.: Data Mining: Practical Machine Learning Tools and Techniques. Morgan Kaufmann Amsterdam (2011). ISBN: 978-0-12-374856-0
16. Lei, Y., Liu, H.: Feature selection for high-dimensional data: A fast correlation-based filter solution. In Proc. Intl. Conf. Mach. Learn. **3**, 856–863 (2003)
17. Benjamini, Y.: HochbergY: Controlling the false discovery rate: a practical and powerful approach to multiple testing. J. Royal Stat. Soc. B **57**(1), 289–300 (1995)
18. Manning, C.D., Raghavan, P., Schutze, M.: Introduction to Information Retrieval. Cambridge University Press (2008)
19. Fawcett, T.: An Introduction to ROC Analysis. Pattern Recognition Letters **7**(8), 861–874 (2006)
20. Hakak, Y., Walker, J.R., Li, C., Wong, W.H., Davis, K.L., Buxbaum, J.D., et al.: Genome-wide expression analysis reveals dysregulation of myelination-related genes in chronic schizophrenia. Proc. Natl. Acad Sci. **98**(8), 4746–4751 (2001)
21. Zong, M., Wu, X.G., Chan, C.W.L., Chio, M.Y., Chan, H.S., Tanner, J.A., Yu, S.: The Adaptor Function of TRAPPC2 in Mammalian TRAPPs Explains TRAPPC2-Associated SEDT and TRAPPC9-Associated Congenital Intellectual Disability. PLOS ONE **6**(8), e23350 (2011)
22. Teixeira, A.L., et al.: Increased serum levels of CCL11/eotaxin in schizophrenia. Prog. Neuropsychopharmacol Biol. Psychiatry **32**, 710–714 (2008)
23. Morawski, M., et al.: Tenascin-R promotes assembly of the extracellular matrix of perineuronal nets via clustering of aggrecan. Philos. Trans. R. Soc. Lond. B. Biol. Sci. **369** (2014)
24. Kahler, A.K., et al.: Candidate gene analysis of the human natural killer-1 carbohydrate pathway and perineuronal nets in schizophrenia: B3GAT2 is associated with disease risk and cortical surface area. Biol. Psychiatry **69**, 90–96 (2011)
25. Lindor, N.M., Sobell, J.L., Heston, L.L., Thibodeau, S.N., Sommer, S.S.: Screening the dystrophin gene suggests a high rate of polymorphism in general but no exonic deletions in schizophrenics. American journal of medical genetics **54**(1), 1–4 (1994)
26. Bowden, N.A., Weidenhofer, J., Scott, R.J., Schall, U., Todd, J., Michie, P.T., Tooney, P.A.: Preliminary investigation of gene expression profiles in peripheral blood lymphocytes in schizophrenia. Schizophrenia research **82**(2), 175–183 (2006)
27. Hattori, K., Tanaka, H., Wakabayashi, C., Yamamoto, N., Uchiyama, H., Teraishi, T., et al.: Expression of Ca2+-dependent activator protein for secretion 2 is increased in the brains of schizophrenic patients. Prog. in Neuro-Psycho. & Biol. Psyc. **35**(7), 1738–1743 (2011)

Mobile Clinical Scale Collection System for In-Hospital Stroke Patient Assessments Using Html5 Technology

Furu Xiang[1,3], Wenxuan Guan[1,3], Xingxian Huang[2],
Xiaomao Fan[1], Yunpeng Cai[1(✉)], and Haibo Yu[2]

[1] Shenzhen Institutes of Advance Technology, Chinese Academy of Sciences,
Shenzhen, People's Republic of China
yp.cai@siat.ac.cn
[2] Shenzhen Traditional Chinese Medicine (TCM) Hospital, Shenzhen, China
[3] University of Science and Technology of China, Hefei, People's Republic of China

Abstract. Clinical scale is a very important means of measuring and recording patient status, especially for capturing features that are not directly reflected by biochemical tests. In this paper, we develop a clinical scale collection system which enables doctors to record patient information during hospital rounds in real-time via different mobile platforms such as Android, iOS or others. The system adopts web technology that is base on the standard of Hypertext Markup Language 5.0 (HTML5) on the client, which solves the issue of platform compatibility of between systems. The technology of web service that uses the style of Representational State Transfer (REST) not only optimizes the logical structure of the system but also increase the system's scalability, and the stable MySQL database increases the security and stability of the system's data storage. The system has been adopted in a traditional Chinese medicine hospital for in-hospital monitoring and assortment of stroke rehabilitation patients and played quite a helpful role in patient management and clinical assertions.

Keywords: Mobile healthcare · Medical scale · In-hospital patient management · Health information systems

1 Introduction

Clinical assessment scales have long been developed in clinical science. In the beginning, a number of medical assessment scales were proposed in the form of index scores. For example, in clinical scales detecting risks of stroke onset, Johnston and his partner made a cohort study on 1707 patients identified with TIA (transient ischemic attack) during the 90 days, which defines the short-term prognosis and risk elements for stroke after TIA, by which they proposed a simple index, the California scores, (vary from 0 to 5 for each risk factor) to help estimate risk [1]. After that, the content of the medical assessment scales have been changed for accurately estimate patient conditions in clinical. As such, through a scoring system with clinical and Magnetic Resonance imaging (MRI) information, risk of a subsequent stroke following an acute TIA (transient ischemic attack) or minor stroke can be predicted accurately [2].

© Springer International Publishing Switzerland 2015
X. Yin et al. (Eds.): HIS 2015, LNCS 9085, pp. 185–194, 2015.
DOI: 10.1007/978-3-319-19156-0_19

And at present, there have been many studies to verify their value to predictive patients' disease progression. As is shown in Johnston's research, the California and ABCD scores can predict the stroke risks at 2 days, 7 days, and 90 days (in each of the four validation cohorts). And compared with the two scores, ABCD(2) score is likely to be most predictive [3].

Meanwhile, the value of medical assessment scales has been gradually accepted by academics and clinicians. For example, in the diagnosis of TIA, Edwards' Qualitative study using semi-structured interviews shows that in two hospital sites in England, 60% Primary care staff (nine GPs and one A&E triage nurse) and 100% Specialist doctors, nurses and administrator do use the ABCD2 risk stratification score as a diagnostic tool and referral pathway facilitator, to help emphasizing urgency to the patient; Meanwhile, analysis of the ABCD2 scores was the core way to communicate about TIA diagnosis in the two sites [4].The effect of clinical scale is reflected in many aspects: to predict disease onset and find the risk factors of diseases, impact on processes of care and clinical outcomes to improve the clinical progress; assessing the development of patients' disease and the effect of rehabilitation to select the clinical therapy. Compared with other form of medical records, clinical scale systems are more powerful in incorporating expert knowledge and judgments as well as providing comprehensive assessments of patient status in systematic rather than isolated way. Hence they are indispensable in real-world clinical applications.

Currently, in most hospitals the patients' clinical scale have to be filled in paper form by health care staff during the course of rounds, before typing into computer database afterwards, which is not only time consuming, but also overwhelming clinicians and having the risk of losing important clinical information due to overloads of working intension. Developing a mobile-based information system which can collect medical scales conveniently on real-time will dramatically help clinicians to better manage and evaluate the situation of patients, and to provide more chances of optimizing the therapy strategies in time.

In order to help health care staff to make accurate judgment of patient's condition and improve the working efficiency of them, we develop a clinical scale collection system with the help of the hospital of Traditional Chinese Medicine of Shenzhen. The clinical scale collection system is composed of two parts: the design and development of scales' web interface and the data Storage and processing of evaluation results. We use the HTML5 technology for the web development in order to compatible with different platforms and use Representational State Transfer (REST), which could reduce the complexity of the development and improve the scalability of the system, to implement the data submitted; and MySQL, a relational database, has been used in clinical scale collection system as its database and in the following we will introduce these technology.

2   System Architecture

Online clinical scale collection system is structured into three parts: the first part is web client which is based on the HTML5 standard. The web client based on HTML5 standard could adapt with different mobile platforms so that health care staff could use their work mobile phone, iPad and computer to evaluate patient condition, view and update evaluation results, and manage history evaluation records. Meanwhile the web client based on HTML5 standard could facilitate modular design of clinical scale so that health care staff could perfect the existing clinical scale in the process of evaluation. The second part is Middle-ware layer, we using web service and REST design style to pack/unpack evaluation data, improve data security and platform compatibility, optimize the system logical structure and facilitate the system development. The third part is database, MySQL be used as the system database to store patient condition assessment information and patient personal information, MySQL is a so mature and stable commercial database that could ensure data security. Fig.1 depicts the system structure of online clinical scale collection System.

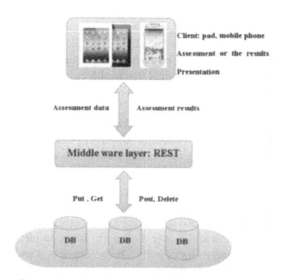

Fig. 1. Architecture of the online clinical scale collection system proposed in this paper. In the client, health care staff could submit, update, delete assessment results, and view the history list of assessment results, middle ware's main function are the assessment data encapsulation and unpacking and standardize health care staff operations.

3   Main Technologies

In this section, we mainly introduce three techniques that are used in the system development, namely, the web client development based on the HTML5 standard, and use web service and REST as middle-ware layer, and use report to represent assessment results. In the following, we will introduce their advantages and how to use them in the system.

3.1   The HTML5 Standard

The HTML5 standard has become one of the hot topics of the Internet and the mainstream browsers all support it. Its advantage is reflected in two aspects, the one is the user of it, it improves user's experience, enhanced visual experience. The standard of HTML5 enables the mobile terminal application to return to the web page, and the functionality can be extended so that the user's operation could be easier. The other one is the developers of application, the standard of HTML5 cross-platform and multi-terminal adapter. Native App of conventional mobile terminal must be developed for different operating systems, while the development of application based on HTML5/JavaScript/CSS don't need to consider the compatibility of the system, it can be distributed into all browsers after the development of the application is completed.

Even take the channels of traditional App Store, we can package underlying applications which is developed on the standard of HTML5 to the App, so that the costs of development is lower.

The web client development of online clinical scale collection system is based on the HTML5 standard because of its powerful features can make the system work so nice in cross-platform and multi-terminal that health care staff can smoothly evaluate and view patient's condition on computer and mobile devices such as iPad and mobile phone.

Meanwhile, we don't need to consider the web client's compatibility, In other words, we do not have to develop client for different platforms so it can reduces unnecessary duplication work during the development of the web client of the system.

3.2   Web Service and REST

The W3C defines a web service as: a software system designed to support interoperable machine-to-machine interaction over a network. It has an interface described in a machine-processable format (specifically Web Service Description Language, WSDL). Other systems interact with the Web service in a manner prescribed by its description using Simple Object Access Protocol (SOAP) messages, typically conveyed using HTTP with an XML serialization in conjunction with other Web-related standards [5]. REST is an architectural style consisting of a coordinated set of architectural constraints applied to components, connectors, and data elements, within a distributed hypermedia system. REST ignores the details of component implementation and protocol syntax in order to focus on the roles of components, the constraints upon their interaction with other components, and their interpretation of significant data elements. In our system, there are four types of action while submitting the results of medical assessment scales [6]:

- "GET": when you want to view clinical scales evaluation history information, the "get" will be triggered to get the information from database.
- "POST": when you want to submit the evaluation results of clinical scale, "post" will be triggered to insert evaluation results into database.

- "PUT": when you want to modify the clinical scale history evaluation information which have been stored into database, "put" wil be triggered to get the information from database and then update the modified information to the database
- "DELETE": if you want to delete useless history evaluation information, "delete" will help you to complete it.

3.3   The Use of Report

To display data from database for medical analysis and research, charts and cross tables are applied into the online clinical scale collection system. NVD3 is a project that builds re-usable charts and chart components for d3.js (a JavaScript library for manipulating documents based on data). Based on d3.js, NVD3 supports datasets, suitable for dealing with a large quantity of patients' data in hospital. Meanwhile, the feature of dynamic behavior for interaction helps the health care staff analyze and investigate patients' condition in the form of chart directly.

4   Functional Design of the System

Before designing of the online clinical scale collection system, we have done a lot of investigations to meet the requirements of health care staffs to the maximum extent. The design goal of the system is simple, stability, practical and scalable, so we did not add complex functionality. The main functions of the online clinical scale collection system are:

Scale assessment results timely presentation; data (including the results of the assessment) synchronization, storage and management; key information extraction and presentation. The following describes the main functions of the system:

4.1   Assessment Results Timely Presentation

Some results of the assessment of complex clinical scales need health care staff to calculate it with the assessment information in accordance with certain rules after the assessment complete. After investigation, we found that these calculations are lightweight computing. So during the design of the system, we put the lightweight calculations on the web client, namely , when the web client detected health care staff fill in the clinical scale, web client will calculate the results of the assessment automatically based on the information that the doctor do. Therefore, health care staff not only don't need spend extra time to get the assessment results, but also they could view the assessment results in real time after filling out the clinical scale. So the system will improve the efficiency of the health care staff and allow health care staff to provide medical advices for the patient's condition in time.

4.2   Data Synchronization, Storage and Management

Health care staff can assess the patient's condition in the online clinical scale collection system on their Pad and other mobile devices and upload them to the database in real time to synchronize the critical information with the hospital's case library. Meanwhile, patient's disease information and assessment information can be retrieved from the hospital library and then be viewed in the form of assessment scales and line chart to obtain the changes of patient's condition; The system database stores the patients personal information, clinical scale assessment information. Each record has a registration number to mark it and registration number is the unique ID for each patient, health care staff could get all the results of the assessment of patients by it so that they could more comprehensive understanding of the patient's condition and provide more accurate follow-up treatment.

We use php-admin, a MySQL management tool which has been widely used, to manage the database rather than independently develop back-end management tool, php-admin is so independent of the database that would not increase the load on the system and reduce development costs. Meanwhile, it could manage the database nicely and easily.

4.3   Key Information Extraction and Presentation

In this system, we provide several retrieval interfaces, where the health care staff can extract the useful information from the database through some key words that provide by the retrieval interfaces. The key words could be divided into two categories, The first category which are presented in each scale and common information is stored in these key words, the others are stored the key information of each scale during the assessment. Through the two kinds of key words doctor can retrieve useful information what they need to understand the condition of patients; In the representation of information, we use report technique which is mentioned in the previous article, the system will show the information in the cross table, graphs or the other forms to present it to the health care staff so that the health care can makes a more intuitive understanding of the patient's condition changes, and in order to facilitate the collection of the clinical data, the information can be exported in the form of excel, based on this information, specialist doctors can make better treatment for the patient, meanwhile, in patients informed, specialist doctors can use the information for clinical research.

5   Applications

The system has been applied in Shenzhen Traditional Chinese Medicine (TCM) hospital, which is one of the best hospitals to treat stroke patients in Shenzhen, which have more than 1000 person-times of stroke patients hospitalized per year. At present, our system has been used for clinicians in Shenzhen TCM hospital to evaluate patients' pathogenic condition with clinical assessment scales. The system in operation comprises altogether 29 types of medical scales in total. The application trail has been carried for one year and during this period 4890 medical scales have been collected from304 in-hospital patients.

Fig.2 show the basic statistics page of the system which can illustrate the number of medical scales collected with respect to patient, doctor or timeline. This page helps hospital managers to keep track of the workload of the doctors and the situation update of patients.

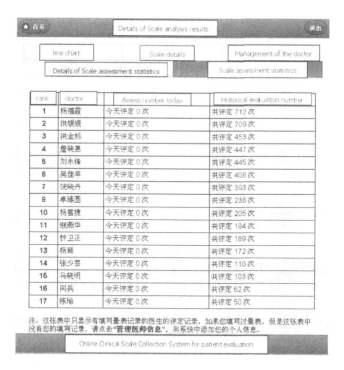

rank	doctor	Assess number today	Historical evaluation number
1	杨福霞	今天评定 0 次	共评定 712 次
2	洪媛媛	今天评定 0 次	共评定 709 次
3	洪金标	今天评定 0 次	共评定 453 次
4	詹晚惠	今天评定 0 次	共评定 447 次
5	刘永锋	今天评定 0 次	共评定 445 次
6	吴佳萃	今天评定 0 次	共评定 408 次
7	饶晓丹	今天评定 0 次	共评定 393 次
9	卓缘圆	今天评定 0 次	共评定 238 次
10	杨雪捷	今天评定 0 次	共评定 205 次
11	娥燕华	今天评定 0 次	共评定 194 次
12	钟卫正	今天评定 0 次	共评定 189 次
13	杨颖	今天评定 0 次	共评定 172 次
14	张少芸	今天评定 0 次	共评定 110 次
15	马晓明	今天评定 0 次	共评定 103 次
16	闰兵	今天评定 0 次	共评定 62 次
17	陈瑜	今天评定 0 次	共评定 50 次

注：这张表中只显示有填写量表记录的医生的评定记录，如果您填写过量表，但是这张表中没有您的填写记录，请点击"管理医师信息"，向系统中添加您的个人信息。

Online Clinical Scale Collection System for patient evaluation

Fig. 2. Basic statistics page of the system displayed on a mobile device. The original interface is in Chinese and the key notations are translated into English. This page helps hospital managers to keep track of the workload of the doctors and the situation update of patients.

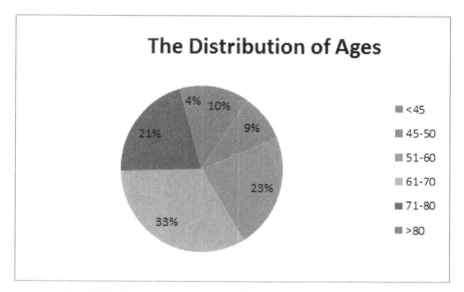

Fig. 3. The distribution of ages in stroke patients enrolled in the system

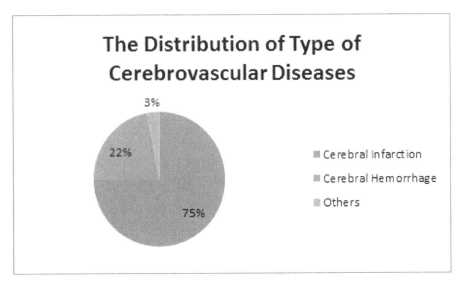

Fig. 4. The distribution of stroke type for patients enrolled in the system

The system also provide survey charts to assert the overall situation of patients enrolled in the studies, including the gender, ages, type of stroke, Body Mass Index, underlying diseases, habits and customs and so on. From the pie charts, we can know more about the characteristics of stroke patients and find out the risk factors of stroke. Fig.3 shows the distribution of ages in enrolled stroke patients, Fig.4 shows the distribution of the stroke subtypes of these patients, and Fig.5 shows the distribution of recurrent history in these patients.

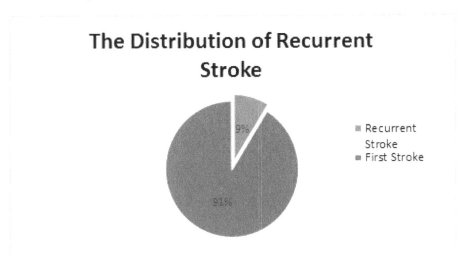

Fig. 5. The distribution of recurrent stroke in enrolled stroke patients

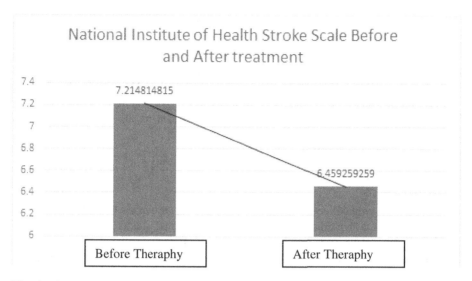

Fig. 6. The curative effect before and after acupuncture treatment with National Institute of Health Stroke Scale (NIHSS). The Chinese contents exist in the original interface is replaced by English notations.

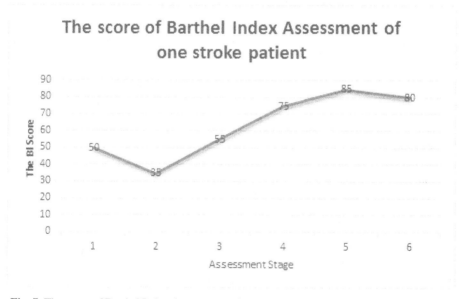

Fig. 7. The score of Barthel Index Assessment of a stroke patient in different assessment stage

An important role of the online medical scale system is to help clinician to study the status change of in-hospital patients and evaluate the quality of treatment timely during hospital rounds. By accessing he assessment result histograms generated in the system from mobile devices, we can know about the curative effect before and after special treatment with clinical scales and make timely decisions. For example, Fig.6 compares the curative effect of a group of patients before and after receiving acupuncture treatments. The average score on multiple patients are displayed. We see that the National Institute of Health Stroke Scale (NIHSS) score of patient drop sharply after therapy, indicating an efficient outcome of the acupunctures. On the other hand, Fig.7 displays the Barthel Index Assessment of a studied stroke patient in different assessment stage, which is another important metric for measuring the rehabilitation status of stroke patients.

6   Conclusion

Online clinical scale collection system is effective for clinicians to evaluate the state of patients' condition. Clinicians could assess the patients' quality of life, psychology, the risk of second attack of stroke with the system. Besides, it is not only convenient for clinicians to take clinical data from patients at their bedside with mobile phones or iPad portable computers, understand the patients comprehensively, guide clinical diagnosis and treatment, but also transform the data to the simplified, visualized statistical charts to assist hospital managements and clinical decision optimizations. In the future, the system would link with hospital information system seamlessly and become an important part of the hospital information system.

Acknowlegements. This work was supported by Shenzhen Municipal Science and Technology Research Development and Funds and Platform Construction Plan Key Laboratory Program (CXB201111250113A), Shenzhen Basic Research Fund (JCYJ2013-0329155553732), the Promotion Funds for Key Laboratory in Shenzhen (ZDSY-20120617113021359) and Shenzhen Innovation Funding for Advanced Talents (KQCX20130628112914291).

References

1. Johnston, S.C., Gress, D.R., Browner, W.S., et al.: Short-term prognosis after emergency department diagnosis of TIA. JAMA **284**(22), 2901–2906 (2000)
2. Coutts, S.B., Eliasziw, M., Hill, M.D., et al.: An improved scoring system for identifying patients at high early risk of stroke and functional impairment after an acute transient ischemic attack or minor stroke. International Journal of Stroke **3**(1), 3–10 (2008)
3. Johnston, S.C., Rothwell, P.M., Nguyen-Huynh, M.N., et al.: Validation and refinement of scores to predict very early stroke risk after transient ischemic attack. (9558) (2007)
4. Edwards, D., Cohn, S.R., Mavaddat, N., et al.: Varying uses of the ABCD2 scoring system in primary and secondary care: a qualitative study. BMJ Open **2**(6), 1–6 (2012)
5. Web Services Glossary W3C. February 11, 2004. (retrieved April 22, 2011)
6. Fielding, R.T., Taylor, R.N.: Principled Design of the Modern Web Architecture (2002)

Comparative Evaluation of Two Systems for Integrating Biometric Data from Self-quantification

Bibin Punnoose and Kathleen Gray[✉]

University of Melbourne, Melbourne, Victoria, Australia
kgray@unimelb.edu.au

Abstract. A layperson can accumulate a large volume of biometric data using the self quantification tools available in the consumer electronics market. However to derive insight, one must be able to integrate data types in order to identify patterns that emerge. This paper compares the practicalities of integrating biometric data from self-quantification, using the TicTrac and HealthVault integration tools. The techniques needed to use such tools may be challenging for many consumers. The aggregated data may have data quality issues. These factors limit the realization of benefits for individual or population health.

Keywords: Consumer health informatics · HealthVault · Quantified Self · Self-tracking · TicTrac

1 Background and Aim

In self-quantification, a layperson can select from a variety of non-standardized consumer electronic devices to measure, record and represent data about their body – biometric data – including one or more of: blood chemistry, blood pressure, body temperature, body weight, heart rate, mood and brain activity, respiratory rate and sleep pattern. These wearable sensing and feedback systems are thought have the potential to produce significant health benefits for individuals and populations (for example, Lupton, 2013; Swan, 2012).

A person can accumulate a large volume of biometric data using self quantification tools such as: Adidas miCoach, Amiigo, Basis, Blipcare, Bodymedia, Cardiio, Emwave2, Fitbit, Happiness, InsideTracker, Lark, Jawbone Up, MercuryApp, Mio, Misfit Shine, Moodjam, MoodPanda, Moodscope, Moves, Myithlete, Nike Fuelband, iHealth, Omron, Polar, RunKeeper, SleepCycle, Strava, Talking20, Tinke, Wakemate, WellnessFX, Withings and Zeo (Technori, n.d). Their use varies according to whether they are static, mobile or wearable; whether they are designed to connect to software on a desktop or laptop computer, to a tablet or smartphone app, directly to a web site or to another device, and whether they need a cable, Bluetooth or Wifi. While some self-quantification tools merely collect and accumulate biometric data, others offer different approaches to integrate and visualize the collected data.

It is hard to derive much insight into health from viewing different biometric data sets separately, as compared to seeing them in relation to each other (Tilahun, 2014). Although recommendations for designing systems to integrate such data using online

X. Yin et al. (Eds.): HIS 2015, LNCS 9085, pp. 195–201, 2015.
DOI: 10.1007/978-3-319-19156-0_20

platforms have been around for some time (Frost 2008), in most cases this still requires a separate set of tools (Almalki et al., 2013), for example Microsoft Excel, Indiemapper, Nineteen, Tictrac (Technori, n.d). Some tools originally designed as a Personal Health Record (PHR) - an electronic application for a member of the public to store all their health data in one place - now offer this functionality, for example Microsoft HealthVault (HealthVault, 2014).

Comparative evaluation of the performance of such tools could be useful to health self-quantifiers and those who work with them. The aim of this paper is to compare the performance of a generic life-logging tool and a personal health record tool for this purpose.

2   Method

Two free online tools were chosen. HealthVault, a PHR, can store a wide variety of data besides biometric data - allergies, appointments, disease conditions, contacts, family history, immunizations, etc. Tictrac, a platform to track lifestyle information grouped under health, wellbeing, entertainment, family, finance, fitness, and social projects, can include data from health and fitness related projects to projects related to daily activities like television watching and holidays (Tictrac, 2014).

This study was undertaken as a self-experiment by one researcher with advice and feedback provided by the other researcher. Since self-quantification is essentially self-experimentation (Fox, 2013), this method was an apt reflection of real-world use of the tools. Further, self-experimentation has been reported previously in this type of research (Smarr, 2012).

Over a four week period, one researcher collected and integrated biometric data routinely in both TicTrac and HealthVault. In addition, the researcher separately maintained a daily log of activities and experiences while using these tools and integrating the data. Four devices widely available in the Australian consumer electronic market were used to collect data:

LARK sleep monitoring system uses the wristband and an iOS 8 compatible app to record sleep data. The wristband was connected to a dock for charging. The alarm time had to be set on the iPad first, turned 'on' and then the wristband removed from the dock and tied on to the wrist. This will activate the system and start recording sleep data from the moment it is disconnected from the dock until the alarm is turned 'off'. The alarm is a silent and vibrating alarm. The data recorded include total hours of sleep, number of times woken up, duration to fall asleep and sleep quality rating (LARK, n.d.).

Fitbit Atria is an electronic weighing scale used to record a person's weight. This device was connected to the local wifi with the help of a computer connected to the same wifi. An account was created in the Fitbit website. Each time the weight was measured, the weight was transmitted through the wifi to the account and it automatically gets updated. (Fitbit, n.d.).

The Polar loop wristband was used to collect the data about daily activity. The data collected was recorded in the Polar Flowsync account by connecting the wristband. This was easy to create and was done using a Windows computer and an Android based smart phone. The wristband was worn all day until going to bed. The data recorded includes: number of steps walked, number of calories burnt, and duration of activity. It also shows time just like a digital watch. The wristband was connected to the laptop using a USB cable and data was transferred to the account. The transfer of data could also be done by opening the app on the mobile and pressing the button on the wristband to enable Bluetooth connection (Polar, n.d.).

The iHealth Non-Invasive Blood Pressure (NIBP) equipment and iHealth app was used to collect data about the blood pressure and heart rate. The app was downloaded on to an iPad using iOS software and an iCloud account was opened. The NIBP equipment was connected to the iPad and controlled through the device via Bluetooth to enable inflation of the cuff. The data collected was saved onto the user's account. (iHealth, n.d.)

Tool performance was compared in terms of usability (a process criterion) and visualization (an output criterion). The approach taken to usability evaluation was the technique of user performance testing, that is, a study conducted on fully complete equipment by a real-life user (Shackel, 2009). The framework for determining usability was based on the perspective of an end user, where effectiveness and efficiency are pragmatic goals and user experience is a hedonic goal (Bevan, 2009). Information visualization was evaluated using the cognitive efficiency model of graphical design, which brings together four concepts (Hullman, 2011): data-ink ratio; information organization; animation; and labelling.

Descriptive data analysis was done by thematically reviewing the content of the log, and by inspecting the resulting visual artifacts that were created using each integrating tool. Themes for data analysis were based on the measures of usability and visualization that were identified from the literature.

3   Findings

3.1   Visualization

In Tictrac biometric data can be viewed as summary of the data up to a date or as a time breakdown as to when the data was recorded each day, or as a line graph (Figure 1); in the latter, all four data sets can be represented with a different colour and viewed simultaneously on the same chart (Figure 2). The data-ink ratio in the line graph is high because the data occupies the majority of the ink viewed in the chart. Information organization is done by having one half of the project page blank where data sets can be dragged one by one for viewing as a summary or a trend or as circular breakdown chart and the other half with tiles of biometric data with their latest readings. It also shows a dropdown box to view as days or weeks or months. Animation of data is not used. The labeling of dates is done by pop-up of the values of the biometric data when a pointer is placed on the node corresponding to each date.

In HealthVault, biometric data are shown as tiles with the names of the data types and their corresponding last reading. Clicking a tile displays all the biometric data from the latest collected. Another tab next can be clicked to view the data as a line graph (Figure 3); however it is not possible to see multiple data trends in one screen simultaneously. The data-ink ratio in the line graph is low in comparison to Tictrac; the majority of the ink viewed in the chart includes the grid lines shown to represent date and value of data, but the information gained is not more than that obtained from the Tictrac chart. The grid lines give an approximation but are not accurate (Bhandari,

2012). Information organization is done using the tabs and tiles; a dropdown box shows days or weeks or months similar to Tictrac. This gives clear insight to the user as to the progress made in each timeframe (Bhandari, 2012). Labelling is done here much more than Tictrac, not only representing dates and but also the values of the data. As with TicTrac, the pointer when placed on the node corresponding to each date shows the data value as a pop-up. There are no legends used in this chart, similar to Tictrac. As with TicTrac, no animation is used.

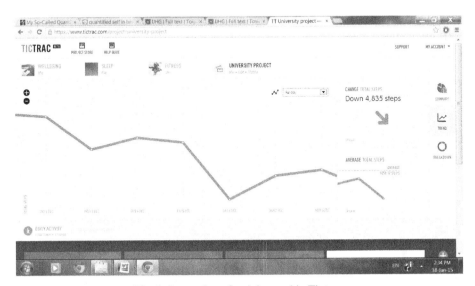

Fig. 1. Screenshot of weight trend in Tictrac

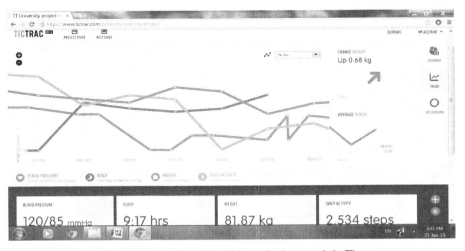

Fig. 2. Screenshot of combined biometric data trends in Tictrac

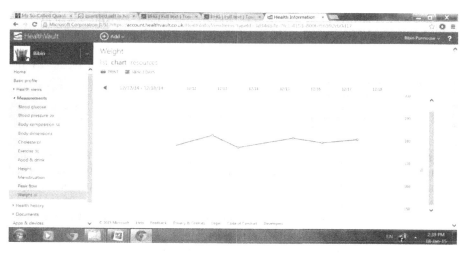

Fig. 3. Screenshot of weight trend in HealthVault

3.2   Usability

In terms of Tictrac effectiveness, the integration of data into the account happened automatically for data from the Fitbit and iHealth apps, once they were connected to Tictrac. However, integration had to be done manually by the user for data from LARK and Polar flowsync devices; the Tictrac account had a format to store these data and the user had to type the readings in. In terms of efficiency, the only time expended on Fitbit and iHealth data was a one-time task to set up this connection, as opposed to the LARK and Polar flowsync apps where logging into the Tictrac account was necessary and then the data had to be entered manually each time the user chose. The average time taken for logging into the account was 25 seconds, 40 seconds per entry for entering activity data and sleep data. The time taken to check an entry on weight and blood pressure was 20 seconds. In terms of satisfaction Tictrac was effective, efficient, and easy to navigate.

In terms of HealthVault effectiveness, the integration of data from the Fitbit app happened automatically once it was connected to the system. The integration of data from iHealth and Polar Flowsync tools had to be done manually by the user; there was a format to store these data and the user had to type the readings in. In the case of LARK, it could neither be connected automatically nor did it have a format to enter the readings. HealthVault had the option to export and import data as an Excel spreadsheet but LARK did not have the option to export data; so the work-around used to was to enter LARK data into Tictrac, export them from Tictrac and then import them into HealthVault. In terms of efficiency, although HealthVault can integrate Fitbit data automatically, as opposed to Tictrac it is not a one-time process: the time expended included the time spent to set up the initial connection; in addition each time the user wanted to integrate the data it was necessary to log into the HealthVault account and go to the Fitbit page and click 'post'. The user had to log into the account each time also to do iHealth and Polar flowsync data entry. The average time taken for logging into the account was 30 seconds, 40 seconds per entry for entering physical activity data and 30 seconds per entry for entering blood pressure data. The time taken to check an entry in weight was 40 seconds. Sleep data entry checking was extenuated by the process described above. HealthVault was effective to some extent, and it was very simple in format and appearance, but it was less time-efficient than Tictrac, so overall it produced lower user satisfaction than Tictrac.

4   Discussion and Conclusions

The researchers acknowledge that the study findings might not be the same for a larger sample of users and data sets, however the use of self-experimentation method had advantages in terms of rapidly and efficiently outlining protocols for conducting a larger study of data collection and integration tool performance.

Several lessons emerged from the experience of working with the two integration tools compared in this study. An integration tool should be able to: interface with the all of the biometric data collection devices used, or at least have appropriate data fields; display data as a graph or a summary, and offer comprehensive and detailed versions of each type of view; and exchange data with other health- and self-management tools.

Usable tools, properly used, can allow individuals to discern biometric data patterns that may help them to set and achieve health improvement goals, with flow on benefits to population health. However, while most tools for collecting a particular type of data follow the same straightforward method irrespective of the brand of tool (for example blood pressure measured using an arm cuff and physical activity recorded using a wristband), the techniques required for the important stage of data integration and information visualization are more complex, less comprehensive and vary considerably from tool to tool. The techniques needed to use integration tools may be challenging and time consuming for many users. Even among persistent users, the need for manual data entry means that their aggregated data may have data quality issues.

Access to an increasing array of devices and services that support self-quantification for health is good in principle. However it is important to understand that many tools do not offer integration or visualization at all. Among those that do, individuals must choose according to their goals and preferences, and a major vendor may not be the source of the most satisfactory product. In practice the potential for individual health and for population health is not likely to be realized until there is a more functional ecosystem for integrating and visualizing biometric data.

References

1. Almalki, M., Sanchez, F., Gray, K.: Self-Quantification: The Informatics of Personal Data Management for Health and Fitness. Institute for a Broadband Enabled Society (IBES). The University of Melbourne (2013). http://www.broadband.unimelb.edu.au/resources/white-paper/2013/Self-Quantification.pdf
2. Bevan, N.: Extending quality in use to provide a framework for usability measurement. In: Kurosu, M. (ed.) HCD 2009. LNCS, vol. 5619, pp. 13–22. Springer, Heidelberg (2009)
3. Bhandari, V.: Enabling programmable self with HealthVault. O'Reilly Media Inc., Sebastopol (2012)
4. Fitbit. (n.d). https://www.fitbit.com/au/aria

5. Fox, S.: The Social Life of Health Information: Pew Internet & American Life Project (2013). http://www.pewinternet.org/2013/01/15/health-online-2013/
6. Frost, J.H., Massagli, M.P.: Social Uses of Personal Health Information Within PatientsLikeMe, an Online Patient Community: What Can Happen When Patients Have Access to One Another's Data. Journal of Medical Internet Research 10(3), e15 (2008)
7. HealthVault (n.d.). https://www.HealthVault.com/au/en
8. Hullman, J.: Benefitting InfoVis with Visual difficulties. IEEE Transactions on visualization and computer graphics 17(12), 2213–2222 (2011)
9. iHealth.   (n.d.).   http://www.ihealthlabs.com/blood-pressure-monitors/wireless-blood-pressure-monitor/
10. Lark.   (n.d.).   http://support.lark.com/hc/en-us/categories/200215850-Lark-and-Lark-Pro-wearable-sleep-device
11. Lupton, D.: Quantifying the body: monitoring and measuring health in the age of mHealth technologies. Critical Public Health. 23(4), 393–403 (2013)
12. Polar. (n.d). http://www.polar.com/au-en/products/get_active/fitness_crosstraining/loop
13. Shackel, B.: Usability – Context, framework, definition, design and evaluation. Interacting with computers 21, 339–346 (2009)
14. Smarr, L.: Quantifying your body: A how-to guide from a systems biology perspective. Biotechnology Journal 7, 980–991 (2012)
15. Swan, M.: Health 2050: The realization of personalized medicine through crowdsourcing, the quantified self, and the participatory Biocitizen. Journal of Personalized Medicine 2, 93–118 (2012)
16. Technori.   (n.d.).   http://technori.com/2013/04/4281-the-beginners-guide-to-quantified-self-plus-a-list-of-the-best-personal-data-tools-out-there/
17. Tictrac (n.d.). https://www.Tictrac.com/
18. Tilahun, B., Kauppinen, T., Kebler, C.: Design and Development of a Linked Open Data-Based Health Information Representation and Visualization System: Potentials and Preliminary Evaluation. JMIR Medical Informatics 2(2), 1 (2014)

Investigating Various Technologies
Applied to Assist Seniors

Pouria Khosravi[✉], Amir Hossein Ghapanchi, and Michael Blumenstein

School of Information and Communication Technology, Griffith University,
Nathan, Queensland, Australia
pouria.khosravi@griffithuni.edu.au,
{a.ghapanchi,m.blumenstein}@griffith.edu.au

Abstract. This study undertakes a systematic literature review to investigate current empirical studies on the assistive technologies applied in aged care. Our systematic review of 54 studies published from 2000 to 2014 examines the role of assistive technologies in seniors' daily lives, from enhancements in their mobility to improvements in the social connectedness and decreases in readmission to hospitals. We found eight key issues in aged care that have been targeted by ICT researchers. We also identified the assistive technologies that have been proposed to overcome those problems, and we categorised these assistive technologies into six clusters. Our analysis showed significant growth in the number of publications in this area in the past few years. It also showed that most of the studies in this area have been conducted in North America.

1   Introduction

The number of old adults in our society is growing: in the Australia, the group of people aged 65 or older comprised 16% of the population in 2012, and by 2040 this percentage will be 25%[1]. This increase in the number of old adults will have a substantial impact on the healthcare system and society such as increasing number of old people with chronic diseases social inclusion and need for more professional caregivers [1].

Information and communication technology (ICT) applied in various field [2-8] and recently have transformed daily life of seniors and offer a great potential to improve the health of these group of people [9]. Various technologies, such as the robot, general ICT and sensor technology have been used to manage specific health problems [10]. These ICTs, which are commonly known as assistive technologies, are defined by Marshal (1997) [11] as "any item, piece of equipment, product or system, whether acquired commercially, off-the-shelf, modified or customized, that is used to increase, maintain or improve functional capabilities of individuals with cognitive, physical or communication disabilities".

Studies demonstrate that ICT has been used for a variety of purposes to help seniors in their daily life. Assistive technologies have a wide range covering from computer use to the most advanced robot technology [12, 13]. Due to the above variability, however,

---

[1] Australian Bureau of Statistics. Available at http://www.abs.gov.au/

© Springer International Publishing Switzerland 2015
X. Yin et al. (Eds.): HIS 2015, LNCS 9085, pp. 202–212, 2015.
DOI: 10.1007/978-3-319-19156-0_21

there is lack of the studies to show the bigger picture and outcome of these technologies. Therefore, in this systematic literature review, we identify assistive technologies that are designed to help seniors in their daily life and relieve their problems. This study aims to fill the gap identified in the literature and provides a broader picture of elderly's problem and the various technology interventions proposed to help them. Therefore, this study poses the following research questions:

RQ1. What problems of the elderly have been targeted and investigated by ICT researchers?
RQ2. What technologies have been proposed for aged care problems?

This study contributes to the literature on assistive technologies in various ways. First, it furthers the attempt to identify seniors' problems and the technologies proposed to assist them. Second, the findings of this study should enable practitioners to better understand the various technologies. With this understanding, practitioners can better advise seniors as to how they might gain an improved quality of life through the use of appropriate assistive technologies.

2   Methodology

To classify, assess and interpret the existing empirical studies and answer our research questions, a systematic literature review was conducted in this study[14]. Many studies have used the same approach [15-21]. Following the guidelines proposed by Kitchenham [14], we conducted the study in three stages, namely, planning, conducting, and reporting the review.

2.1   Search Terms

We undertook systematic searches using keywords of publications between 2000 to the present in the following databases: ScienceDirect, PubMed, ProQuest and IEEE Explore. The following keywords were used: ("elderly" or "older" or "aged" or "senior" or "elders") AND ("technology" or "adoption" or "benefits" or "information and communication technology" or "intervention") in the publication's titles, keywords, abstracts or full texts.

2.2   Inclusion/Exclusion Criteria

We included studies involving seniors aged 60 or older with different types of study designs. The studies had to include technologies related to aged care problems. We included studies that applied to help seniors and provide evidence of changes ranged in seniors' daily life. Studies in languages other than English were excluded.

2.3   Data Extraction and Synthesis

First, two authors independently reviewed the abstracts of the retrieved sources and agreed on the included articles. In total, 2069 titles and abstracts were screened to find the qualified studies for the review. Full papers of 248 studies were retrieved and evaluated by the authors. Based on the predefined criteria, 54 articles were included in this review (Fig 1). In addition, an independent reviewer independently evaluated the paper against the inclusion criteria. Subsequently, the key details were extracted and synthesised from the 54 studies included in our systematic review. For the analysis of the data and to draw diagrams we used Microsoft Excel.

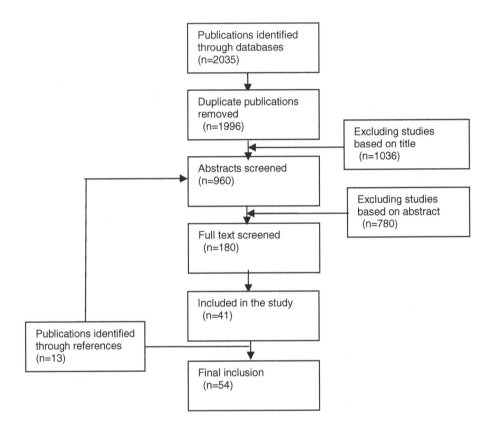

Fig. 1. Study selection procedures

3   Results

3.1   Trends

The distribution of the included studies per year is shown in Figure 2. The number of studies noticeably increased in the past few years; this suggests that this area is increasingly attracting the attention of academics and practitioners because of the growth of the older population.

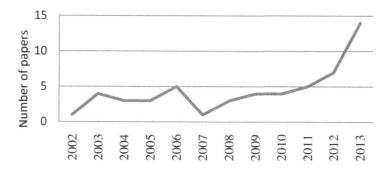

Fig. 2. Frequency of publications per year

Figure 3 shows that most of the included studies were conducted in North America and Canada (N=27, 50%) and Asia (N=13, 24%). The rest of the studies were conducted in Europe (N=10, 19%) and Australia (N=4, 7%).

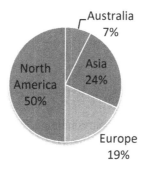

Fig. 3. Number of publications per continent

3.2   Seniors' Problems

The analysed outcomes differed widely between the various studies. We found that the studies target eight older adults' problems: (1) independent living, (2) fall risk (3) chronic disease, (4) dementia, (5) social isolation, (6) depression, (7) wellbeing, and (8) medication management (Figure 2).

The highest level of research attention was paid to wellbeing (with thirteen publications in the final set), which covers many aspects of positive functioning including happiness, life satisfaction and subjective wellbeing.

Independent living and Social isolation are the next two highest categories (with 9 and 8 publications, respectively). The majority of older adults want to continue living independently and technologies may enable them to stay in their own home longer before moving to nursing facilities. This preference is particularly facilitated by sensor technologies and robotics that can help seniors to live independently.

206 P. Khosravi et al.

General ICT used to reduce social isolation and increase social connectedness. Studies report that the experience of social isolation in older people has increased and clearly has negative effects on older adults' health, wellbeing and quality of life [22, 23].

The next highest category is chronic disease (Seven publications). As population aging has accelerated, one of the challenges is dealing with chronic conditions. Innovative and cost-effective ways are required to meet the healthcare needs of older adults.

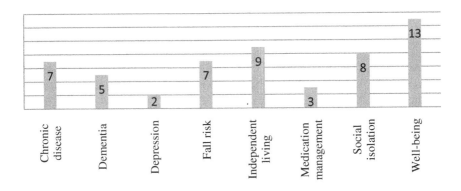

Fig. 4. Seniors' problems targeted by ICT researchers (and number of publications)

To monitor the elderly with chronic conditions in their own residence, telemedicine can be used as a cost-effective way to reduce unnecessary hospitalisation and to ensure that patients receive urgent care in a timely fashion.

Falls are a costly and unresolved safety issue for older adults and seniors who fall usually need medical attention. Researchers have tried to reduce the fall risk using technologies such as sensors and video games. Seven publications in the final pool dealt with fall risk.

Dementia is the next highest category of research on technology that provides benefits for older adults (with five publications in the final pool). The ageing population has led to a surge in the number of people with dementia. Dementia has implications for the individual's quality of daily life [24]. Seniors with dementia need suitable supportive living environments in which they can live safely.

Medication management is the next category (with three publications). Reminding older adults to take the right dosage of medicine at the right time especially those who suffer from chronic disease is very significant and has been one of the significant aids of technology for older adults [25].

Depression is the last category (with two publications in the final pool). The lack of communication and emotional support among older adults may result in depression. Technologies such as the internet may reduce depression by engaging seniors in social interaction.

3.3   Technologies Used to Assist Seniors

We categorised the technological interventions reported in the 54 studies into six categories, namely, general ICT, robotics, telemedicine, sensor technology, medication management applications, and video games. Table 1 provides a summary showing which technologies were applied to address the eight categories of seniors' problems.

Robotics is a rapidly growing area of technology that provides services such as the operation of appliances and various other tasks that support the elderly's daily living.

The main purpose of telemedicine is to provide specialist consultations to distant patients including diagnosing and treating through telecommunication devices [26]. Telemedicine is used in a more restrictive sense at home and involves the use of ICT to monitor the patient's status at a distance [26].

Table 1. Various assistive technologies proposed for seniors' issues

	Sensor Technology	Robotics	Telemedicine	ICT	Video games	Medication dispensing device
Fall risk	[27] [28] [29] [30] [31] [32]				[33]	
Independent living	[34-36] [37]	[38]	[39]			
Chronic disease			[40-42] [43] [44] [1] [45]			
Dementia	[46]			[47] [48]		
Social isolation		[49] [9] [50] [51]		[23] [22] [52] [53]		
Depression		[54]		[55]		
Wellbeing		[56] [57] [58] [59]	[60]	[61] [62, 63] [64] [65] [12]	[66] [67]	
Medication management				[68]		[69] [70]

Sensor technologies are designed to identify and alert caregivers and patients about critical events such as falling out of bed. The two goals that have lead to the fast development of various types of sensor technologies are independent living and fall prevention.

General ICT includes technologies such as using the computer and the internet. The selected studies focus on how the use of these successful technologies impacts on different aspects of senior life.

Seniors face the complex task of medication management, especially those with chronic disease. To enhance the accuracy of medication administration, medication management applications are designed through reminder services. These tools include medication dispensers and smart phone applications.

The last category is video games. The interactive nature of video gaming means that it can be used as a therapy tool and for relaxation and entertainment. Video games can improve the central processing speed and movement by brain training.

4   Discussion

This study showed the importance of assistive technology uptake by older people and its positive impact not only on the individuals but also on those who work with them, including healthcare professionals, family members and the broader society. To encourage seniors and other stakeholders to accept and use new technologies, researchers and practitioners should promote the anticipated benefits such as independent living, increased safety, increased social connectedness and advances in mobility.

There is a need for medical researchers to be involved in ICT research projects to categorise the significant clinical benefits as well as the cost-effectiveness of using assistive technologies. Therefore, multidisciplinary research is needed to find and assess an approach to evaluating the impact of assistive technologies on older adults' daily life.

It is essential for ICT research to be based on theoretical frameworks and models to provide a justification for hypothesised relationships [71]. The lack of a theoretical approach prevents the researcher from following a systematic approach. However, few studies in this review were based on a theoretical framework. Therefore, future studies should develop a theoretical model that is specific to the context of aged care.

Most of the studies suffer from small sample size; therefore, future studies should use larger samples in order to validate the outcomes.

5   Implications for Practice

The findings of this study provide a number of implications for practice by showing the benefits of assistive technologies. First, policy-makers and governments should financially support new technologies and increase ICT literacy among seniors. Therefore, governments should recognise and promote the use of new technologies and the positive impact of these technologies on society, healthcare and the quality of life among seniors. This is because the use of assistive technologies not only elevates the quality of the senior individual's life but also has a positive impact on the healthcare system overall by reducing costs, readmissions and the length of hospital stays. In addition, this study showed how assistive technologies offer various possibilities which could support seniors to live independently and have a better quality of life. Therefore, practitioners should integrate appropriate technologies and combinations of technologies based on older adults' needs either in their own residences or in nursing homes.

6   Conclusion

Assistive technologies are a reality and can be applied to improve quality of life, especially among older age groups. A combination of various assistive technologies provides promising results in supporting the elderly in daily life. By conducting a systematic literature review, this study identified various assistive technologies proposed by ICT researchers to assist the elderly. This review shows that, it is vital to develop systems and devices that suit seniors' needs and limitations with clear benefits.

References

1. Pinto, A., et al.: Home telemonitoring of non-invasive ventilation decreases healthcare utilisation in a prospective controlled trial of patients with amyotrophic lateral sclerosis. Journal of neurology, neurosurgery, and psychiatry **81**(11), 1238 (2010)
2. Ghapanchi, A.H., Aurum, A.: The impact of project licence and operating system on the effectiveness of the defect-fixing process in open source software projects. International Journal of Business Information Systems **8**(4), 413–424 (2011)
3. Ghapanchi, A.H., Aurum, A.: Competency rallying in electronic markets: Implications for open source project success. Electronic Markets **22**(2), 117–127 (2012)
4. Ghapanchi, A.H., Aurum, A.: The impact of project capabilities on project performance: Case of open source software projects. International Journal of Project Management **30**(4), 407–417 (2012)
5. Ghapanchi, A.H., Aurum, A., Daneshgar, F.: The Impact of Process Effectiveness on User Interest in Contributing to the Open Source Software Projects. Journal of software **7**(1), 212–219 (2012)
6. Ghapanchi, A.H., Jafarzadeh, M.H., Khakbaz, M.H.: An application of data envelopment analysis (DEA) for ERP system selection: case of a petrochemical company. In: Proceedings of the ICIS 2008, p. 77 (2008)
7. Ghapanchi, A.H., et al.: A methodology for selecting portfolios of projects with interactions and under uncertainty. International Journal of Project Management **30**(7), 791–803 (2012)
8. Zarei, B., Ghapanchi, A.: Guidelines for government-to-government initiative architecture in developing countries. International Journal of Information Management **28**(4), 277–284 (2008)
9. Bickmore, T.W., et al.: 'It's just like you talk to a friend'relational agents for older adults. Interacting with Computers **17**(6), 711–735 (2005)
10. Heerink, M., et al.: Assessing acceptance of assistive social agent technology by older adults: the almere model. International journal of social robotics **2**(4), 361–375 (2010)
11. Marshall, M.: State of the art in dementia care (1997)
12. Demiris, G., et al.: Using informatics to capture older adults' wellness. International journal of medical informatics **82**(11), e232–e241 (2013)
13. Broadbent, E., Stafford, R., MacDonald, B.: Acceptance of healthcare robots for the older population: review and future directions. International Journal of Social Robotics **1**(4), 319–330 (2009)
14. Kitchenham, B.: Procedures for performing systematic reviews (2004)

15. Ghanbarzadeh, R., et al.: A Decade of Research on the Use of Three-Dimensional Virtual Worlds in Health Care: A Systematic Literature Review. Journal of medical Internet research 16(2) (2014)

16. Najaftorkaman, M., et al.: A taxonomy of antecedents to user adoption of health information systems: A synthesis of thirty years of research. Journal of the Association for Information Science and Technology (2014)

17. Ghapanchi, A.H., Aurum, A.: Antecedents to IT personnel's intentions to leave: A systematic literature review. Journal of Systems and Software 84(2), 238–249 (2011)

18. Amrollahi, A., Ghapanchi, A.H., Talaei-Khoei, A.: A systematic literature review on strategic information systems planning: Insights from the past decade. Pacific Asia Journal of the Association for Information Systems 5(2), 4 (2013)

19. Ghanbarzadeh, R., Ghapanchi, A.H., Blumenstein, M.: Application areas of multi-user virtual environments in the healthcare context. Studies in health technology and informatics 204, 38–46 (2013)

20. Najaftorkaman, M., et al.: Recent research areas and grand challenges in electronic medical record: A literature survey approach. International Technology Management Review 3(1), 12–21 (2013)

21. Najaftorkaman, M., Ghapanchi, A.H.: Antecedents to the user adoption of electronic medical record

22. Blažun, H., et al.: Information and communication technology as a tool for improving physical and social activity of the elderly. In: NI 2012: Proceedings of the 11th International Congress on Nursing Informatics. American Medical Informatics Association (2012)

23. Ballantyne, A., et al.: 'I feel less lonely': what older people say about participating in a social networking website. Quality in Ageing and Older Adults 11(3), 25–35 (2010)

24. Moyle, W., et al.: Factors influencing quality of life for people with dementia: a qualitative perspective. Aging & Mental Health 15(8), 970–977 (2011)

25. Budnitz, D.S., et al.: Emergency hospitalizations for adverse drug events in older Americans. New England Journal of Medicine 365(21), 2002–2012 (2011)

26. Ekeland, A.G., Bowes, A., Flottorp, S.: Effectiveness of telemedicine: a systematic review of reviews. International journal of medical informatics 79(11), 736–771 (2010)

27. Diduszyn, J., et al.: Use of a wireless nurse alert fall monitor to prevent inpatient falls. JCOM 15(6) (2008)

28. Bressler, K., Redfern, R.E., Brown, M.: Elimination of Position-Change Alarms in an Alzheimer's and Dementia Long-Term Care Facility. American journal of Alzheimer's disease and other dementias 26(8), 599–605 (2011)

29. Rantz, M.J., et al.: Sensor technology to support aging in place. Journal of the American Medical Directors Association 14(6), 386–391 (2013)

30. Cumming, R.G., et al.: Cluster randomised trial of a targeted multifactorial intervention to prevent falls among older people in hospital. Bmj 336(7647), 758–760 (2008)

31. Ferrari, M., et al.: Clinical feasibility trial of a motion detection system for fall prevention in hospitalized older adult patients. Geriatric Nursing 33(3), 177–183 (2012)

32. Maki, B.E., et al.: Preventing falls in older adults: new interventions to promote more effective change-in-support balance reactions. Journal of electromyography and kinesiology 18(2), 243–254 (2008)

33. Schoene, D., et al.: A randomized controlled pilot study of home-based step training in older people using videogame technology. PloS one 8(3), e57734 (2013)

34. Alexander, G.L., et al.: Passive sensor technology interface to assess elder activity in independent living. Nursing research 60(5), 318 (2011)

35. Van Hoof, J., et al.: Ageing-in-place with the use of ambient intelligence technology: Perspectives of older users. International journal of medical informatics **80**(5), 310–331 (2011)
36. Miller, S.J.: Sensor Technology to Support Aging in Place. JAMDA **14**, 386–391 (2013)
37. Demiris, G., et al.: Older adults' attitudes towards and perceptions of 'smart home' technologies: a pilot study. Informatics for Health and Social Care **29**(2), 87–94 (2004)
38. Shimada, H., et al.: Effects of a robotic walking exercise on walking performance in community-dwelling elderly adults. Geriatrics & gerontology international **9**(4), 372–381 (2009)
39. Mahoney, D.F.: An evidence-based adoption of technology model for remote monitoring of elders' daily activities. Ageing international **36**(1), 66–81 (2011)
40. Sicotte, C., et al.: Effects of home telemonitoring to support improved care for chronic obstructive pulmonary diseases. Telemedicine and e-Health **17**(2), 95–103 (2011)
41. Giordano, A., et al.: Multicenter randomised trial on home-based telemanagement to prevent hospital readmission of patients with chronic heart failure. International journal of cardiology **131**(2), 192–199 (2009)
42. Chau, J.P.-C., et al.: A feasibility study to investigate the acceptability and potential effectiveness of a telecare service for older people with chronic obstructive pulmonary disease. International journal of medical informatics **81**(10), 674–682 (2012)
43. Shea, S., et al.: A randomized trial comparing telemedicine case management with usual care in older, ethnically diverse, medically underserved patients with diabetes mellitus. Journal of the American Medical Informatics Association **13**(1), 40–51 (2006)
44. West, S.P., et al.: Goal setting using telemedicine in rural underserved older adults with diabetes: experiences from the informatics for diabetes education and telemedicine project. Telemedicine and e-Health **16**(4), 405–416 (2010)
45. Gellis, Z.D., et al.: Outcomes of a telehealth intervention for homebound older adults with heart or chronic respiratory failure: a randomized controlled trial. The Gerontologist **52**(4), 541–552 (2012)
46. Aloulou, H., et al.: Deployment of assistive living technology in a nursing home environment: methods and lessons learned. BMC medical informatics and decision making **13**(1), 42 (2013)
47. Leuty, V., et al.: Engaging older adults with dementia in creative occupations using artificially intelligent assistive technology. Assistive Technology **25**(2), 72–79 (2013)
48. Lancioni, G.E., et al.: Supporting daily activities and indoor travel of persons with moderate Alzheimer's disease through standard technology resources. Research in developmental disabilities **34**(8), 2351–2359 (2013)
49. Wada, K., Shibata, T.: Social effects of robot therapy in a care house-change of social network of the residents for two months. In: 2007 IEEE International Conference on Robotics and Automation. IEEE (2007)
50. Kanamori, M., Suzuki, M., Tanaka, M.: Maintenance and improvement of quality of life among elderly patients using a pet-type robot. Nihon Ronen Igakkai zasshi. Japanese journal of geriatrics **39**(2), 214–218 (2002)
51. Beer, J.M., Takayama, L.: Mobile remote presence systems for older adults: acceptance, benefits, and concerns. In: Proceedings of the 6th International Conference on Human-Robot Interaction. ACM (2011)
52. Bradley, N., Poppen, W.: Assistive technology, computers and Internet may decrease sense of isolation for homebound elderly and disabled persons. Technology and disability **15**(1), 19–25 (2003)

53. Blažun, H., Saranto, K., Rissanen, S.: Impact of computer training courses on reduction of loneliness of older people in Finland and Slovenia. Computers in Human Behavior **28**(4), 1202–1212 (2012)
54. Wada, K., et al.: Effects of robot assisted activity to elderly people who stay at a health service facility for the aged. In: Proceedings of the 2003 IEEE/RSJ International Conference on Intelligent Robots and Systems, (IROS 2003). IEEE (2003)
55. Cotten, S.R., et al.: Internet use and depression among older adults. Computers in human behavior **28**(2), 496–499 (2012)
56. Wada, K., Shibata, T.: Living with seal robots—its sociopsychological and physiological influences on the elderly at a care house. IEEE Transactions on Robotics **23**(5), 972–980 (2007)
57. Wada, K., Shibata, T.: Robot therapy in a care house-its sociopsychological and physiological effects on the residents. In: Proceedings of the 2006 IEEE International Conference on Robotics and Automation, ICRA 2006. IEEE (2006)
58. Wada, K., et al.: Effects of robot-assisted activity for elderly people and nurses at a day service center. Proceedings of the IEEE **92**(11), 1780–1788 (2004)
59. Kanamori, M., et al.: Pilot study on improvement of quality of life among elderly using a pet-type robot. In: Proceedings of the 2003 IEEE International Symposium on Computational Intelligence in Robotics and Automation. IEEE (2003)
60. Chou, C.-C., et al.: Technology Acceptance and Quality of Life of the Elderly in a Telecare Program. Computers Informatics Nursing **31**(7), 335–342 (2013)
61. Salovaara, A., et al.: Information technologies and transitions in the lives of 55–65-year-olds: The case of colliding life interests. International journal of human-computer studies **68**(11), 803–821 (2010)
62. Campbell, R.J., Nolfi, D.A.: Teaching elderly adults to use the Internet to access health care information: before-after study. Journal of medical Internet research **7**(2) (2005)
63. Karavidas, M., Lim, N.K., Katsikas, S.L.: The effects of computers on older adult users. Computers in Human Behavior **21**(5), 697–711 (2005)
64. Shapira, N., Barak, A., Gal, I.: Promoting older adults' well-being through Internet training and use. Aging & mental health **11**(5), 477 (2007)
65. Berkowsky, R.W., et al.: Attitudes towards and limitations to ICT use in assisted and independent living communities: Findings from a specially-designed technological intervention. Educational gerontology **39**(11), 797–811 (2013)
66. McKay, S.M., Maki, B.E.: Attitudes of older adults toward shooter video games: An initial study to select an acceptable game for training visual processing. Gerontechnology **9**(1), 5–17 (2010)
67. McLaughlin, A., et al.: Putting fun into video games for older adults. Ergonomics in Design: The Quarterly of Human Factors Applications **20**(2), 13–22 (2012)
68. Stojmenova, E., et al.: Assisted living solutions for the elderly through interactive TV. Multimedia tools and applications **66**(1), 115–129 (2013)
69. Reeder, B., Demiris, G., Marek, K.D.: Older adults' satisfaction with a medication dispensing device in home care. Informatics for Health and Social Care **38**(3), 211–222 (2013)
70. Marek, K.D., et al.: Nurse Care Coordination and Technology Effects on Health Status of Frail Older Adults via Enhanced Self-Management of Medication: Randomized Clinical Trial to Test Efficacy. Nursing research **62**(4), 269–278 (2013)
71. March, S.T., Smith, G.F.: Design and natural science research on information technology. Decision support systems **15**(4), 251–266 (1995)

Characteristics of Research on the Application of Three-Dimensional Immersive Virtual Worlds in Health

Reza Ghanbarzadeh, Amir Hossein Ghapanchi$^{(\boxtimes)}$, and Michael Blumenstein

School of Information and Communication Technology, Griffith University,
Gold Coast, Queensland, Australia
reza.ghanbarzadeh@griffithuni.edu.au,
{a.ghapanchi,m.blumenstein}@griffith.edu.au

Abstract. Three-dimensional immersive virtual worlds (3DVW) offer research-ers and health professionals the opportunities to experiment with their rich communication, collaboration, virtual and 3D content creation integrated tools. This study presents the results of a systematic literature review conducted on the adoption of 3DVWs in the health care sector. Our systematic review began with an initial set of 1088 studies from five major and top-ranking scientific da-tabases published from 1990 to 2013 which have used 3DVWs in health. We found a large quantity of application areas for the 3DVWs in health care, and classified them into two main categories: educational and non-educational ap-plications. We also analyzed different 3DVW platforms and virtual environ-ments which have been used in health care, as well as the avatar-mediated roles these applications, and frequency of papers in different countries. Our findings can be very insightful for the health care community and researchers.

Keywords: Three dimensional virtual worlds · 3DVW · Healthcare · Health

1 Introduction

Web 2.0, as a new technology, facilitates various applications and activities such as collaboration, interaction, social networking, and participation among users [1, 2]. One of the major applications of Web 2.0 is three dimensional immersive virtual worlds (3DVW). A 3DVW is a computer-generated, simulated, collaborative, interactive, networked, graphic, and multimedia environment, running on the web, and designed so that their users may 'live in' and interact using their own digital and graphical self-representations known as 'avatar' [3, 4]. Avatars have the ability to communicate with each other through text or voice tools, either privately or publicly, inside the virtual environments of 3DVWs. These 3D worlds mostly share the sufficiency and capabili-ties and of virtual reality technologies, especially the rendering of 3D environments, and they are accessible to the users through Internet-connected and high-speed PCs. 3DVWs also have capabilities that make them different from virtual reality and other web-based technologies. In particular, these worlds are collaborative and persistent

© Springer International Publishing Switzerland 2015
X. Yin et al. (Eds.): HIS 2015, LNCS 9085, pp. 213–224, 2015.
DOI: 10.1007/978-3-319-19156-0_22

(they exist even when users are not online and logged in) and, as a multi-user environment, they support social networking and interactivity [5, 6]. Importantly, the ability of customizing a personal avatar and using it to communicate with other avatars contributes to a new way of supporting people's embodied subjectivity.

Information technology has made significant advancements which have impacted various aspects of human being life. So far, numerous research studies have been conducted on different effects of IT in a wide variety of fields [16-26] .Over the last decade, there has been a growing interest in the health care communities in using information technologies, especially, 3DVWs for medical purposes. 3DVWs currently feature a lot of medical and health-related projects, and they offer opportunities for different groups such as patients, physicians, providers, educators and health care institutions for improving the quality and efficiency of their care, treatment and education. They offer improved experiences to users and patients seeking health care information, skill building, health care education, group support, and individual consultation in terms of health. It is very important for the health care community and researchers to understand the impacts of using 3DVWs in their specific field, so they can consider the application of this technology in their own research, business or profession.

Previously several studies have been conducted related to this topic and we address some of them as follows. In [7], 3DVWs and their educational potential to health and medical educators and librarians have been introduced. Another study, [8], provides an overview of 3DVWs which are currently used in healthcare professional education and medicine. A survey of activities related to health on Second Life (www.secondlife.com) is conducted in [9]. The opportunities which are available for nursing students inside the multi-user virtual environment are presented by Peck and Miller (2010) [10]. The application areas of three-dimensional virtual worlds in the health care sector have been investigated in [12] and [13].

This paper conducts a systematic review of current studies into the application of 3DVWs in healthcare and medical contexts. This literature review helps us to shape the future direction of research by providing an understanding of previous studies, and recurring themes in the literature, and identifies gaps in the existing body of knowledge to date. This study seeks to respond to these research questions:

RQ1: For which medical purposes have 3DVWs been used by researchers and health professionals?
RQ2: What 3DVW platforms have been used by researches in health care?
RQ3: What kinds of environments have been developed using 3DVWs in health care researches?
RQ4: Which avatar roles have been simulated by 3DVWs in health care?
RQ5: In which countries have the studies related to applications of 3DVWs in health care been conducted mostly?

The remainder of this paper is organized as follows: Section two explains the applied research methodology for our systematic review. Section three presents the results, and section four concludes the article.

2   Research Methodology

In this study, we follow systematic literature review guidelines to achieve our research objectives. A systematic literature review is a methodical approach to identify, evaluate, and interpretation of the previous studies conducted on a specific research topic [11]. Previously, several studies have used this method to conduct a review on literature [14, 15]. The current section explains the research methodology of this study and identifies the inclusion and exclusion processes of papers, data extraction and analysis.

2.1   Search and Select Procedures

The search for relevant literature in the current study was performed in 6 stages. Fig. 1 indicates the stages of study selection for systematic review in this study according to Kitchenham [11] guidelines.

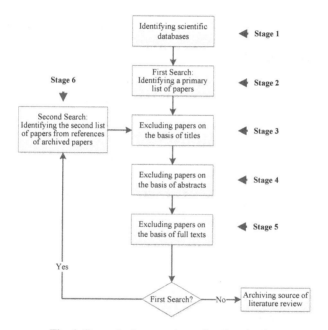

Fig. 1. Stages in the procedure of study selection

In the first stage the scientific databases (see Section B) have been identified to search the key words. In Stage 2, a search of 42 keywords (see Section C) on those databases was carried out. As of July 20, 2013, our searches resulted in 1088 primary studies. As can be seen from the diagram in fig. 1, Stages 3 to 5 were undertaken two times in the search process. In the first iteration, in Stage 3, 789 papers were eliminated on the basis of their titles. In Stage 4, from the remaining 299 papers, 262 papers were excluded on the basis of their abstracts. The total number of relevant papers was 37. In order to increment the comprehensiveness of the study, we tried to increase the number of relevant papers. Therefore, we investigated the reference papers of those of 37 papers in Stage 6 which resulted in an additional 1183 papers. 1152 papers were excluded on the basis of their titles. Another six papers were excluded based on their abstracts, resulting in 25 remaining papers. Altogether, as of 20 Aug 2013, we found 2271 papers, of which 2209 were eliminated for being unrelated to our topic. Eventually, the total number of relevant papers in our systematic review was 62. There was not any paper elimination on the basis of the full text in either iterations. Table 1 represents a comprehensive summary of our search and paper selection process in each stage.

Table 1. Total number of remaining papers

	First Search	References Included
Initial number of papers	1088	1183
Discarded by title	789	1152
Discarded by abstract	262	6
Number of remaining papers	37	25
Total number of remaining papers	62	

2.2   Resources Searched

Five main scientific databases were selected for the searching process: PubMed, ScienceDirect, ProQuest, IEEE Explore and ACM Digital Library.

2.3   Search Terms

The advanced search or expert search service provided by each scientific database's search engine was used to carry out the search operations. Based on the search patterns offered by each database's search engine, the title, abstract, key words and in some of the cases, the full text of articles, were sourced using the 42 various search terms including the keywords related to 'three dimensional', 'virtual world', and 'health'.

2.4   Inclusion and Exclusion Criteria

In the current systematic review, in order to select materials, two inclusion and exclusion criterion were considered:

1) During the search process in all of the above-mentioned databases, a publication date filtration was carried out and we included studies published between January 1990 and July 2013.

2) The studies in languages other than English were excluded.

2.5   Data Extraction

Two kinds of data were extracted from 62 studies in this systematic review: 1) Application areas of 3DWV in healthcare. 2) 3DVW platforms, virtual environment, avatar-mediated roles, year of publication and country of studies. Microsoft Excel 2010 and Microsoft Visio 2010 were used for data collection and analysis, drawing diagrams and designing the tables.

2.6   Data Analysis

In order to accomplish a data analysis, we read the title, abstract and full text of the 62 extracted papers. Our goal was to classify these papers into meaningful categories. Therefore, we tried to insert each paper in an appropriate category based on the main area of research of that article. At the end of the first stage, all the articles were classified according to different categories. To clarify our classification, we revised our categorizing operation several times and finally we grouped all of the extracted papers to two major research categories. After that, we attempted to extract additional information from the articles required for our systematic review, such as health contexts, 3DVW platforms, avatar roles, virtual environments, year of publication, and country of publication. Fig. 2 demonstrates the procedure undertaken to achieve the data analysis process.

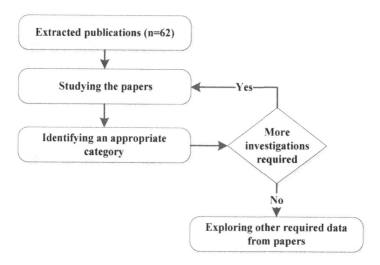

Fig. 2. Stages in the data analysis procedure

3   Results

As mentioned previously, this study seeks to answer five research questions in conjunction with the application areas of 3DVWs in the health care sector. Below are the research questions and discussion.

3.1   RQ1: For Which Medical Purposes have 3DVWs been Used by Researchers and Health Professionals?

3DVWs have been used in a vast majority of application areas in the health care sector and health-related activities. In order to gain a general understanding of 3DVW research, as previously mentioned, we classified all the studies on 3DVW into two categories: educational and non-educational application. Fig. 3 shows the number of published studies in each category. As can be seen from the chart, the education category includes the largest number of papers, namely 34. In contrast, 24 papers are related to non-educational application of 3DVWs in health care. From the total of 62 papers, 4 papers conducted surveys and literature reviews on this field [7-10].

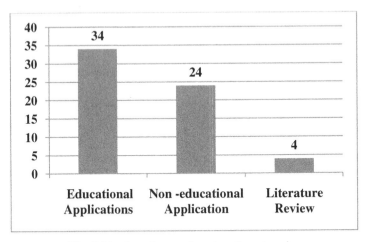

Fig. 3. Number of papers based on the categories

A. Educational Applications

As mentioned, from the total number of 62 papers, 34 studies have used 3DVWs for pedagogical and educational applications in health care. These studies mostly focused on academic and professional education programs which are related to training programs for students and staff in educational communities and universities as well as education in professional health care communities such as training programs for physicians, nurses, and hospital staff for different health contexts like public health, radiotherapy, emergency, safety, pharmacy and clinical medical etc.

B. Non-educational Applications

Studies in this group mostly discuss the use of 3DVWs in several areas such as simulation, treatment and assessment in health. In some studies, patients, nurses, physicians or other medical staff had their own avatars entered in a specific environment in 3DVWs and patients were treated using specialized techniques. Other studies have applied 3DWVs for simulating a replica of hospital, health care logistics, e-health marketing, and public health. For example, a replica of a university lab, a hospital, a ward, an emergency ward, or an operating room has been created virtually inside the various islands of the 3DVWs. Other studies have used these worlds for evaluation and assessment of a particular proficiency in specific groups like nurses and sergeants, or measurement of a factor in emergency services, or investigating a rate of improvement in a patient.

3.2   RQ2: What Platforms have been Used by 3DVW Researches in Health?

In particular, the highest number of papers used Second Life as their study's 3DWV platform, 77.42%. Of the remaining 22.58% of platforms, 16.13 % of studies applied their own self developed virtual world, and the other 6.45% used different platforms like Open Simulator, Virtual-U, Active Worlds and 3D ICS, each 1.61%. These statistics show that Second Life is the most well-known of the 3D virtual worlds which have been used in health care. Fig. 4 demonstrates percentages of different 3DWV platforms applied in the literature.

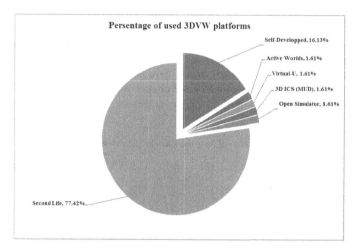

Fig. 4. Percentage of applied 3DWV platforms in health care

3.3   RQ3: What Types of Environments have been Developed Using 3DVWs in Health Researches?

In all of the studied articles in the two application areas of 3DWVs, different virtual environments have been designed, developed and used. We divided them into the following six environments:

- Gaming environments
- Virtual training environments
- Virtual medical environments
- Special islands inside the virtual worlds
- Virtual houses
- Other virtual environments

The most applied environments in the literature were virtual medical environments with 29% of all. These environments were virtual health-related areas built inside the 3DVWs for medical purposes such as virtual hospitals, virtual ICUs, virtual emergency wards, virtual physician's offices, and virtual pharmacies.

The virtual training environments, with 26% of all environments, are the next kind of these areas which were locations such as virtual classrooms, virtual campuses, virtual board room, or a virtual replica of a university campus for educational and training purposes in health care.

14% of the studies used the existing virtual islands in 3DVWs in their works for health specific purposes. Popular 3D virtual worlds like Second Life have several built-in islands for various purposes and users of these worlds can teleport there and use them for their own related works.

7% of all the papers studied in our literature review, created virtual house environments for their health-related works in a house-like environment.

Gaming environments are other kinds of virtual environments which have been applied by 3% of studies. In these environments, the users of 3DVWs mostly play a specific game which is designed inside the virtual worlds to learn about a particular concept.

The remainder of the studies, 21%, used other virtual environments in their works. Some of these environments were virtual exhibitions, virtual parking lots, virtual meeting rooms, virtual accidents, and virtual chat rooms.

Fig. 5 depicts the distribution of the papers across the virtual environments.

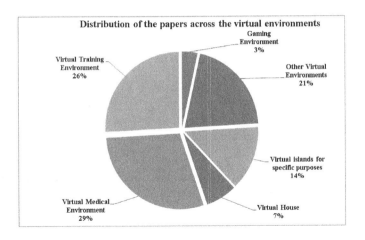

Fig. 5. Distribution of the papers across the virtual environments

3.4   RQ4: Which Medical and Non-medical Roles have been Simulated Avatars by 3DVWs in Health?

3DVW environment are most often populated by avatars, which are controlled by users of the virtual worlds. Avatars are users' own digital and graphical self-representations and people can 'live in' these worlds and interact using their own avatars. Avatars can be represented in humanoid form, as an animal, a mythical figure, an imaginary or contrived figure or object.

In various applications of 3DVWs, different roles of participants may be implemented using avatars. In our systematic literature review, we tried to identify the roles of participants in each study and classify them into meaningful classifications.

According to the roles in each application area which played with avatars, we catego-rized them into two main groups; user participant avatars and instructor participant avatars.

User participant avatars mostly play roles such as medical professionals, patients, students and other avatars which get some health care and educational services in the applications. In contrast, instructor participant avatars undertake the roles that provide health care and educational services for other avatars. We divided these roles to medi-cal professional, instructor, patient, supervisor and other avatars. Some studies didn't need to have instructor participant avatars.

In the first category, 28 studies had avatars in the role of a student who participated in educational health care services in 3DVWs. Eleven studies used avatars for the role of patient and 13 studies used medical professional roles for avatars in their works. Six papers used avatars in other roles such as veterans, teens, common visitors and volunteers.

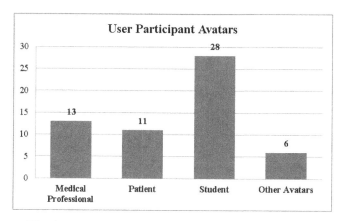

Fig. 6. Distribution of user participant avatars in the literature

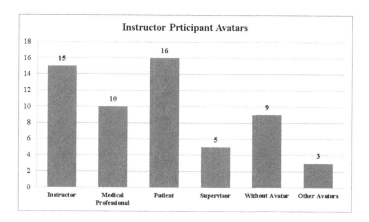

Fig. 7. Distribution of instructor participant avatars in the literature

In the second category, avatars with the role of instructor and medical professionals were used in 15 and 10 studies respectively. Authors in 16 papers applied patient avatars in their studies. Ten studies didn't have instructor participant avatars, while 3 studies used other avatars such as virtual human agents.

Fig. 6 and Fig. 7 show the user and instructor participant avatars and their distribution in the studies, respectively.

3.5 RQ5: In Which Countries have the Studies Related to Applications of 3DVWs in Health Care been Conducted Mostly?

Fig. 8 shows a percentage of the extracted papers in different countries around the world. Most of the articles relate to authors affiliated with the United States of America, which is around 60% of total studies. The United Kingdom, with 13% of

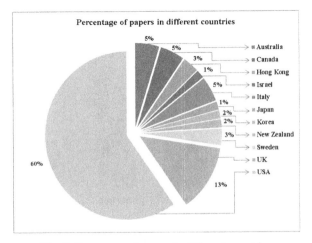

Fig. 8. Frequency of papers in different countries

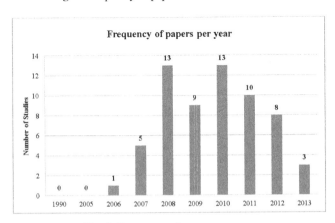

Fig. 9. Frequency of papers per year

publications, is the next largest source of papers in this field. In the third ranking, with 5% of publications each, are Australia, Canada and Italy. The remaining 12% of papers came from Japan, Sweden, Korea, Hong Kong, New Zealand and Israel.

Fig. 9 illustrates the number of published papers per year. As can be seen from the chart, between 1990 and 2005 there are no papers related to 3DVWs in healthcare contexts. The number of published papers per year increased significantly from 1 to 13 between 2006 and 2010 decreasing to 9 in 2009. There is a decline to 10 papers in 2011 and to 8 in 2012. As our research was in July 2013, 3 papers were published in this year prior to this date.

4   Conclusion

3D Virtual Worlds offer several innovative ways to carry out health-related activities. In this study we developed two main categories to explain the application of 3DVWs in various healthcare contexts: Educational and Non-educational applications. We also classified the different applied 3DVW platforms, virtual environments, and avatar-mediated participant roles which have been used in the literature. We found that Second Life is the most used 3DVW in health care application. We also found that most of the studies relate to this topic have been conducted in the United States of America. Our findings can be used to provide an overview of the application of 3DVWs in healthcare and medical research which professional health communities and academic institutions can use in their professions, researches, implementations and studies.

References

1. Eysenbach, G.: Medicine 2.0: social networking, collaboration, participation, apomediation, and openness. Journal of Medical Internet Research **10**(3) (2008)
2. Boulos, M.N.K., Wheeler, S.: The emerging Web 2.0 social software: an enabling suite of sociable technologies in health and health care education1. Health Information & Libraries Journal **24**(1), 2–23 (2007)
3. Bell, M.W.: Toward a definition of "virtual worlds". Journal of VirtualWorlds Research **1**(1), 2–5 (2008)
4. Boulos, M.N.K., Burden, D.: Web GIS in practice V: 3-D interactive and real-time mapping in Second Life. International Journal of Health Geographics **6**(1), 51 (2007)
5. Morie, J.F., Chance, E.: Extending the reach of health care for obesity and diabetes using virtual worlds. Journal of diabetes science and technology **5**(2), 272–276 (2011)
6. Montoya, M.M., Massey, A.P., Lockwood, N.S.: 3D collaborative virtual environments: exploring the link between collaborative behaviors and team performance. Decision Sciences **42**(2), 451–476 (2011)
7. Boulos, M.N.K., Hetherington, L., Wheeler, S.: Second Life: an overview of the potential of 3-D virtual worlds in medical and health education. Health Information & Libraries Journal **24**(4), 233–245 (2007)
8. Hansen M.M.: Versatile, Immersive, Creative and Dynamic Virtual 3-D Healthcare Learning Environments: A Review of the Literature (2008)
9. Beard, L., Wilson, K., Morra, D., Keelan, J.: A survey of health-related activities on second life. Journal of Medical Internet Research **11**(2) (2009)

10. Peck, B., Miller, C.: I think I can, I think I can, I think I can... I know I can Multi-user Virtual Environments (MUVEs) as a means of developing competence and confidence in undergraduate nursing students An Australian perspective. Procedia-Social and Behavioral Sciences **2**(2), 4571–4575 (2010)
11. Kitchenham, B.: Procedures for performing systematic reviews, p. 33. Keele University, Keele (2004)
12. Ghanbarzadeh, R., Ghapanchi A.H., Blumenstein M., Talaei-Khoei. A.: A Decade of Research on the Use of Three-Dimensional Virtual Worlds in Health Care: A Systematic Literature Review. Journal of medical Internet research **16**(2) (2014)
13. Ghanbarzadeh, R., Ghapanchi, A.H., Blumenstein, M.: Application areas of multi-user virtual environments in the healthcare context. Studies in health technology and informatics **204**, 38–46 (2013)
14. Amrollahi, A., Ghapanchi, A.H., Talaei-Khoei, A.: A systematic literature review on strategic information systems planning: Insights from the past decade. Pacific Asia Journal of the Association for Information Systems **5**(2) (2013)
15. Ghapanchi, A.H., Ghapanchi, A.R., Talaei-Khoei, A., Abedin, B.: A Systematic Review on Information Technology Personnel's Turnover. Lecture Notes on Software Engineering **1**(1), 98–101 (2013)
16. Ghapanchi, A.H., Jafarzadeh, M.H., Khakbaz, M.H.: An Application of Data Envelopment Analysis (DEA) for ERP system selection: Case of a petrochemical company. In: Proceedings of the ICIS 2008, p. 77 (2008)
17. Ghapanchi, A.H., Aurum, A.: Measuring the effectiveness of the defect-fixing process in open source software projects. 2011 44th Hawaii International Conference on System Sciences (HICSS). IEEE (2011)
18. Ghapanchi, A.H., Aurum, A.: The impact of project capabilities on project performance: Case of open source software projects. International Journal of Project Management **30**(4), 407–417 (2012)
19. Zarei, B., Ghapanchi, A.H.: Guidelines for government-to-government initiative architecture in developing countries. International Journal of Information Management **28**(4), 277–284 (2008)
20. Ghapanchi, A.H., Aurum, A., Low, G.: Creating a Measurement Taxonomy for the Success of Open Source Software Projects, First Monday **16**(8) (2011)
21. Ghapanchi, A.H., Aurum, A., Daneshgar, F.: The Impact of Process Effectiveness on User Interest in Contributing to the Project. Journal of software **7**(1), 212–219 (2012)
22. Merati, E., Zarei, B., Ghapanchi, A.H.: Project Process Re-engineering (PPR): A BPR Method for Projects. International Journal of Information Systems and Change Management **4**(4), 299–313 (2010)
23. Ghapanchi, A.H., Aurum, A.: Competency Rallying in Electronic Markets: Implications for Open Source Project Success. Electronic Markets **22**(2), 117–127 (2011)
24. Ghapanchi, A.H., Aurum, A.: The Impact of Project License and Operating System on the Effectiveness of the Defect-Fixing Process in Open Source Software Projects. International Journal of Business Information Systems **8**(4), 413–424 (2011)
25. Najaftorkaman, M., Ghapanchi, A.H., Talaei-Khoei, A., Ray, P.: Recent Research Areas and Grand Challenges in Electronic Medical Record: A Literature Survey Approach". The International Technology Management Review **3**(1), 12–21 (2013)
26. Najaftorkaman, M., Ghapanchi, A.H., Talaei-Khoei, A., Ray, P.: A Taxonomy of Antecedents to User Adoption of Health Information Systems: A Synthesis of Thirty Years of Research. Journal of the Association for Information Science and Technology (2014)

Trend Prediction of Biomedical Technology
by Semantic Analysis

Xiaomeng Sun[1,3], Kexu Zhang[2], Peng Nan[3(✉)], and Lei Liu[1(✉)]

[1] Fudan University, No.138, Medical School Road, Shanghai, China
liulei@fudan.edu.cn
[2] Shanghai Ebuinfo Co., Ltd., No. 170, Lane 277, Chen Hui Road, Shanghai, China
kexu.zhang@ebuinfo.com
[3] Fudan University, No. 2005, Songhu Road, Shanghai, China
nanpeng@fudan.edu.cn

Abstract. This paper proposes a solution to establish a biomedical technology analysis platform to laying foundation for an expert knowledge-based biomedical system, which aims to give intelligent medical decision in the end. It curates 23.44 million biomedical articles since 1970 for serving as repository to supporting as knowledge base. Based on the platform, trend prediction in biomedical technology has been made by semantic analysis.

1 Introduction

Scientific researches lead great progress on human race in all ages, especially the science of health and medicine. With the explosive growth of digitized data in the past few decades, remarkable development has been achieved in the realm of biomedicine study, computational technology and their crossing domain. Transforming experience based biomedical knowledge into computer sensitive language, developing logical algorithm to learn the pattern and give optimized diagnosis, building intelligent autonomic learning knowledge-based systems are of great interest today [1,2,3,4].

An expert knowledge-based system (KBS) stores, organizes, manages and utilizes complex structured and unstructured domain-specific information to give valuable knowledge from mass data, and therefore solves complex problems that we can't deal with before the era of information explosion. Medical library is the most widely used KBS which contains full text or abstract of medical research articles [5,6]. It normally provides multiple search interfaces, grouping and sorting feedback, citation indexes and knowledge network graphs for user retrieval request [7,8]. It represents the simplest model of KBS and settles the basis for more advanced knowledge integrated and decision making models.

Below, we elaborate on the challenges facing effective knowledge discovery from mass data and describe a biomedical technology analysis system that contains 23.44 million articles in the field of biomedical research. At the core of this platform is technical classification and hotspot keywords analysis so far. Both results are based on word frequency statistics.

© Springer International Publishing Switzerland 2015
X. Yin et al. (Eds.): HIS 2015, LNCS 9085, pp. 225–230, 2015.
DOI: 10.1007/978-3-319-19156-0_23

2   Biomedical Technology Analysis Platform

This platform has collected large amount of biomedical articles from different open source databases on the Internet from February 1970 to February 2015. Considering the quality of the data, we eventually selected the biomedical articles of recent ten years, which is from February 2005 to February 2015, as our analysis object. Data of these ten years includes 0.5 million Chinese articles and 22.94 million English articles. All of the Chinese information is gathered from the WANFANG MED ONLINE (http://www.wanfangdata.com.cn) website with only abstracts, headings, keywords, authors and some other related data. English information is downloaded mainly from PubMed (http://www.ncbi.nlm.nih.gov/pubmed/) and BioMed Central (http://www.biomedcentral.com) in the same form, along with 0.8 million full text among them.

Again, building on the biomedical library, we employed word frequency statistics to yield accurate technical classification and keyword analysis. An important component of this platform is the ability to automatically capture technical keywords and roughly cluster articles in different technical categories. The platform illustrates each technical classification and its article amount in percentage. Also important for this platform use is the ability to acquire research hotspots through keyword frequency statistics. This result is especially useful for industry development analysis, which helps us better understanding the ongoing biomedical research territory.

3   Trend Prediction of Biomedical Technology by Semantic Analysis

3.1   Method

Gaining and reediting biomedical research spheres information from UMLS system (http://www.nlm.nih.gov/research/umls/), we summarized a list of widely used biomedical technologies in the recent decade. This list of words then served as search keys by scanning the library to cluster articles into technical classifications and give their corresponding distribution probabilities. This process requires repeatedly integration and optimization according to the distribution result to approach the most reasonable and balanced classification result.

To verify and support this biomedical technology taxonomy, we simultaneously conducted content analysis based on keyword. Word frequency statistics is the analytic method of giving list of keywords grouped by frequency of occurrence within the giving text corpus. By extracting and sorting keywords from Chinese and English library, we generated 3512 Chinese keywords and 440,650 English keywords, with total frequency amount of 87932 and 1,693,163 times respectively.

3.2   Result

At the beginning, we chose the top 500 keywords in both languages as raw data for further discussion. For Chinese library, in contrast to the fact that 500 only account for 14.24% of total keyword amount, they contain 67% of total frequency, which means that they represent 67% of all Chinese articles. Both figures for English library are 0.11% and 18.16% respectively. These indexes strongly indicate these 1000 keywords could reflect the overall biomedical study in both languages.

Combining evidences from both technical classification and keyword analysis, screening obscure content, connecting categories with detailed high frequency keywords, we exhibit top 3 technical classification results and their high frequency subcategory keywords in English language (Table 1).

Table 1. Top three technical classifications and their keywords with frequency

Category	Keyword	Frequency
Genomics Technology	Genome wide association study (GWAS)	38534
	Next generation sequencing (NGS)	20473
	Single cell transcriptome sequencing	19695
	Chromatin structural genomics	13527
	Haplotype analysis	11289
Proteomics Technology	Western blot	60275
	Immunofluorescence	23688
	Protein microarray	14470
	Isoelectric focusing (IEF)	12681
	Bioinformatics analysis	6185
Glycomics Technology	Glyco-catch method	5357
	Fluorophore-assisted carbohydrate electrophoresis (FACE)	4440
	Two-step proteolytic digestion combined with sequential microcolumns technology	1726
	Chemoselective glycoblotting	1500
	Mass spectrum	1444

Since the announcement of the essentially complete human genome a decade ago, various omics subjects welcome a booming generation by benefitting from the rapid progress of biotechnology and computer science. GWAS, NGS, different kinds of electrophoresis and GC-MS technology are shared a comparative short history and rapid development speed in general. Among every top three well-studied omics areas, these technologies are all widely used, that we can tell from the investigated frequency showed in table 1. In this statistical result, articles related to genomics, proteomics and glycomics study amount to 21.30% of the English library, accounted for a large proportion of biomedical research in recent ten years. This article will give extra analysis of genomics study and its relevant crucial technologies.

4   Discussion

Genomics study dedicates on solving problems of genome in two directions: structure and function. Therefore the field includes efforts to determine the entire DNA sequence of organisms and fine-scale genetic mapping, which could be inducted as structural genomics, and to understand the intragenomic phenomena and other interactions between loci and alleles within the genome, which can be deemed to functional genomics or postgenome study.

Table 2. Genomics technology major sub-classifications with frequency

Category	Keyword	Frequency
	Genome wide association study (GWAS)	38534
	Next generation sequencing (NGS)	20473
	Single cell transcriptome sequencing	19695
	Chromatin structural genomics	13527
	Haplotype analysis	11289
Genomics Technology	Pan genomics technology	10827
	Immune genomics technology	9438
	Epigenetics technology	5974
	Nutrigenomics technology	5161
	Pharmacogenomics related technology	3950
	Metagenomics technology	2564
	Druggable genome discovery technology	1107

Next generation sequencing (NGS), chromatin structural genomics and single cell transcriptome sequencing focus on the first question. NGS technologies enable us to parallelize the sequencing process, producing millions of sequences concurrently, lower the cost of DNA sequencing to a great extent and make sequencing much more convenient and more accurate than ever before. NGS sets a lower base for conducting genomics study today and helps to accelerate the knowledge discovery routine. One important purpose of getting genome sequences is to find out the connection between human genome and drug susceptibility rules of gene expression and interpreting transcriptional bursting phenomenon. Beyond DNA studies, single cell transcriptome sequencing gives information about different kinds of RNA molecules of a specified cell population. With that, the processes of cellular differentiation and carcinogenesis can be learned in depth. Articles clustered under these keywords verify our research hotspot analysis.

Genome wide association study (GWAS) and haplotype analysis, on another direction, belong to the fundamental functional genomics research. If structural genomics is about gathering information, functional genomics works to make sure of these vast produced data turning into valuable knowledge wealth. GWAS exams common genetic variants in different individuals to test if any variant is associated with a trait, mainly focused on associations between single nucleotide polymorphisms (SNPs) and traits like major diseases. Haplotype analysis also proceeds with SNPs and polymorphic sites to provide valuable evidence for investigating the genetics of common diseases. Relevancy to medical care and drug delivery explains the high frequency of both technologies.

Besides, there are some other areas of expertise in our statistical list: pan genomics technology, immune genomics technology, epigenetics technology, nutrigenomics technology, metagenomics technology and druggable genome discovery technology. Each keyword mirrors an aspect of genomics study and numerous neoteric technologies, combined to form a tip of the iceberg in biomedical research today. To better understand the trend in biomedical industry, we furthermore looked into the top five most studied sub-classifications in genomics technology.

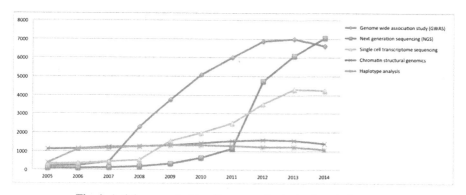

Fig. 1. Article amount of top five genomics technology in last years

Figure 1 concludes the article amount of top five genomics technologies of past ten years, while genomics study has faced huge improvement by means of technology advancement. GWAS' application experiences rapidly growth since 2007, peaks in 2013, and still holds leading position of genomics study this year. NGS also sees a quick growth stage around 2013 with even higher rates of increase and surpasses GWAS last year to becoming the most widely used genomics technology today. Single cell transcriptome sequencing starts to becoming a research hotspot in 2008, gently increases and remains steady last year. Chromatin structural genomics and haplotype analysis, on the other hand, shares much smoother curves in last ten years, indicated fundamental status of them in genomics industry. All these figures indicates that structural genomics embraces a significant milestone after the accomplishment of Human Genome Project in May 2006, and succeeding genomics study starts to focus on intragenomic phenomena afterwards: heterosis, epistasis, pleiotropy, other interactions within genome and their roles in etiopathology. Functional genomics is welcoming great development opportunity today to give more clue to personal medicine and intelligent medical treatment, which would revolutionize our healthy care industry in the long run, and corresponding technologies will similarly be extensively applied over the coming decades.

This article only discusses the most widely studied genetics technology in English language. Thus far, we can summarize and demonstrate industry hotspot analysis report of all biomedical fields in both languages on the biomedical technology analysis platform website. Integrality of Chinese library and more accurate technical classification for English library still require further efforts. This work would lay a foundation for establishing a reasonable structured knowledge-based system in biomedical realm.

Acknowledgement. This work is part of a larger project "The development of a medical knowledge and clinical decision support system" under the National High Technology Research and Development Program of China (863 Program), award 2012AA02A602.

References

1. Kuru, K., Niranjan, M., Tunca, Y., Osvank, E., Azim, T.: Biomedical Visual Data Analysis to Build an Intelligent Diagnostic Decision Support System in Medical Genetics. Artificial Intelligence in Medicine **62**(2), 105–118 (2014)
2. Peek, N., Swift, S.: Intelligent Data Analysis for Knowledge Discovery, Patient Monitoring and Quality Assessment. Methods of Information in Medicine **51**(4), 318–322 (2012)
3. Torralba-Rodrigueza, F.J., Bixquert-Montagud, V., Fernandez-Breis, J.T., Martinez-Bejar, R.: An Incremental Knowledge Acquisition-Based System for Supporting Decisions in Biomedical Domains. Computer Methods and Programs in Biomedicine **98**(2), 161–171 (2010)
4. Gonzalez-Velez, H., Mier, M., Julia-Sape, M., Arvanitis, T.N., Garcia-Gomez, J.M., Robles, M., Lewis, P.H., Dasmahapatra, S., Dupplaw, D., Peet, A., Arus, C., Celda, B., Van Huffel, S., Lluch-Ariet, M.: Healthagents: Distributed Multi-Agent Brain Tumor Diagnosis and Prognosis. Applied Intelligence **30**(3), 191–202 (2009)
5. Cain, T.J., Rodman, R.L., Sanfilippo, F., Kroll, S.M.: Managing Knowledge and Technology to Foster Innovation at the Ohio State University Medical Center. Academic Medicine **80**(11), 1026–1031 (2005)
6. Chen, P., Verma, R.: A query-based medical information summarization system using ontology knowledge. In: Proceedings 19th Ieee International Symposium on Computer-Based Medical Systems, pp. 37–42 (2006)
7. Montani, S.: How to Use Contextual Knowledge in Medical Case-Based Reasoning Systems: A Survey on Very Recent Trends. Artificial Intelligence in Medicine **51**(2), 125–131 (2011)
8. Ranky, P.G.: A 3d Web-Enabled, Case-Based Learning Architecture and Knowledge Documentation Method for Engineering, Information Technology, Management, and Medical Science/Biomedical Engineering. International Journal of Computer Integrated Manufacturing **16**(4-5), 346–356 (2003)

SMS *for Life* in Burundi and Zimbabwe: A Comparative Evaluation

Gerardo Luis Dimaguila[✉]

School of Information, University of Melbourne, Melbourne, Victoria, Australia
g.dimaguila@student.unimelb.edu.au

Abstract. Several benefits of mobile health (mHealth) technologies have been documented in the literature. However, available literature is not as "extensive" as those in developed countries, particularly on implementation issues and challenges of mHealth interventions. This is worrying, as addressing the usefulness and appropriateness of a mHealth program before implementation is essential. This paper comparatively assessed the ease and appropriateness of implementing a Short Messaging Service (SMS)-based mHealth technology in developing countries of similar settings. The framework of Marshall, Lewis and Whittaker, based on the Bridges' criteria, was chosen for the comparison. It was found that Burundi has many challenges that need to be addressed first before implementing a mHealth intervention. Zimbabwe enjoys a better funding model with more 'experience' in eHealth projects and initiatives, and a successful mHealth intervention is more plausible. This paper highlights the importance of critically assessing the mHealth intervention and the target community before implementation.

Keywords: *SMS for life* · Bridges' criterion · mHealth evaluation · eHealth evaluation · mHealth implementation · eHealth implementation · mHealth africa · mHealth burundi · mHealth zimbabwe · mHealth malaria

1   Introduction

Disease burden in developing countries is high [37] due to limited resources and infrastructure [3, 5, 37] and lack of medical expertise, technology and corresponding technical support [5]. This leads to health services being focused on urban areas [37].

Mobile health (mHealth) is the use of mobile technologies to support healthcare [37], and can be described as eHealth with a particular focus on mobile technologies. mHealth is useful in "removing physical barriers to care and service delivery and by improving weak health system management, unreliable supply systems, and poor communication" [37].

Mobile health is increasing in viability because of the rising ubiquitousness of mobile phones. Mobile phones are 'everywhere' [24, 37], sometimes more than other basics such as clean water [11]. This highlights the potential that mHealth has in developing countries.

© Springer International Publishing Switzerland 2015
X. Yin et al. (Eds.): HIS 2015, LNCS 9085, pp. 231–240, 2015.
DOI: 10.1007/978-3-319-19156-0_24

Several benefits of mHealth in developing countries have been documented, and there is evidence of successes [11].

However, despite the increase in mHealth applications and projects, there is still a relative dearth of literature in the area. The literature of mHealth in developing countries is particularly not as "extensive" as those in developed countries [5]. There are "minimal formal evaluation of mHealth" [37] and limited evidence of its successes beyond the pilot stage [11, 24]. In fact, about two-thirds of mHealth implementations are only pilot studies [24]. It is clear that any implementation of mHealth have to be carefully evaluated, as the success stories are mostly in their infancy.

There is also a lack of frameworks for implementation of mHealth technologies [23], and correspondingly, literature on the implementation of a mHealth intervention. This is unfortunate as it is important to clearly identify the challenges faced by health stakeholders in developing countries; unique as they are in different countries and different areas within those countries. "Forms and related practices" vary "because of different or very different situations" [27].

2   Objectives

This paper will assess the ease and appropriateness of implementing *SMS for Life*, a Short Messaging Service (SMS)-based mHealth technology for developing countries of similar settings: Burundi and Zimbabwe.

There is a need to address the usefulness and appropriateness of a mHealth program before implementation [23, 24]. It is important to assess implementaions prior to execution in order to address challenges that relate to "people, process, technology, mobile devices, computing standard, security and privacy and electromagnetic conformity" [24]. This is especially true in developing countries, which often are not able to develop the technology needed themselves, and therefore rely on the proper selection of the best suited technology to quickly "achieve economic and social development goals" [5]. Developing countries have a low tolerance for failure or instability [20].

SMS for Life is a collaboration between public and private partners, led by Novartis, an international pharmaceutical company. It is listed as an initiative of the global Roll Back Malaria Partnership. It seeks to solve problems related to malaria medicine distribution, and uses "mobile phones, SMS messages, the Internet and electronic mapping technology" for tracking medicine stocks in health facilities [26, 29] "to: Eliminate stock-outs, increase access to essential medicines, reduce the number of deaths from malaria" [26].

There are many other mHealth applications, but assessing the ease of implementation of more than one tool is out of the scope of this paper. *SMS for Life* has been chosen as a focus because of documented successes, and/or strong partnerships for implementation gained with government and/or non-governmental agencies, in Tanzania, Ghana, Kenya, Cameroon and the Democratic Republic of Congo [26]. Some examples include *SMS for Life* in Tanzania that resulted in 95% stock count data provided (accuracy of 94%), and with stock-outs falling from 78% to

26% in twenty-one (21) weeks [2]. Meanwhile in Kenya, the response rate was 97% (accuracy of stock-outs 93%), with stock-outs going down by 38% in twenty-six (26) weeks [8]. Novartis also reports quick deployment of the technology, reaching "5000 health facilities in 7 months" [26].

The two (2) countries included in this comparative evaluation are Burundi and Zimbabwe, which both have problematic cases of Malaria and are the two countries with the lowest GDP in Sub-Saharan Africa [27].

3   Methodology

3.1   Evaluation Framework

There were four frameworks analysed for appropriateness to meet the objectives of this paper.

- Mburu, Franz, and Springer (2013, July) developed a 'Conceptual framework for designing mHealth solutions for developing countries'. Its main focus however is to determine the potential usefulness of a mHealth intervention, and not on the ease of implementation.
- The paper of Wall, Vallières, McAuliffe, Lewis, and Hederman (2014) entitled 'Implementing mHealth in Low-and Middle-Income Countries: What Should Program Implementers Consider?' focused on practical considerations of implementing mHealth. Although it is a useful reference, it is not really a framework.
- Chan and Kaufman (2010) developed a 'technology selection framework for supporting delivery of patient-oriented health interventions in developing countries'. It is a good framework that would do well as a guide to selecting the type of technology that would fit a health problem in developing countries. It takes into account social and cognitive sciences. However, it is slightly broader and is more appropriate for determining the category of technology appropriate, and does not focus too much on specific implementation issues.

The chosen framework is the work of Marshall, Lewis and Whittaker (2013). Their paper entitled 'mHealth technologies in developing countries: a feasibility assessment and a proposed framework' presents a framework based on the Bridges' criteria that evaluates the "appropriateness of mHealth technologies, in the context to which they are being proposed". It is a comprehensive framework that takes into account the technical, political, economical and social factors that would impact the ease and effectiveness of eHealth interventions.

The framework is divided into twelve (12) main categories. The descriptions and importance of each category is described in the findings section, alongside relevant comparative data gathered for *SMS for Life,* Burundi and Zimbabwe. The descriptions have been edited to make them more concise for the purposes of this paper, than was originally presented in the paper of Marshall, Lewis and Whittaker (2013).

3.2   Search Strategy

To search for the appropriate evaluation framework, the following keywords were used: 'mHealth', 'eHealth', 'developing countries', 'evaluation framework', and 'implementation'. The words were combined several times; 'mHealth' and 'eHealth' were interchanged and combined, while 'developing countries' was always used.

To search for eHealth applications related to Burundi and Zimbabwe, the following general search terms were used: 'eHealth', 'mHealth', 'mobile health', and 'malaria'. They were interchanged and combined with the specific terms 'Burundi' or 'Zimbabwe' during the search. Links and information offered/mentioned by the results of the search were also followed.

The search resulted in many examples of eHealth applications implemented in Burundi, Zimbabwe, or more generally in Sub-Saharan Africa, Africa or developing countries. However, most did not discuss implementation issues. To gather data relevant for Category-specific terms, other search terms were used. The search terms were 'mobile phone', 'access', and 'implementation'; and combined with 'Burundi' or 'Zimbabwe'. The search results provided a lot of information regarding the socio-cultural, political and mobile phone access of Burundi and Zimbabwe.

The Global Observatory for eHealth and Global Health Observatory webpages of the World Health Organization, which include country fact sheets, were also used as a source of reference. Data and information from the websites of World Bank and the International Telecommunications Union were also used. These provided country- and region-specific information relating to health (i.e., malaria) status, eHealth policies, mobile phone activity, and GDP, among other things.

To search for information related to the features, application and corresponding results of *SMS for Life*, the websites of Novartis – *SMS for Life* [26] and Roll Back Malaria – *SMS for Life* [29] initiatives were investigated for information and leads to conferences, reports and/or research papers. The website of Greenmash, the company behind the platform used by *SMS for Life*, was also used as a source. Moreover, the term '*SMS for Life*' was used as a search term for PubMed, Biomed Central and Google Scholar. The previous search results for the evaluation framework, Burundi and Zimbabwe were also investigated for information leads on *SMS for Life*.

Lastly, only English-written papers were considered.

4   Results and Findings

Table 1 outlined in the next pages present the findings as mapped to the framework used.

Table 1. Evaluation of the ease of implementation of SMS for Life in Burundi and Zimbabwe, based on the framework of Marshall, Lewis and Whittaker (2013)

Bridges Criterion	Burundi	Zimbabwe
Criterion 1: Physical access to mobile technology Is the mobile technology available and accessible by target populations and field workers? Consider the: • availability of infrastructure, such as mobile networks • existence of barriers (e.g. poor signal coverage) • accessibility of the mobile phones themselves, particularly to disadvantaged populations.	• Mobile subscriptions at 24.96% [13]. • Burundi reports that underdeveloped infrastructure **is not** a barrier to mHealth [36]. • A member of the International Medical Informatics Association, which "promotes the effective use of informatics within healthcare, the dissemination of knowledge and health informatics education, and translation of research into practice" [28]. BOTH (Burundi and Zimbabwe): Fluctuating network and electricity coverage were common problems of mobile data surveillance. Some solutions identified were recording of information via paper then sending later on [1].	• 96.35% mobile subscriptions [13]. • 12% have access to the Internet, and mobile phone communications rate at 78.5%. However, there is load shedding as long as 8 hours/day every day [38]. • Zimbabwe reports that underdeveloped infrastructure **is** a barrier to mHealth [36]. • There is a lack of national/international standards use for interoperability [38]. • Has Observer membership with the ISO technical committee 215 (ISO TC 215) [28], which works on standardization in health informatics (International Standards Organization) [12].
Criterion 2: Appropriateness of mobile technology We must now examine whether the chosen mHealth program is suitable to local needs. Undertake a more technical evaluation of the mobile technology: • What is its capacity? • What operating system does it require (this is particularly relevant to smartphones and PDAs)? • Is it a user-friendly application, or will people need significant training? • Can it be translated into appropriate local languages, or is it only available in English? Will the target population be able to read and understand the messages they receive? • Will the mobile technology function independently, or will it require a comprehensive (i.e. expensive) supporting network of computers and other ICT measures? • What energy sources are required? For example, can mobile phones easily be charged? • Are there cheaper / simpler options available that will provide the same function?	BOTH: • *SMS for Life* uses the Mango platform by Greenmash (http://www.greenmash.com/). The platform has three plans. The Basic plan allows only a maximum of ten (10) users per month. Standard allows for an average of ten (10) to two hundred (200) users. Finally, Enterprise allows an average of more than one thousand (1,000) users per month [9]. • Mango works on 'smart' devices, basic handsets such as the old Nokia phones, web forms, and other complementary systems [9]. • Health workers who would use the system to send stock reports attended only one-day trainings, which was deemed to be sufficient and produced effective results [8]; indicative of the ease of use of the system. District health officers were also given a half-day training on how to view the system, along with coaching on supporting health workers [2]. • The health workers need to use specific, simple codes in sending stock count messages. The codes are A = AL 6, B = AL 12, C = AL 18, D = AL 24 and T = RDT; which are then to be followed by the number of those specific stocks left. • The system has only two (2) components, basic mobile phones and at least one (1) Internet-enabled PC in the national/regional health district [26]. • The proliferation of mobile devices in both Burundi and Zimbabwe are indicative of the feasibility of charging the phones. The pilot tests in the five countries mentioned in the introduction aid in this assumption. Health workers used their own mobile phones and numbers – which means that they already had phones and were using them, prior to the project being implemented [2, 8]. • High weekly response rates so far (97%), low formatting error rates (3%) and good accuracy of stock counts (79%) and stock outs (93%) [8]. • Other SMS-based eHealth initiatives have been implemented before, including one in Zambia which tracked malarial diagnoses; however *SMS for Life* is the first to track stock levels locally [2].	
Criterion 3: Affordability of mobile technology and technology use • Can we afford it? • Start-up costs may be significant, but do costs remain high over the long term? • Is the technology expected to become widely used, mass produced and, therefore, cheaper and more affordable for the local population?	BOTH: • Basic, cheap phones will do [2, 9]. • Many projects did not continue or never scaled because of lack of sustainable funding [1]. • A survey conducted on public health professionals from developing countries including Southern Africa indicated that lack of funds for credit purchase can serve as a challenge for mobile health [22]. • However, Burundi reports that perceived high costs of mHealth technologies is **not** a barrier [36]. • This is not really an issue: the stock messages could be sent by the health workers to the designated number free of charge [2].	• Duty free importation of ICT tools present [38]. • Informal economy with regards to sale of prepaid phones, trading and rental of mobile phones and so on shows affordability; and even helps the economy [7]. • However, Zimbabwe reports that perceived high costs of mHealth technologies is considered a barrier to mHealth [36].
Criterion 4: Human capacity and training Consider people's capacity for understanding and using the mobile technology: Who will be using the mHealth program? • Will it be used only by healthcare workers, or will the general public also use it? • At this stage, it is important to examine the technical and literary capacities of the target user population. • Will the program require a technical expert and frequent IT support or will the program be relatively self-sustaining? • Are training programs available, or will they need to be created?	• Students in health sciences are given ICT training at tertiary institutions, however, lack of knowledge of applications and technical expertise were considered a barrier to implementing mHealth initiatives [36]. BOTH: • Only health workers use the system [2, 8, 26]. • The short time of training needed [2, 8] and simple codes required [2] make it ready easy to use. • Difficulties recorded in keeping health staff motivated because of the additional work burden [1].	• 'Best' with good skills are leaving the country [38]. • Increase in banking transactions when SMS banking were introduced in Zimbabwe [32] may be indicative of literacy. • Students in health sciences are given ICT training at tertiary institutions. Moreover, institutions also offer continuing education in ICT for health professionals, and lack of knowledge of applications nor technical expertise were not considered a barrier to implementing mHealth initiatives [36].
Criterion 5: Locally relevant content, applications, and services • Does the program come with pre-packaged messages and/or questions that may not be locally relevant? • Is there opportunity to edit and adapt messages and/or questions to local customs and needs?	BOTH: The program requires the use of structured codes; however they are simple to learn and use [2].	
Criterion 6: Integration into daily routines It is important to consider how the chosen technology will integrate into the daily lives of its users: • Will it take a lot of extra time to use or complete? • Will it require travel to an inconvenient location?	BOTH: A maximum of two (2) to three (3) hours' walk to get a network coverage (in areas with low or no coverage) was observed as "acceptable", although a fifteen- (15) to thirty- (30) minute walk would be best [2]. Aside from that, it does not take too much time to count the stocks and send the message.	
Criterion 7: Socio-cultural factors Implementation of mobile technology can be impeded by socio-cultural factors if the local cultural context has not been properly evaluated. Some things to consider: • Are women allowed to carry mobile phones? • What is the interest level of the elderly? Are they generally considered too old to be included? • Will the mobile technology only be accessible by richer populations (e.g. people with smartphones)?	• It appears that sex is not a determining factor of involvement in e-learning activities. However, younger people are more active [4]. BOTH: • Mobile phones are an "aspirational status symbol" within affordable reach" [34]. • Rapid growth of mobile phones in developing countries are "egalitarian" [15].	BOTH: • Preliminary evidence of mobile phones being gender neutral in Africa [19]. • Mobile phones shows some "optimism" of increasing

Table 1. Evaluation of the ease of implementation of SMS for Life in Burundi and Zimbabwe, based on the framework of Marshall, Lewis and Whitaker (2013)

Bridges Criterion	Burundi	Zimbabwe
• What can program/policy managers do to overcome these restrictions and avoid discrimination? • Is there room to communicate with political and religious leaders to aid in implementation?		women's empowerment in developing countries [14].
Criterion 8: Trust in mobile technology When addressing this criterion, it is important to understand people's historical use and experience with data collection and technology. • What is the level of confidence in mobile networks and existing mHealth programs? • What does the target population know about data sharing and technology issues? • What can program/policy leaders do to build people's trust in the project?	• Some eHealth implementations in Burundi include a mobile technology for disease surveillance [25] and the biggest community of open source hospital management information flow software OpenClinic GA [18]. However, focus are on effectiveness, (which are positive) and not implementation. • However, in a survey of key European ESTHER Alliance partners from Francophone Africa, which included Burundi, 64% reported never having any involvement in e-learning activities [4]. • Burundi's reports that there are no mHealth project initiatives [36]. What 'initiatives' mean are not clear however; perhaps it means initiatives by Burundi's government, and not from outside agencies/groups. • Laws for privacy of personally identifiable data present; but no laws specifically for EMR/EHRs [36].	• Some eHealth implementations in Zimbabwe include the District Health Information System (DHIS), which captures data from all 67 districts in the country and supported by mobile apps; also, the Human Resource Information Systems to track human resources for health [38]. • WHO notes Zimbabwe's claim of existence of mHealth project initiatives, but no formal evaluation or publication exists [36]. What 'initiatives' mean are not clear however; perhaps it means initiatives by Zimbabwe's government, and not from outside agencies/groups. BOTH: Mandatory registration of mobile numbers will increase privacy concerns and fear. There are also "insufficient data protection rules" [16].
Criterion 9: Local economic environment Relating to criterion 3 (affordability), it is important to consider the appropriateness of the technology in the local economic context. • Is the economy in a state of growth? What is the cost of mobile phone handsets, mobile phone calls, and/or SMS? • Is the economy expected to grow? • Will the new technology assist in creating new jobs, facilitate economic growth by streamlining processes, and existing mobile technology uptake in the community? Or will it replace jobs, thereby creating unemployment and distrust in the program?	• Burundi has a mixed financing model for health. Most of its funds come from international donors, and it has strong private-oriented practices. This means that it receives a high level of international support. Although this sounds good on the surface, it lends to problems; rendering "the identification of functioning modes difficult. The existence of a plethora of donors weakens health system's coordination, and characterizing funding modes in such situations is almost impossible." [27]. • Burundi is therefore categorised as having a Low Human Development index for the reasons mentioned above [27]. • Burundi's GDP growth is expected to decline from 4.0% this year to 3.0% in 2016 [31]. • Contribution of mobile telecommunications to annual GDP of Burundi is 0.12%. As a comparison, the average of high income countries is 0.20% [10].	• Zimbabwe is categorised as having a High Human Development Index as its health financing model, a mix of national funds and strong private-oriented practices [27], allows for better coordination. • Zimbabwe's GDP growth is expected to decline from 2.0% this year to 0.6% in 2016 [31]. • Contribution of mobile telecommunications to annual GDP of Zimbabwe is 0.091%. The average of high income countries is 0.20% [10]. • A thriving informal economy, particularly in the sale of mobile phone cards, served as a "coping strategy" for Zimbabwe's "various crises" [7]. BOTH: • Positive correlation of mobile technology with economic growth can be deduced [21]. • Prepaid system matches Sub-Saharan Africa's economic situation "perfectly." There are also indications some evidences that it helps revitalise their economy [19], reduce price disparities of products in the market (through price information sharing) and grow their GDP [30].
Criterion 10: Macro-economic environment In the same way that it is important to understand the political and cultural factors impacting technology uptake, we must examine the national economic environment of the country. • What are the taxation policies? • Do policies support technology use?	• WHO's Global Observatory for eHealth [36] noted that Burundi has a National eGovernment policy, a National eHealth Policy and a National ICT procurement policy for the health sector. However, upon checking, none of the policies could be found in the Directory of eHealth policies in the same page. Neither can such policies be found in government websites [4]. • Lack of policy frameworks is considered a barrier to mHealth implementation [36].	• Zimbabwe has an eHealth Strategy (2012-2017) developed by Zimbabwe's Ministry of Health and Child Welfare that aims to "support, promote and advocate for the provision of quality and efficient health information technology in Zimbabwe, while maximising the use of available resources. A national ICT policy is already in place and efforts are being made to incorporate numerous sector-wide policies including eHealth" [36]. A draft can be found at the Directory of eHealth policies. • Has an existing national ICT policy according to the Zimbabwe Ministry of Health and Child Welfare (2012). However, in a World Health Organization (2014) report, the country responds that they do not. They are also noted to not have a national ICT procurement policy for the health sector. • Lack of policies for coordinated eHealth efforts exists. Lack of policy frameworks is considered a barrier for mHealth implementation [36].
Criterion 11: Legal and regulatory framework • Do current laws and policies promote or hinder the use of the mobile technology? Consider the legal responsibilities, and what implications the laws (or lack thereof) have for future liabilities.	• Lack of legal policies or regulation reported as a barrier [36]. BOTH: • Mandatory registration reduces the penetration growth of mobile subscriptions due to increase in cost, and difficulties in gathering sufficient identification information [16]. • Laws for privacy of personally identifiable data present; but no laws specifically for EMR/EHRs [36]. • No laws or policies present regarding sharing of health-related data between health care staff through EMR/EHR [36].	• Lack of legal policies or regulation not considered a barrier to mHealth [36].
Criterion 12: Political will and public support • It is important to assess whether the public supports the program and whether their preferences have been communicated to local government. • Opportunities for collaborating with stakeholders, and developing e-strategies and public-private partnerships to reduce operational costs should be examined.	• Top 2 lowest GDP in Sub-Saharan Africa, but not part of top ten lowest % GDP allocated to health [27]. There is demand for mHealth initiatives [36]. • For e-Learning activities, partnerships between local health institutions and national, African, American and European institutions are reported to be high in Francophone Africa [4]. 60% however, have not ben in direct contact with their partner colleagues.	• Top 1 lowest GDP in Sub-Saharan Africa, but % GDP allocated to health is higher than Congo, which is the richest among the group [27]. There is demand for mHealth initiatives [36]. • National ICT policy and National eHealth Strategy exists [36]. • Their National eHealth strategy notes that the government is seeking to increase collaboration through Public-Private Partnership initiatives [38].

5   Discussion and Conclusions

SMS for Life is a simple, effective and cheap eHealth tool. It matches the needs of developing countries in that they require only the most basic, cheapest technologies, and is easy to learn. It can be gathered that the difficulties of implementing it lies on the economic, political and infrastructure challenges of the country in which it will be implemented.

Implementing *SMS for Life* in Burundi presents several challenges. First of all, it requires that health workers use their own mobile phones. This is good in principle, as it ensures that it avoids the extra expense of buying mobile phones for health workers, thus making it more cost-effective to implement and feasible to scale-up. However, Burundi's mobile subscription rate is very low. This presents problems implementing the technology in a health facility with some, if not all, health workers not having their own phones. Buying phones for every health worker would be expensive. It may present more risks of incurring further costs if the phone is lost and/or stolen, and reduces the sense of ownership and responsibility of the device from the health worker. Moreover, if health workers without phones are given one, it might cause conflicts between them and those who were not given phones because they already have one. It might even lead to health workers pretending that they do not have phones.

The current structure of *SMS for Life*, which rewards health workers with a few cents' credit to send stock counts, is shown to be an effective motivation - even when some users need to walk for hours to send the stock count. It is not clear whether Burundi will be able to sustain it on their own, as most of their health funding comes from international donors, especially with the expected decline of their GDP growth. The fact that younger people are more active in eHealth might also be a cause for concern in health facilities where there are elderly health workers. They might not only have a hard time using the system, but may also feel left out. The simple codes used by *SMS for Life* gives hope that this will be a minimal issue, however.

There is no mention of *SMS for Life* using standards for interoperability with other systems. It may not be really relevant in Burundi as the use of standards is weak, however, it is important to assess the system's ability to interoperate when the need arises.

Implementing *SMS for Life* in Burundi will be met with many different challenges, and it seems that the country needs more assistance in the areas of economics, infrastructure and livelihood. Perhaps a compromise can be achieved - carefully implementing the intervention in the hardest-hit areas in Burundi, and in health facilities with workers who own mobile phones, and focusing more assistance in other areas. For this, however, strong private-public partnerships are required. International donors would have to keep communication lines open as much as possible, in order to deliver the most important interventions as soon as possible, and without duplicating efforts, and challenges.

Great care would also have to be taken when including elderly health workers. Their willingness to learn and use the messaging service will have to be assessed and addressed prior to implementation, and especially during training.

In Zimbabwe, the ease of implementation appears more promising, as they have very high mobile subscription rates and tax-free ICT importations. However, similar with Burundi, their infrastructure in terms of network and electricity coverage is not good. Be that as it may, they still enjoy more experience with eHealth projects and initiatives than Burundi. Their funding model is also better, as it is more dependent on public funds than external donors - indicative of a more stable financing model. Although the prospects of implementing *SMS for Life* and scaling it up later on is better in Zimbabwe, it must still be assessed whether the motivational structure of the intervention is feasible.

It would be good to monitor the long-term, scaled-up implementations of *SMS for Life* in the five (5) countries it is in now, to determine if the motivation and success of the implementation of *SMS for Life* persists through time and scope. Moreover, there might be issues related to the complete turnover of the project to the health departments which are not yet known; the issues encountered after turnovers are less known still. All these will be a good area of work and research in order to facilitate the implementations of the technology in other areas and countries.

References

1. Barnett, I., Gallegos, J.: Using mobile phones for nutrition surveillance: A review of evidence. Institute of Development Studies (2013)
2. Barrington, J., Wereko-Brobby, O., Ward, P., Mwafongo, W., Kungulwe, S.: SMS for Life: a pilot project to improve anti-malarial drug supply management in rural Tanzania using standard technology. Malaria Journal **9** (2010)
3. Black, J.: Low-cost technology for health in developing countries. Lecture, Nossal Institute for Global Health, Melbourne School of Population and Global Health (2014)
4. Blake, C., Cartana, L., Castro, G., Zahorka, M.: E-Learning and continuous education within the health facility setting, March 2013
5. Chan, C., Kaufman, D.: A technology selection framework for supporting delivery of patient-oriented health interventions in developing countries. Journal of Biomedical Informatics **43**, 300–306 (2010)
6. Chen, P.: Well Blog. The New York Times, July 26 2012. http://well.blogs.nytimes.com/2012/07/26/what-we-can-learn-from-third-world-health-care/?_r=1 (retrieved November 3 2014)
7. Chiumbu, S., Nyamanhindi, R.: Negotiating the crisis: mobile phones and the informal economy in Zimbabwe. In: Chiumbu, S., Musemwa, M. (eds.) CRISIS! WHAT CRISIS? The multiple dimensions of the Zimbabwean crisis, pp. 62–80. HSRC Press (2012)
8. Githinji, S., Kigen, S., Memusi, D., Nyandigisi, A., Mbithi, A., Wamari, A., et al.: Reducing stock-outs of life saving malaria commodities using mobile phone text-messaging: SMS for Life study in Kenya. PloS ONE, January 17 2013
9. Greenmash. Plans. Greenmash (2013). http://greenmash.com/products/pricing/ (retrieved November 27 2014)
10. Gruber, H., Koutroumpis, P.: Mobile telecommunications and the impact on economic development. Economic Policy **26**(67), 387–426 (2011)
11. Hall, C., Fottrell, E., Wilkinson, S., Byass, P.: Assessing the impact of mHealth interventions in low- and middle-income countries - what has been shown to work?. Global Health Action 2014 (2014)

12. International Standards Organization. (n.d.). ISO/TC 215 Health Informatics. ISO. http://www.iso.org/iso/iso_technical_committee?commid=54960 (retrieved December 09 2014)
13. International Telecommunications Union. Statistics. International Telecommunications Union: Committed to connecting the world (2013). http://www.itu.int/en/ITU-D/Statistics/Pages/stat/default.aspx (retrieved November 27 2014)
14. Jacobsen, J.: The role of technological change in increasing gender equity with a focus on information and communications technology. ACSPL Working Paper Series **1**(2) (2011)
15. James, J.: The distributional effects of leapfrogging in mobile phones. Telematics and Informatics **29**(3), 294–301 (2012)
16. Jentzsch, N.: Implications of mandatory registration of mobile phone users in Africa. Telecommunications Policy **36**(8), 608–620 (2012)
17. Kallander, K., Tibenderana, J., Akpogheneta, O., Strachan, D., Hill, Z., Asbroek, A., et al.: Mobile health (mHealth) approaches and lessons for increased performance and retention of community health workers in low- and middle-income countries: A review. Journal of Medical Internet Research **15**(1) (2013)
18. Karopka, T., Schmuhl, H., Demski, H.: Free/Libre Open Source Software in Health Care: A Review. Healthcare Informatics Research **20**(1), 11–22 (2014)
19. Kefela, G.: The impact of mobile phone and economic growth in developing countries. African Journal of Business Management **5**(2), 269–275 (2011)
20. Labrique, A., Vasudevan, L., Kochi, E., Fabricant, R., Mehl, G.: mHealth innovations as health system strengthening tools: 12 common applications and a visual framework. Global Health: Science and Practice **1**(2), 160–171 (2013)
21. Lee, S., Gardner, L.: Does the spread of mobile phones promote economic development? Empirical evidence from South Asia and Sub-Saharan Africa regions. Southwestern Economic Review **38**, 15–26 (2011)
22. Machingura, P., Adekola, O., Mueni, E., Oaiya, O., Gustafsson, L., Heller, R.: Perceived value of applying Information Communication Technology to implement guidelines in developing countries; an online questionnaire study among public health workers. Online Journal of Public Health Informatics **6**(2) (2014)
23. Marshall, C., Lewis, D., Whittaker, M. mHealth technologies in developing countries: a feasibility assessment and a proposed framework. University of Queensland, School of Population Health. Health Information Systems Knowledge Hub (2013)
24. Mburu, S., Franz, E., Springer, T. A conceptual framework for designing mHealth solutions for developing countries. In: Proceedings of the 3rd ACM MobiHoc Workshop on Pervasive Wireless Healthcare, pp. 31–36. ACM (2013)
25. Mwabukusi, M., Karimuribo, E., Rweyemamu, M., Beda, E.: Mobile technologies for disease surveillance in humans and animals. Onderstepoort Journal of Veterinary Research. 81. AOSIS OpenJournals (2014)
26. Novartis. Novartis Malaria Initiative. Novartis (2014). http://malaria.novartis.com/innovation/sms-for-life/index.shtml (retrieved November 26 2014)
27. Parnaudeau, M., Garcia, H.: Designing simulations for health managers in sub-saharan african countries: adherence to eHealth services. In: Ma, M., Jain, L., Anderson, P. (eds.) Virtual, Augmented Reality and Serious Games for Healthcare I, vol. 68, pp. 93–109. Springer, Heidelberg (2014)
28. Payne, J.: The state of standards and interoperability for mHealth among low- and middle-income countries. mHealth Alliance (2013)
29. Roll Back Malaria. SMS for Life: An RBM initiative. Roll Back Malaria (2010). http://rbm.who.int/psm/smsWhatIsIt.html (retrieved December 4 2014)

30. Samarajiva, R., Stork, C., Kapugama, N., Zuhyle, S., Perera, R.: Mobile phone interventions for improving economic and productive outcomes for farm and non-farm rural enterprises and households in low and middle-income countries. International Initiative for Impact Evaluation, November 2013
31. The World Bank. Data. The World Bank (2014). http://data.worldbank.org/income-level/LIC (retrieved December 06 2014)
32. Thulani, D.: Adoption and use of SMS/mobile banking services in Zimbabwe: An exploratory study. Journal of Internet Banking and Commerce 16(2) (2011)
33. Wall, P., Vallieres, F., McAuliffe, E., Lewis, D., Hederman, L.: Implementing mHealth in low-and middle-income countries: What should program implementers consider?. In: Adibi, S. (ed.) mHealth Multidisciplinary Verticals, pp. 259–275. CRC Press (2014)
34. Wasserman, H.: Mobile Phones, Popular Media, and Everyday African Democracy: Transmissions and Transgressions. Popular Communication: The International Journal of Media and Culture 9(2), 146–158 (2011)
35. World Health Organization. Global Health Observatory. World Health Organization (2012). http://www.who.int/gho/malaria/epidemic/cases/en/ (retrieved November 26 2014)
36. World Health Organization. Global Observatory for eHealth. World Health Organization (2014). http://www.who.int/goe/policies/countries/zwe/en/ (retrieved November 26 2014)
37. Yang, J., Kahn, J.S., Kahn, J.G.: 'Mobile' Health Needs and Opportunities in Developing Countries. Health Affairs 29(2), 252–258 (2010)
38. Zimbabwe Ministy of Health and Child Welfare. Zimbabwe's E-Health strategy 2012-2017 (2012)

Healthcare Data Validation and Conformance Testing Approach Using Rule-Based Reasoning

Hira Jawaid[1(✉)], Khalid Latif[1], Hamid Mukhtar[1],
Farooq Ahmad[2], and Syed Ali Raza[1]

[1] School of Electrical Engineering and Computer Science, NUST, Islamabad, Pakistan
{hira.jawaid,khalid.latif,
hamid.mukhtar,ali.raza}@seecs.nust.edu.pk
[2] Department of Computer Science,
College of Computer Sciences and Information Technology (CCSIT),
King Faisal University, Alahssa 31982, Kingdom of Saudi Arabia
hfahmad@kfu.edu.sa

Abstract. HL7 community is profoundly involved in the development of standards in order to exchange, share and retrieve health related in-formation. FHIR is an emerging standard of HL7 that encourages use of JSON as a data serialization approach. Validation of healthcare data is crucial task because errors in data can result serious consequences. Currently there does not exist a validator that can validate and conform data as per FHIR. This paper presents an approach to validate health-care data embodied in JSON documents and to test its conformance with FHIR standard. We first developed Description Logic (DL) based schema of the FHIR. JSON data is then translated to RDF and we ap-ply rule-based reasoning to validate data. As verified by results, design of the validation algorithm ensures that validation step is performed in sub seconds and overall system remains efficient. Further, the rule based reasoning provides aid in identifying incompatibilities in data which should be fixed to bridge the gaps in achieving interoperability.

Keywords: HL7 · FHIR · Ontology · Validation · Conformance · Reasoning

1   Introduction and Background

Validation is necessary to ensure that data is in accordance with a standard and can be processed without causing any erroneous implication [1]. According to Shanks et al [2], after constructing a conceptual model, it should be validated with requirements of stakeholders. ISO/IEC specify that conformance testing is attainment of a service [3]. Javascript Object Notation (JSON) is serialization format in the form of attribute-value pairs [5]. Different approaches are used for JSON validation. JSON Lint [6], is a reformatter and is an inline JSON validator. Logic reasoner is used to infer consequences from set of axioms. These inference rules are specified by means of Web ontology language (OWL). Reasoning can be performed on large ontologies using DLs [7]. Health Level 7 (HL7), is involved in development of standards for exchange

© Springer International Publishing Switzerland 2015
X. Yin et al. (Eds.): HIS 2015, LNCS 9085, pp. 241–246, 2015.
DOI: 10.1007/978-3-319-19156-0_25

of medical information. Fast Healthcare Interoperability Resources (FHIR) is an HL7 content standard [8]. It supports JSON based content payloads. JSON-LD is JSON based serialization format and is acronym for JSON for Linked Data. Currently there is no validator that can validate FHIR data. FHIR specifications are available in JSON and XML. For JSON, no language schema exists. This paper presents an approach for validation of FHIR data in JSON format. Semantic model of FHIR's resources is developed in OWL. In order to validate FHIR JSON against semantic model, JSON is converted into JSON-LD. Afterwards rule-based reasoning is applied to validate the data against standard data model, FHIR.

Rest of the paper is organized as follows: Proposed framework is explained in Section 2. Details of FHIR Semantic Structure is described in Section 3. In Section 4 we have described validation approaches. Evaluation strategy is explained in Section 5 and finally we conclude our work in Section 6.

2   Proposed Framework

For validation of FHIR JSON against schema of FHIR, we have proposed an architecture of validator that validates FHIR JSON data. The validation process is depicted in Figure 1. The validator takes FHIR JSON as an input and translates FHIR JSON into JSON-LD that is validated by using FHIR ontology, FHIR primitive types and resoner. The validator gives response in the form of valid or invalid data. An example of FHIR JSON is shown in Figure 2 and its translated JSON-LD is shown in Figure 3.

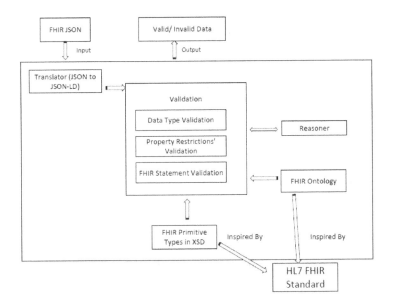

Fig. 1. Validation Process for FHIR JOSN

```
[
"name" :
"Organization",
"publisher" : "FHIR
Project",
"status" : "draft",
"date" : "2013-11-26",
}
```

Fig. 2. FHIR JSON

```
    "Profile.mapping" : [ "_:t2", "_:t9" ],
    "http://hl7.org/fhir#Profile.name" : {
       "@type" : "http://hl7.org/fhir#string",
       "@value" : "organization"
    },

"http://hl7.org/fhir#Profile.publisher" : {
       "@type" : "http://hl7.org/fhir#string",
       "@value" : "FHIR Project"
    },

    "http://hl7.org/fhir#Profile.status" : {
       "@type" : "http://hl7.org/fhir#code",
       "@value" : "draft"
                              },

    "@id" : "_:t10",
    "http://hl7.org/fhir#Profile.date" : {
       "@type" : "http://hl7.org/fhir#dateTime",
       "@value" : "2013-11-26"
    },
```

Fig. 3. JSON-LD

3   FHIR Schema in OWL

Ontology provide aid in inference through axioms. FHIRs semantic structure (ontology) is developed by using DL because DL provides aid in inferring. A FHIR resource of RelatedPerson is shown in Figure 4.

FHIR contains two kinds of data types. These include primitive and complex types. Primitive data types are predefined types of data. Some examples of primitive data types include date, dateTime, instant, oid, uuid. In ontology it is modelled as follows:

```
<xs:simpleTypename="oid">
<xs:restrictionbase ="xs:anyURI">
<xs:patternvalue="urn:oid:(0|[1-9][0-9]*)(\(0|[1-9][0-9]*))*"/>
<xs:minLengthvalue ="1">
</xs:restriction>
</xs:simpleType>
```

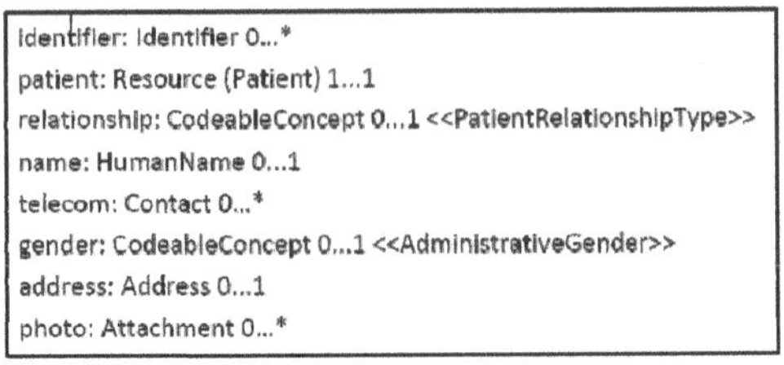

```
Identifier: Identifier 0...*
patient: Resource (Patient) 1...1
relationship: CodeableConcept 0...1 <<PatientRelationshipType>>
name: HumanName 0...1
telecom: Contact 0...*
gender: CodeableConcept 0...1 <<AdministrativeGender>>
address: Address 0...1
photo: Attachment 0...*
```

Fig. 4. Practitioner Resource in FHIR

This is an example of string data type oid. Several complex types are also used in FHIR. As Identifier in Figure 4 is complex type. Quantity, a complex type, is shown in Figure 5. If we consider Figure 4 then in this figure, property identifier contains cardinality of 0 to many. These restrictions are modelled in the following manner in ontology

```
1. fhir:Practitioner.identifier rdf:type owl:ObjectProperty;
   rdfs:domain fhir:Practitioner ;
   rdfs:range fhir:Identifier.
```

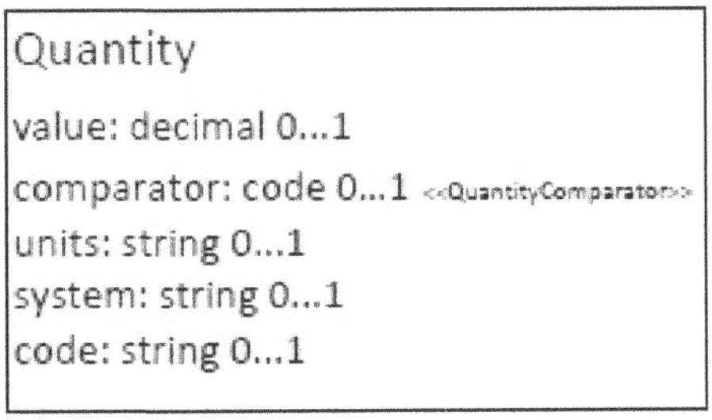

```
Quantity
value: decimal 0...1
comparator: code 0...1 <<QuantityComparator>>
units: string 0...1
system: string 0...1
code: string 0...1
```

Fig. 5. Complex Data Type Example

Ontology is developed by following modular approach where all resources are implemented as sub-classes of "Resource" and all the dependent resources are implemented as sub-classes of "DependentResource" followed by name of Re-source.

4   Data Validation

Data is passed into validator that results in valid or invalid data. After conversion of JSON into RDF it is validated against FHIR schema. Rule based reasoning is performed to validate data as per ontology. Initially data type validation is performed that verifies individual characters are consistent with expected characters of data types that are defined in schema. For example, for instant, valid value will be 2013-04-03T15:30:10+01:00. All other values as 2013-04-03T15:30 will be invalid. After data types validation, cardinality validation is performed that checks whether data values are according to cardinalities de ned in FHIR schema. If cardinality is 1 to 1 then exactly one value should be there. We have applied reasoner that checks different types of validity scenarios according to inference rules that are defined in FHIR ontology. Some of these rules are defined below:

1. `(patient:Patient(1 to 1) )`
   `∃x∃y(RelatedPerson(x)⇒ Patient(y)∧(x=y))`.
2. `name:HumanName (0 to 1)`
   `∀x (RelatedPerson(x)∧ Name(x))⇒ Name(x)`.

Finally FHIR statement validation checks that all the attributes of data are as per FHIR standard. Conformance testing is performed by us in order to find out whether system validates the correct data as per FHIR standard.

5   Evaluation and Results

Evaluation of the system is performed on the basis of parameter that shows all valid documents are declared as valid and only valid documents should be declared as valid. Validation and conformance is performed on 266 examples of FHIR documents, out of which 221 are correct and are available on FHIR website. These examples vary in complexity from low to medium and high. The complexity is calculated on the basis of number of attribute-value pairs. Examples having more number of attribute-value pairs are considered to be more complex. Conformance and validation for 45 examples is also performed by introducing errors in valid FHIR documents. These errors include addition of extra property and data against cardinality. The evaluation is performed on a regular desktop that is Core i5, 2.53GHz, 4 GB memory, 64 bit Windows OS, Hard Disk 300 GB.

FHIR JSON is passed on to validator where Pellet reasoner is used to infer over JSON data by using FHIR schema. For any resource, that is going to be validated, its time is calculated by executing it 10 times and then average time is calculated. Validation time is shown in Table 1. Efficiency of system was measured by calculating response time using J-Meter. Out of 221 examples, 49 FHIR resources of high, medium and low complexity were selected and response time was calculated. Initially system was hit by 10 users and number of users are kept on increasing till 40,000. Figure 6 shows response time.

Table 1. Validation Time

FHIR Resource	Complexity Level	Validation Time (sec)
Patient	Medium	126.8
Organization-Pro le	High	135
Location	High	133

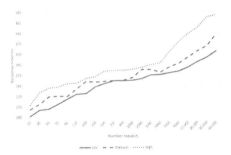

Fig. 6. Response Time

6   Conclusion

This paper presents a validation approach that is feasible for healthcare data to test its conformance as per standard. Proposed validator enables healthcare data to be validated against FHIR. Our work aims to provide accurate and consistent data among healthcare entities. It takes JSON and test its conformance with FHIR. Efficiency of this system is evaluated on the basis of validation time and response time of multiple requests that access the system simultaneously.

References

1. HIMDataValidation http://library.ahima.org/xpedio/groups/public/documents/ahima/bok1_049164.hcsp?dDocName=bok1_049164
2. Shanks, G., Tansley, E., Weber, R.: Using ontology to validate conceptual models. Communications of the ACM **46**(10), 85–89 (2003)
3. Rout, T.P.: ISO/IEC 15504 evolution to an international standard. Software Process: Improvement and Practice **8**(1), 27–40 (2003)
4. Rosenthal, L., Skall, M., Carnahan, L.: White paper: Conformance testing and certication framework (2001)
5. The application/json media type for javascript object notation (json) (2006) http://www.ietf.org/rfc/rfc4627.txt?number=4627/
6. JSON lint. http://zaach.github.io/jsonlint//
7. Turhan, A.-Y.: Description logic reasoning for semantic web ontologies. In: Proceedings of the International Conference on Web Intelligence, Mining and Se-mantics, p. 6. ACM (2011)
8. FHIR standard, September -30, 2014. http://www.hl7.org/implement/standards/fhir/overview.html/

Author Index

Ahmad Fauzi, Mohammad F.   165
Ahmad, Farooq   241
Aickelin, Uwe   45
Alem, Leila   31
Ally, Mustafa   1
Awad, Ali Ismail   92

Blumenstein, Michael   202, 213
Browne, James   104
Bruder, Ilvio   154

Cai, Yunpeng   174, 185
Chen, Anjun   123
Chen, Lei   56
Chen, Tao   79
Cheng, Taoran   133

de Courten, Maximilian   104
Dimaguila, Gerardo Luis   231
Duan, Changjiang   7

Escall, Aileen   104

Fan, Xiaomao   185
Feng, Ling   133

Gao, Hongchao   111
Ghanbarzadeh, Reza   213
Ghapanchi, Amir Hossein   202, 213
Gokozan, Hamza N.   165
Gray, Kathleen   195
Guan, Wenxuan   185
Guo, Zhaoyang   45
Gurcan, Metin N.   165

Hallam, Karen T.   104
Heuer, Andreas   154
Hua, Yuncheng   123
Huang, Jing   133
Huang, Renwei   7
Huang, Weidong   31
Huang, Xingxian   185

Jawaid, Hira   241
Jia, Jia   133
Jia, Liya   7
Jones, Andi   104

Karopka, Thomas   154
Khosravi, Pouria   202
Kosche, Kerstin   154

Latif, Khalid   241
Li, Jane   31
Li, Qi   133
Li, Xin   69
Liu, He   79
Liu, Lei   123, 225
Liu, Yuhang   7

Malki, Ouçamah Mohammed Cherkaoui   37
Mazouz, Sanae   37
Mukhtar, Hamid   241

Nan, Peng   225
Nfaoui, El Habib   37
Ni, Hongbo   56
Nie, Zedong   7

Okoh, Ebenezer   92
Otero, Jose J.   165

Pierson, Christopher R.   165
Punnoose, Bibin   195

Raza, Syed Ali   241
Reps, Jenna   45
Rissanen, Marjo   146

Schuldt, Juliane   154
Soar, Jeffrey   1
Song, Luping   69
Sun, Xiaomeng   225

Vimalachandran, Pasupathy   17

Wang, Hua   17
Wang, Lei   7, 79
Wang, Yingying   174
Wang, Zhu   56
Wlodarczak, Peter   1

Xiang, Furu   185
Xie, Juanying   111
Xie, Jue   123
Xing, Chunxiao   69
Xu, Shuangqing   133
Xue, Yuanyuan   133

Yang, Jun   56
Yu, Haibo   185

Zeng, Zichun   174
Zhang, Guigang   69
Zhang, Kexu   225
Zhang, Qingna   79
Zhang, Tong   69
Zhang, Yanchun   17
Zhao, Tingzhi   56
Zhou, Xingshe   56
Zhu, Haoyue   45

Printed in the United States
By Bookmasters